THE HUMAN CARDIOVASCULAR SYSTEM

Facts and Concepts

The Human Cardiovascular System

Facts and Concepts

John T. Shepherd, M.D., M.Ch., D.Sc., F.R.C.P.
Professor of Physiology and Dean
Mayo Medical School
and Director for Education
Mayo Foundation
Rochester, Minnesota

Paul M. Vanhoutte, M.D., Ag.E.S.
Professor of Pharmacology and Pathophysiology
Department of Medicine
Universitaire Instelling Antwerpen
University of Antwerp
Wilrijk, Belgium

Raven Press ▪ New York

Raven Press, 1140 Avenue of the Americas, New York, New York 10036

Made in the United States of America

Library of Congress Cataloging in Publication Data

Shepherd, John Thompson, 1919–
The human cardiovascular system.

Includes bibliographies and index.
1. Cardiovascular system. I. Vanhoutte, Paul M., joint author. II. Title.
QP102.S52 612'.1 79–64083
ISBN 0–89004–367–1

Second Printing, February 1980

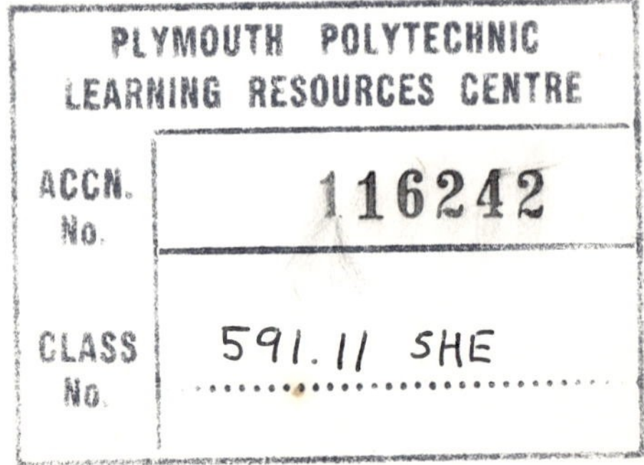

Dedication

To Dr. L. Vandendriessche, formerly Rector of the Universitaire Instelling Antwerpen, and the Board of Trustees of the Francqui Foundation, Brussels: the former for sponsoring Dr. Shepherd for an International Francqui Chair at the University of Antwerp and the latter for providing the award. These events permitted two long-time colleagues to continue their collaboration in research and to develop the groundwork for this overview of the cardiovascular system.

Prologomenon

The prologue to any textbook demands of the authors the reasons why it merits publication. In this endeavor, we were reminiscing, in congenial circumstances, about our combined total of over fifty years of research on the cardiovascular system, and over ten in collaborative studies. These ranged from the analysis of the behavior of the circulation in human limbs, the hemodynamic events in the human heart studied by heart catheterization, the role of the veins in circulatory control, the regulation of arterial blood pressure by the cardiovascular reflexes, and the responses of isolated blood vessels to local, humoral, and nervous stimuli. All of this reminded us of the complexity of the cardiovascular system and the difficulties faced by scholars of any age, confronted with the outpouring of years of information in original and review articles, symposia and textbooks, from which they must identify key facts. We decided to challenge ourselves to write a clear and concise description of the current knowledge of cardiovascular function which would relate the physiology and pharmacology of the circulatory system to its common diseases and which would endeavor to separate facts from concepts, and hopefully, from personal bias.

The text is designed for use by medical students, graduate students, residents, and other medical professionals desiring a modern review of the circulation. Based on our own experience in research and teaching, we have tried to summarize the most important aspects of cardiovascular function and have stressed the continuous interaction between the components of the system. We have tried to make each statement understandable to both of us, on the supposition that if this were achieved, anyone who reads the text would comprehend it.

The text is extensively illustrated with original diagrams that serve to summarize important components and events within the system. Particular attention has been paid to the index and to cross-references in the text so that the reader can rapidly gain access to the pertinent facts. All discussion of methodology has been placed in the final chapters so that the reader's thought processes are not as easily interrupted by complex mathematical derivations as are those of the authors. Selected references are cited at the end of each chapter; the majority are reviews by outstanding investigators of specific aspects of the circulation in health and disease and provide the advanced student with a key to further reading.

As for the reasons why this book merits publication, others must make the judgment. We offer no apologia. Suffice it to say we have enjoyed the challenge of this transatlantic overview of the cardiovascular system and if those who read it become as fascinated as we are by its intricacy and are stimulated to become active in its affairs, this will be our reward.

Acknowledgments

Our special thanks are due to Robert R. Lorenz and Tony J. Verbeuren, long-time friends and collaborators in research, who combined their knowledge of the circulation with artistic skills to transform our ideas for the illustrations of the text into graphic realities. In addition, many friends and colleagues kindly gave permission to reproduce classic illustrations selected from their work. We are indebted to Nancy J. Rusch and R. Clinton Webb for constructive criticism of the text. We also thank Liliane Van den Eynde and Joan Y. Krage for their patience in typing version after version of the manuscript. We acknowledge the pleasure we have had in the scientific collaboration and social interchange with the many Research Fellows with whom we have worked both at the Mayo Graduate School of Medicine and at the University of Antwerp. We are grateful to Raven Press and especially to Dr. Diana Schneider and Ms. Rita Scheman for the efficient way in which they collaborated with us, and for proceeding rapidly and smoothly from the typescript to the final product.

Contents

1

From Historical Hallmarks to Modern Concepts of Cardiovascular Control

> "Coepi egomet mecum cogitare, an motionem quandam quasi in circulo haberet"
> *William Harvey*[1]

William Harvey, who discovered the basic principles of the circulation of the blood, was so impressed by its complexity that he stated in the first chapter of his classic book *Exercitatio Anatomica de Motu Cordis et Sanguinis in Animalibus* (1628) that he almost felt that the motion of the heart and blood was to be comprehended only by God. Indeed, when studying the cardiovascular system it is easy to become so engrossed with its complexity that one overlooks its primary role, namely to ensure at every moment the survival of all cells of the body.

For unicellular organisms the problem is a simple one. Surrounded by water, these cells can take up nutrients directly from and eliminate waste directly into their environment; in this way they ensure the constancy of the intracellular conditions necessary for their proper function. As evolution proceeded, multicellular complexes developed whereby groups of cells emerged to fulfill the various functions which initially were performed within the single cell. This organization of cells has reached its most advanced development in the higher vertebrates. Regardless of the function they subserve, all cells of the organism, just as their single cell predecessors, must receive nutrients and eliminate their waste prod-

[1] Translation: I began to think within myself whether it [the blood] might have a sort of motion, as it were, in a circle."

ucts. Each living cell of the organism is surrounded by a small amount of extracellular fluid. For each cell to function properly the composition of this fluid, the *milieu intérieur,* may vary only within narrow limits (Claude Bernard, 1866). To achieve this there must be a continuous stream of nutrients from the outside world to the extracellular fluid, and a continuous stream of waste products from the cells to the outside world. Therefore the organism needs specialized tissues for exchange (lung, gut, and kidney) and a transport system (blood and cardiovascular system) to link these tissues with the individual cells.

CIRCULATION OF THE BLOOD

Harvey's classic experiments dispelled the concept that the blood ebbed and flowed in the vascular system, an idea which had dominated medical thinking from the time of Galen 15 centuries earlier. Harvey recognized that the blood returning from the peripheral tissues and organs through the great veins enters a thin-walled collecting chamber (atrium) of the right heart, and that when this chamber is filled it contracts and forces the blood into a thicker-walled chamber (right ventricle). The subsequent contraction of this ventricle expels the blood through the pulmonary artery into the lungs, from which it returns to the left heart. A similar succession of events brings the blood from the left atrium to the thick-walled left ventricle (Fig. 1–1). The latter propels the blood into a large channel (aorta), which conveys it to the peripheral organs of the body (Fig. 1–2). The forward motion of the blood through the various cavities of the heart is made possible by the presence of valves between the atria and the ventricles, and between the ventricles and the great vessels which leave them. The alternating sequence of contraction (emptying) and relaxation (filling) of the heart chambers, known as systole and diastole, respectively, permits the heart to function as a pump. Harvey also recognized the important role of the valves in the venous system of the extremities in assisting the forward movement of the blood from periphery back to the heart.

A century later Hales (1733) measured the postmortem capacity of the left ventricle. By assuming that the whole ventricular content was expelled with each systole, and by knowing the frequency of contraction from measuring the pulse rate, he estimated that each ventricle expels about 4.5 liters of blood per minute (cardiac output), a value surprisingly close to that measured directly with modern technology in living subjects (p. 289). Since both sides of the heart are in series in the same circuit (Fig. 1–1), both ventricles must pump the same average amount of blood per unit of time. The cardiac output is determined by the number of times the heart beats per minute (heart rate) multiplied by the amount of blood pumped out per beat (stroke volume). The remarkable performance of the cardiovascular system is illustrated by the fact that in the human at rest the heart beats about 100,000 times a day, and the ventricles move approximately 16,000 liters of blood around the vascular tree. During strenuous exercise this amount may increase temporarily by as much as four or five times.

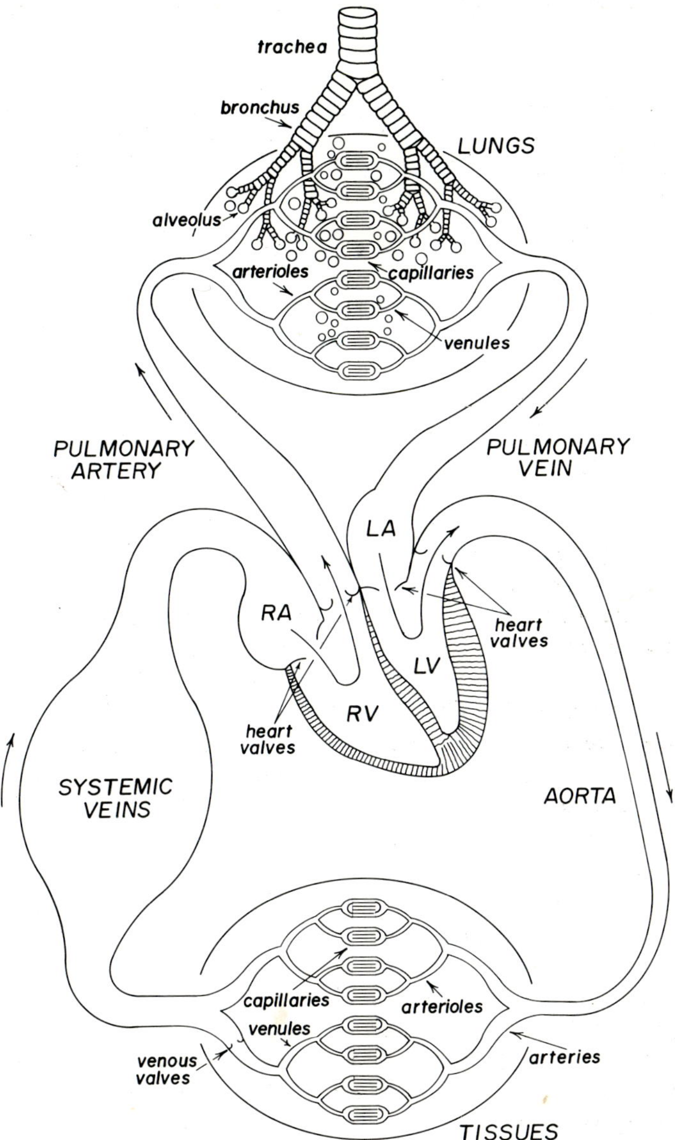

FIG. 1–1. The cardiovascular system. The heart, blood vessels, and lungs provide for exchange of gases between the atmosphere and the tissues. The right and left side of the heart are two pumps arranged in series on the same circuit. The oxygenated blood (arterial blood) returning from the lungs by the pulmonary veins enters the left atrium (LA) and the left ventricle (LV). Contraction of the latter expels the blood into the aorta, which ramifies into numerous arteries for distribution of the blood to the tissues. The end branches of the arteries (arterioles) give rise to the exchange vessels (capillaries) where oxygen and foodstuffs pass to the tissues and carbon dioxide and waste products are taken up by the blood (venous blood). The capillaries reunite to form the venules and veins, which return the venous blood to the right atrium (RA) and right ventricle (RV). The contraction of the right ventricle propels the blood into the pulmonary artery and its branches. In the pulmonary capillaries the carbon dioxide diffuses to the small air sacs (alveoli), and oxygen is taken up from the latter by the blood. The alveoli are connected to the atmosphere by the bronchial tree and the trachea. The presence of valves in the heart and the limb veins ensures forward movement of the blood.

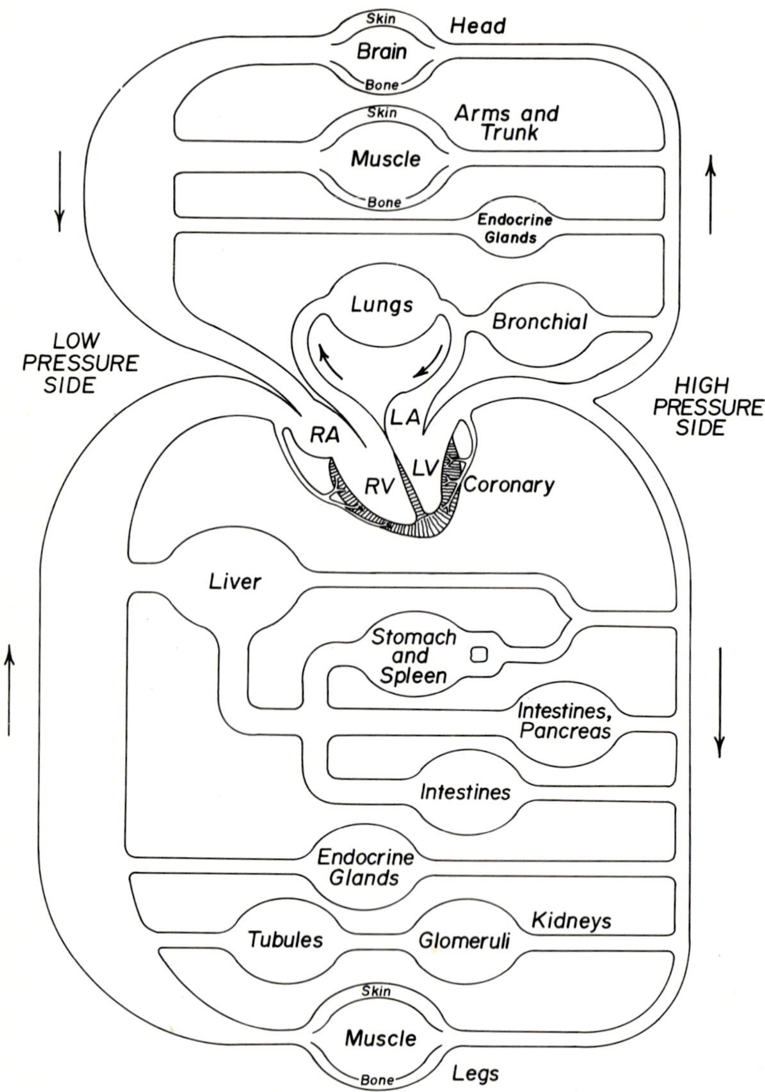

FIG. 1–2. Distribution of blood to the systemic vascular beds. The various vascular beds are arranged in parallel. Within each bed the consecutive sections (arteries, arterioles, capillaries, venules, and veins) are arranged in series. In the kidney the blood passes through two consecutive capillary beds. Venous blood from the spleen and gastrointestinal organs passes through a second capillary network, the portal circulation, in the liver. The greater proportion of the blood volume resides within the venous side of the circulation.

The completion of the description of the cardiovascular circuit came when the communication channels between arteries and veins, assumed to exist by Harvey, were described by Malpighi in 1661 and called capillaries. The capillaries, in the lungs and other organs, soon were recognized as the sites of exchange between the body cells and the transport system (the blood) and between the latter and the outside world. Lower (1669) showed that the function of the pulmonary capillaries is to replenish the blood with oxygen. Starling (1896) demonstrated that the direction and the quantity of the fluid which moves across the capillary wall are determined mainly by the balance between the pressure of the blood which tends to push fluid into the tissues (capillary hydrostatic pressure) and the attraction of fluid exerted by the plasma proteins (colloid osmotic pressure).

PRESSURES AND FLOWS WITHIN THE VASCULAR SYSTEM

Prior to Harvey, Vesalius (1543) had recognized that the contraction of the heart creates the arterial pulsation. Although Harvey understood that the high arterial pressure provides the driving force for the circulation, it remained for Hales to make the first direct measurement of arterial blood pressure, which he did by determining the height that blood rose in a vertical tube inserted

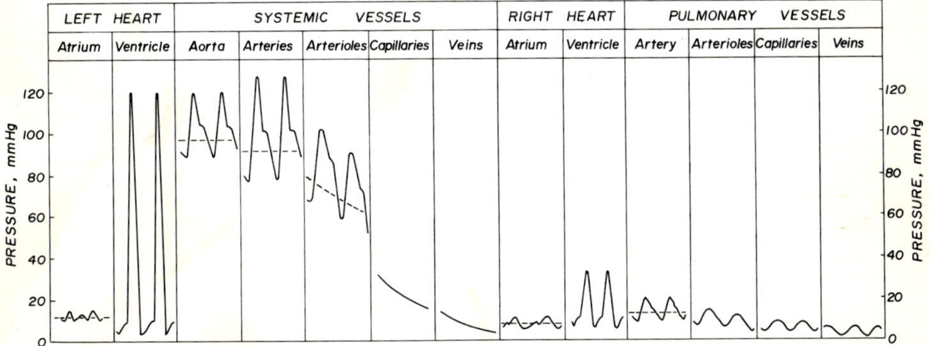

FIG. 1–3. Pressure changes in the human cardiovascular system. In the left atrium the pressure is low but pulsatile because of the rhythmic contractions of the atrial muscle. The main generator of pressure is the muscle of the left ventricle; in the latter cavity the pressure alternates with each cardiac cycle from near zero (diastole) to about 120 mm Hg (systole). When the pressure in the ventricle exceeds that in the aorta, the aortic semilunar valves open, the ventricle and aorta become a common chamber, and the pressure in both rises in unison. The rise in aortic pressure causes an expansion of the aorta and the large arteries because of their elasticity and because blood enters the arterial tree faster than it leaves it through the small-bore arterioles. When the ventricle starts to relax, the aortic valve closes. As the ventricle continues to relax, the pressure within it drops quickly to near zero, but the pressure in the aorta falls slowly throughout ventricular diastole as the distended arterial tree recoils and blood continues to flow to the capillaries through the arterioles. The major loss of pressure occurs at the arterioles because of the high resistance to flow they offer. The pressure in the capillaries and veins decreases further to approximate zero in the great veins entering the right atrium; the flow in the systemic capillaries and veins is relatively nonpulsatile. The right side of the heart generates a pressure pattern similar to that in the systemic circulation, but the systolic pressure in the pulmonary artery is about six times less than that of the aorta, and the flow in the pulmonary capillaries is pulsatile. Mean pressures are indicated by dotted lines. In the large arteries the mean pressure is lower than in the aorta although the systolic pressure is higher owing to reflection of the pulse waves.

into one of the main arteries of a mare. Years later the use of the mercury manometer and modern manometers allowing exact measurement of dynamic changes in pressure (p. 288), as well as the ability to pass catheters into all parts of the cardiovascular system (p. 287), has permitted precise determination of the pressure changes throughout the circulatory system (Fig. 1–3) (Table 1—Appendix). Although the same amount of blood is pumped by the two ventricles, the pressure generated by the left is about six times greater than that generated by the right. The high pressure in the aorta ensures adequate delivery of blood to all organs; the low pressure in the pulmonary artery ensures that no fluid leaves the lung capillaries, which would cause flooding of the air sacs of the lung and prevent adequate uptake of oxygen from the outside air.

By contrasting the intermittent flow from the ventricles with the steady flow in the veins, Hales deduced that the large arteries, because of their distensibility

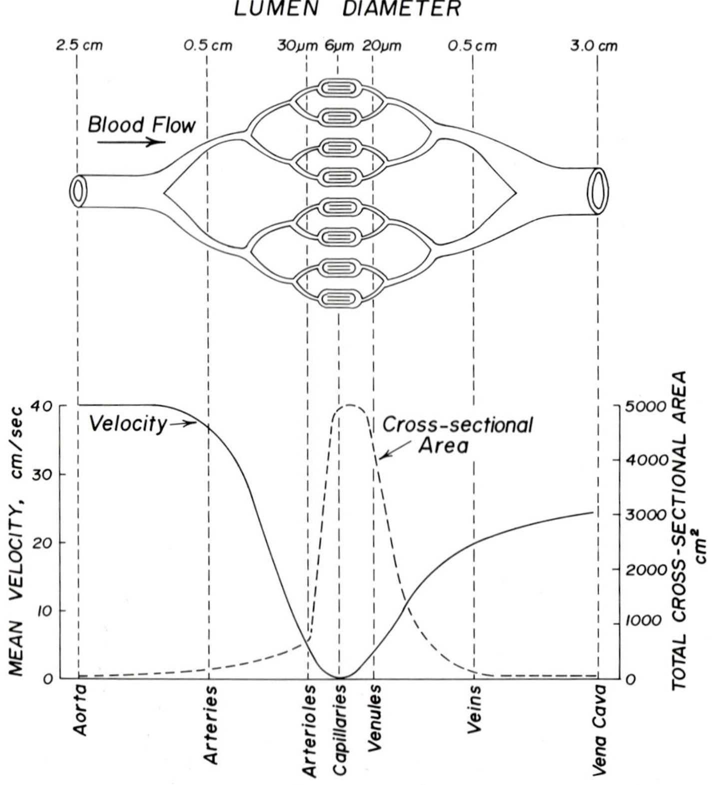

FIG. 1–4. Changes in estimated total cross-sectional area *(dotted line)* and mean velocity of flow *(solid line)* in consecutive segments of the systemic blood vessels. Since the flow through each segment is the same, the velocity is highest in the aorta and the caval veins, which have the smallest cross-sectional area, and lowest in the capillaries where the cross-sectional area is very large. This favors the exchange between blood and tissues.

(elastic properties), act as a depulsator to dampen the pulsatile output of the heart into a continuous flow of blood to the tissues and organs of the body. As the main arteries pass to the latter, they branch and become progressively smaller; the smallest branches are called arterioles, from which the capillaries originate. Although the individual vessels become smaller in diameter as the branching occurs, their number multiplies to such an extent that the total cross-sectional area of each consecutive section of the vascular tree increases, to reach a maximum at the capillary level. When the capillaries reunite to form venules, and the latter to form veins, there is a progressive decrease in total cross-sectional area. Since the amount of blood passing per unit of time through each cross-section is the same, the velocity of flow decreases progressively toward the

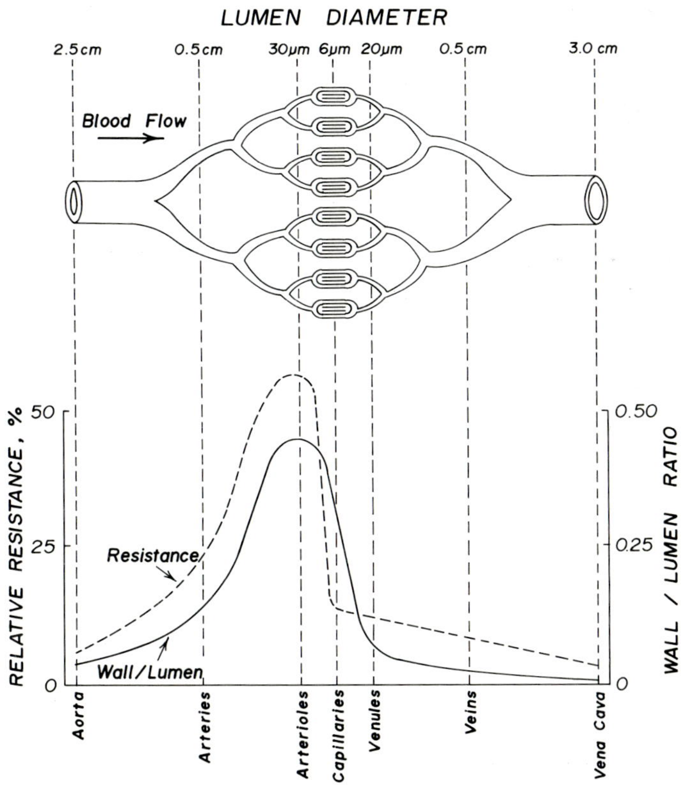

FIG. 1–5. Changes in the wall-to-lumen ratio *(solid line)* and in relative resistance to blood flow *(dotted line)* of the systemic blood vessels. The arterioles have the greatest wall-to-lumen ratio because of the large amount of smooth muscle in their wall relative to their size. Variations in the degree of contraction of this muscle permit control of the blood supply to the individual vascular beds and of the total resistance to flow through the systemic vascular bed. The low wall-to-lumen ratio of the capillaries is due to the absence of muscle in their walls, and that of the veins to their large diameter relative to the amount of muscle they contain.

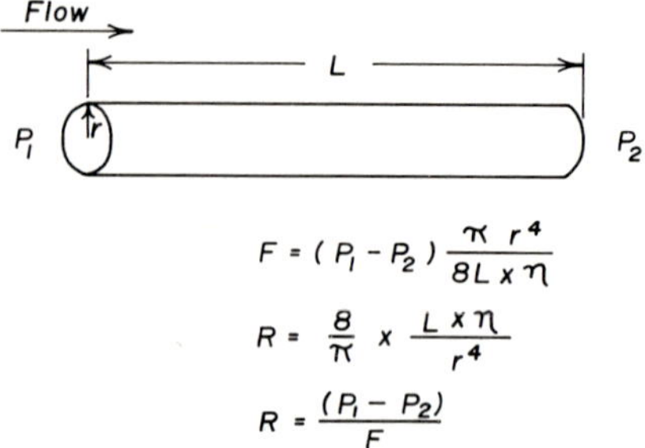

Flow
L
P_1
r
P_2
$F = (P_1 - P_2)\dfrac{\pi r^4}{8L \times \eta}$
$R = \dfrac{8}{\pi} \times \dfrac{L \times \eta}{r^4}$
$R = \dfrac{(P_1 - P_2)}{F}$

FIG. 1–6. Relations between pressure, flow, and resistance derived from Poiseuille's (1842) work on cylindrical tubes. R = resistance (dyne-sec/cm^5). L = length (mm). η = viscosity (poise). r = radius (mm). P = pressure (mm Hg). F = flow (ml/min). Strictly speaking, these equations apply only for Newtonian fluids flowing in a nonpulsatile manner through rigid tubes, whereas in the vascular system a pulsatile non-Newtonian fluid flows through distensible tubes. However, they illustrate the importance of alterations in diameter as the key determinant of the resistance to flow in blood vessels because the resistance is inversely proportional to the fourth power of the radius.

periphery and is lowest at the capillary level; when returning toward the right heart the velocity of flow augments progressively. This creates optimal conditions for exchange in the capillaries (Fig. 1–4).

Hales, in another important discovery, established that the major resistance to flow is offered by the minute vessels of the tissues, the arterioles (resistance vessels), and hence that they are the site of the greatest pressure drop between the arteries and the veins (Fig. 1–3). He showed that water and brandy at different temperatures can affect the resistance of the arterioles and thus demonstrated that the blood vessels can undergo active changes in diameter (vasomotion), as was confirmed 150 years later by Claude Bernard. Indeed the arterioles combine a small diameter with an abundance of muscle in their wall (Fig. 1–5). When this muscle contracts or relaxes, the diameter of the arteriole decreases or increases, respectively. The work of Poiseuille (1842) predicts that such changes in diameter profoundly affect the resistance to flow since in cylindrical tubes this is inversely proportional to the fourth power of the radius (Fig. 1–6). Changes in arteriolar diameter affect the quantity of blood flowing to the capillaries subserved by the arterioles and the pressure within the capillaries. On the other hand, the resultant of all arteriolar resistances (systemic vascular resistance), together with the cardiac output, dictates the level of arterial blood pressure because the latter is determined by the product of the former two (Figs. 1–7 and 1–8).

BLOOD VOLUME, VENOUS RETURN, AND CARDIAC FILLING

Early experiments, including those in which blood was drained from decapitated criminals, indicated that the blood volume approximates 1/14th the body

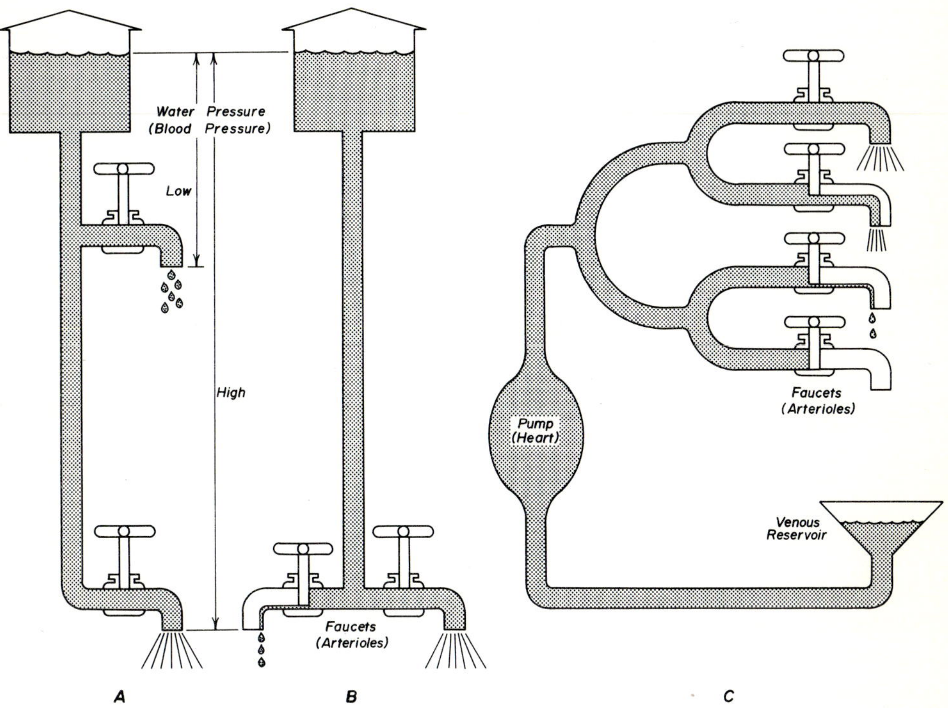

FIG. 1–7. A: If a different pressure head is applied to identical resistances (faucets of the same diameter, fully open), the circuit with the highest pressure (lower faucet) will allow the greatest flow. This means that for an identical degree of opening of a given arteriole, the flow through it is directly proportional to the pressure head (mean blood pressure). **B:** For a constant-pressure head the amount of fluid flowing through a circuit depends directly on the encountered resistance (e.g., identical faucets with different degrees of opening). The circuit with the lowest resistance *(right)* allows the most flow. This means that, provided the mean blood pressure is kept constant, the degree of opening of the arteriole determines the amount of flow through it. **C:** For a given output of the pump, the pressure is determined by the resultant of the individual resistances. If more faucets close, the pressure increases and vice versa. If the total resistance changes, the only way to maintain a constant pressure in the system is to alter the pumping rate.

weight, a value close to the 5 to 6 liters obtained for an average adult by modern methods. Thus in the human, as in most mammals, the heart at rest pumps the equivalent of the total blood volume per minute. The greater part of the blood volume is contained in the low-pressure side of the circulation, which includes the postcapillary systemic veins, the right heart, the pulmonary vessels, and the left atrium (Figs. 1–2 and 1–3). The work of Frank (1895) and Starling (1914) showed that the degree of filling of the heart is an essential factor in determining its stroke volume. The systemic veins (capacitance vessels) play the dynamic role of ensuring the filling of the heart. Like the arterioles, the veins contain muscle in their walls, and this muscle permits active alterations of vascular capacity (Fig. 1–9).

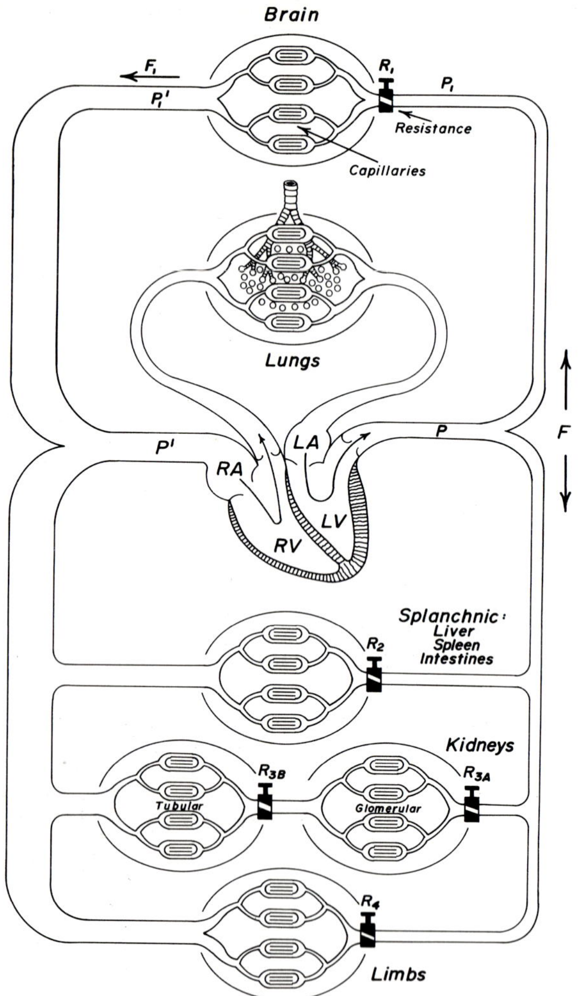

FIG. 1–8. Interdependence of pressure, flow, and resistance to flow. For the systemic circulation as a whole, the arterial pressure (P) is determined by the product of the cardiac output (F) and the resistance to flow (R) offered by the various vascular beds arranged in parallel ($1/R = 1/R_1 + 1/R_2 + 1/R_3 + 1/R_4 + \ldots . 1/R_x$). When two resistances are arranged in series (e.g., in the kidney) their total resistance equals the sum of the individual resistances ($R_3 = R_{3a} + R_{3b}$). Since the systemic arterial blood pressure remains relatively constant, the flow through the individual beds is inversely proportional to the resistance they offer, which is determined mainly by their arterioles.

CONTROL OF THE CIRCULATION

Claude Bernard (1851) recognized that integration of the function of the cardiovascular system depends mainly on the nervous system. Loewi (1921) demonstrated that the signals from the nerve cells to the muscle cells is transmit-

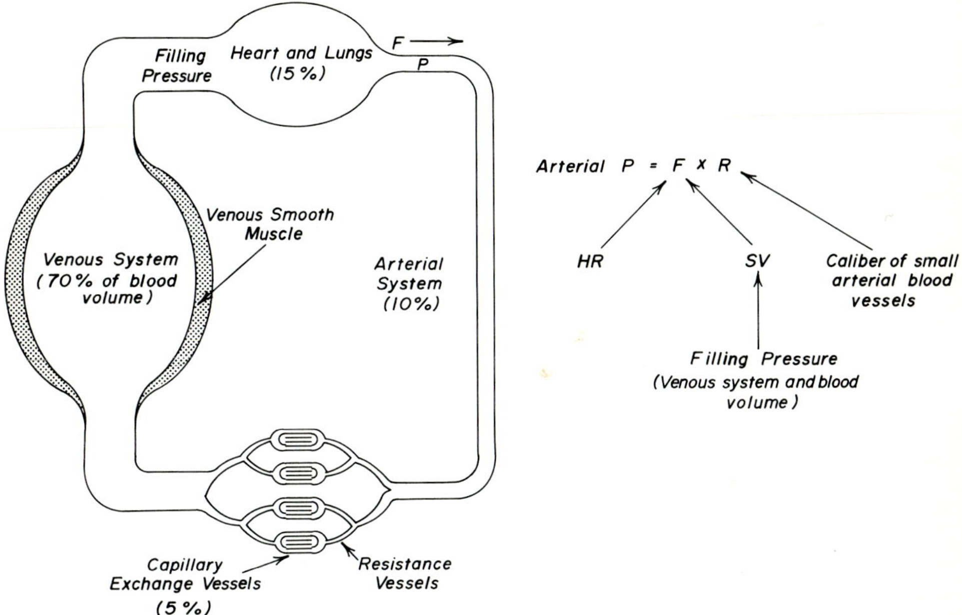

FIG. 1–9. Distribution of blood volume and the role of the venous system in regulating the filling of the heart. The normal values for total blood volume in humans range from 5 to 6 liters. The largest part of the blood volume is contained in the systemic veins. The capacity and pressure in this venous reservoir is continuously adjusted by contraction and relaxation of the smooth muscle in the venous wall. This permits the filling pressure of the heart to be continuously regulated so that an appropriate stroke volume is maintained. F = cardiac output. P = arterial blood pressure. R = total systemic vascular resistance. HR = heart rate. SV = stroke volume.

ted by chemical substances (neurotransmitters). It has been established that the sympathetic nerves cause cardiovascular activation by release of norepinephrine from their endings (von Euler, 1946). Selected parts of the cardiovascular system, in particular the heart, are controlled by an inhibitory system as well; these inhibitory cholinergic nerves liberate acetylcholine at their endings (Dale, 1914; Loewi, 1921). The activity of the nerves is regulated by centers in the brainstem (Ludwig, 1873), which in turn are influenced by peripheral receptors that sense pressures within the system and chemical changes in the blood. In certain circumstances hormones such as epinephrine, first demonstrated by Oliver and Schäfer (1894), are liberated into the bloodstream and modify the behavior of muscle cells in the heart and blood vessels. The metabolism and contractile activity of these cells can also be influenced by numerous alterations in their immediate environment. All of these regulatory factors combine in normal conditions to maintain adequate perfusion of the tissues and thus to ensure a proper *milieu intérieur* (Fig. 1–10).

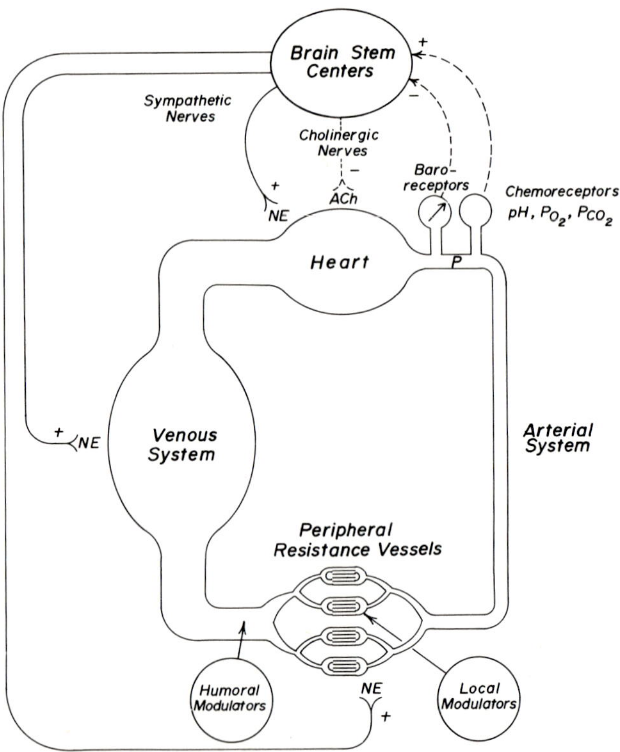

FIG. 1–10. Nervous, humoral, and local regulation of the cardiovascular system. Peripheral receptors sense either changes in blood pressure (mechanoreceptors) or variations in the chemical composition of the blood (chemoreceptors). The degree of activity of these receptors is conveyed by afferent nerves to centers in the brainstem which control the function of the heart and blood vessels by altering the activity of the sympathetic and cholinergic nerves. When the activity of the former is increased, the neurotransmitter norepinephrine (NE) is released, which stimulates the heart and constricts the blood vessels (+). When the cholinergic nerves are activated, the released acetylcholine (ACh) depresses the heart (—). The activity of both heart and blood vessels is also modulated by substances released into the circulation from endocrine glands (e.g., epinephrine from the adrenal medulla). In the tissues products of metabolism (e.g., adenosine) regulate the local blood flow in accordance with their needs. P = pressure.

SELECTED REFERENCES

Fishman, A. P., and Richards, D. W. (1964): *Circulation of the Blood. Men and Ideas.* Oxford University Press, New York.

Heymans, C., and Neil, E. (1958): *Reflexogenic Areas of the Cardiovascular System.* Churchill, London.

Leake, C. D. (1962). The historical development of cardiovascular physiology. In: *Handbook of Physiology, Sect. 2: Circulation,* Vol. 1, p. 11. American Physiological Society, Washington, D.C.

2

Components of the Cardiovascular System: How Structure Is Geared to Function

Having discussed the general concepts governing cardiovascular function, it is appropriate to examine how the components of the system are designed to make their particular contribution to the functioning of the whole. This is most easily done by examining in sequence the role played by the blood, the lining of the heart and vessels, the muscle elements in the cardiac and vascular walls, their supporting structure, the tissues surrounding them, and the ways by which their metabolic requirements are met.

THE BLOOD

The blood is a suspension of erythrocytes (red blood cells), leukocytes (white blood cells), and platelets in plasma; the proportion of cells to plasma (hematocrit) approximates 45% (see Appendix, Table 8). The red cells contain hemoglobin (approximately 15 g/100 ml blood), a complex protein which has the ability to bind with oxygen. One molecule of hemoglobin can combine with four mole-

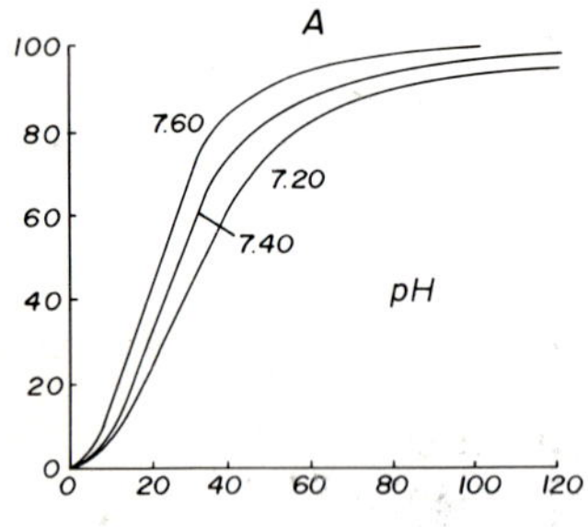

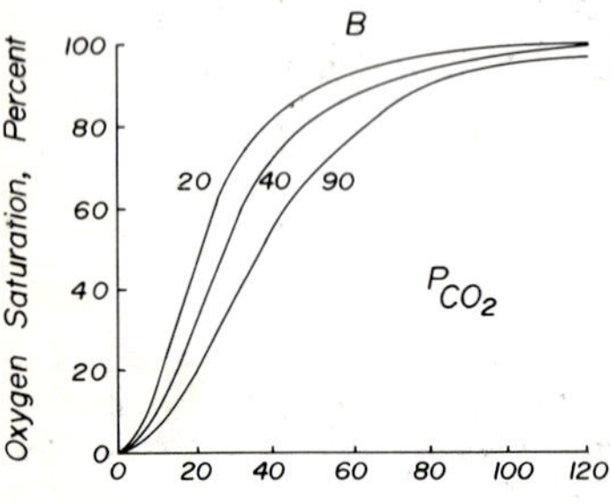

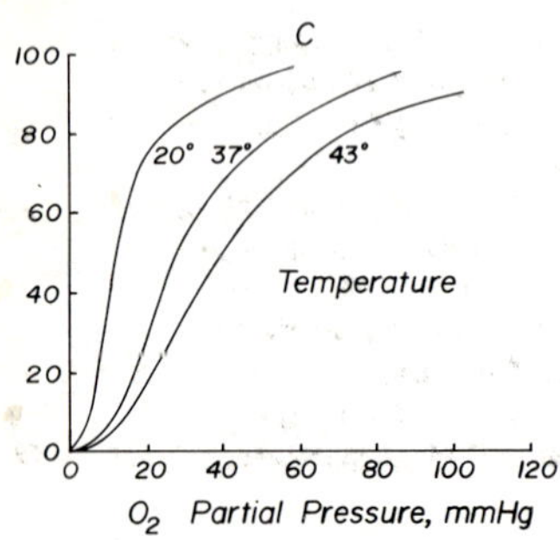

FIG. 2–1. Characteristics of the binding of oxygen to hemoglobin. If the oxygen content of hemoglobin solution is measured after equilibration at different partial pressures of the gas (Po_2) and the results are plotted as percent saturation (oxygen content divided by oxygen capacity multiplied by 100, *ordinate*) versus the Po_2 *(abscissa)*, a sigmoid curve, called the oxyhemoglobin dissociation curve, is obtained. The dissociation for whole blood is similar to that of hemoglobin solutions. The properties of hemoglobin, which are reflected in the S-shape of the oxyhemoglobin dissociation curves, permit almost complete saturation of the blood at the oxygen concentration normally present in the alveolar air (Po_2 = 100 mm Hg). The steepness of the dissociation curve illustrates the ability of hemoglobin to release large amounts of oxygen for small decreases in partial pressure of the gas, as happens in the tissues.

Various conditions alter the binding properties of oxygen to hemoglobin, which is reflected in a shift of the dissociation curve. **A:** A decrease in pH shifts the oxygen dissociation curve to the right, whereas an increase has the opposite effect. **B:** An increase in carbon dioxide tension from normal values shifts the dissociation curve to the right, and a decrease to the left (Bohr effect). This facilitates the uptake of oxygen in the lungs as carbon dioxide is released, and the release of oxygen to the tissues as carbon dioxide enters the blood. The carbon dioxide promotes release by increasing the acidity of the blood and by forming carbamino compounds with hemoglobin. Carbamino hemoglobin has less affinity for oxygen than hemoglobin. The pH change contributes about 80% to the Bohr effect. As a consequence the amount of oxygen the blood holds at a given oxygen pressure decreases and more oxygen is available to the tissues. When the venous blood passes through pulmonary capillaries, the Pco_2 decreases from 46 to 40 mm Hg and the pH rises from 7.37 to 7.40; both factors contribute to enhance the uptake of oxygen. **C:** An increase in temperature shifts the oxygen dissociation curve to the right and a decrease to the left. This facilitates the transfer of oxygen to active cells around which the temperature is highest.

cules of oxygen. The amount of oxygen bound to the hemoglobin, and thus the amount of oxyhemoglobin present in the red cell, depends on the local oxygen concentration (partial pressure). Almost complete saturation (97.5%) of the hemoglobin is reached at a partial pressure of oxygen (Po_2) of 100 mm

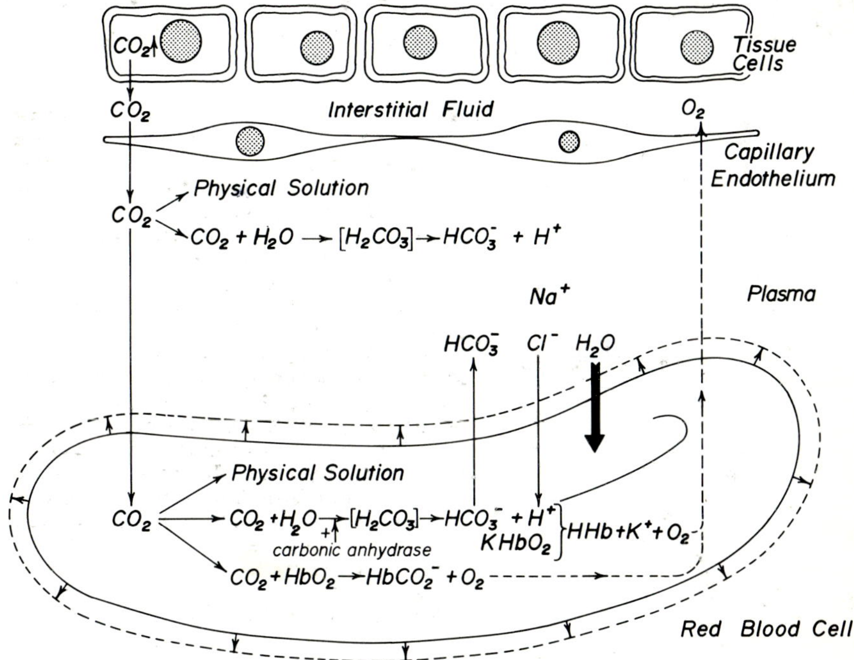

FIG. 2–2. Passage of carbon dioxide from the tissues into the blood, where it is transported to the lungs in the plasma and red cells. The carbon dioxide produced during cell metabolism diffuses through the interstitial fluid and the capillary endothelium into the plasma. In the plasma some is present in physical solution and some combines slowly with water to form the unstable carbonic acid (H_2CO_3), which immediately dissociates into hydrogen and bicarbonate ions. The carbon dioxide also diffuses into the red cells. Here some is transported in physical solution and some by formation of carbamino components, mainly carbamino hemoglobin. Most of the carbon dioxide is hydrolyzed rapidly to carbonic acid by the enzyme carbonic anhydrase. The carbonic acid dissociates into bicarbonate ions (which diffuse to the plasma) and hydrogen ions (which are buffered by the oxyhemoglobin). The binding of hydrogen ions to the latter facilitates the release of oxygen as does the formation of carbamino hemoglobin. The amounts of carbon dioxide transported in physical solution and as carbamino components and bicarbonate, average 8%, 27%, and 65%, respectively.

The loss of negative charges (HCO_3^-) from the erythrocyte is compensated for by an inward movement of chloride ions, which preserves electrical neutrality (chloride shift). The binding of hydrogen ions to the hemoglobin (Hb) liberates potassium ions, which balance the chloride ions diffusing from the plasma. To compensate for the increased osmolarity of the cell content due to the chloride and potassium ions, water penetrates the cells, which increase in volume by approximately 3%; this explains in part the difference in hematocrit between arterial and venous blood. In the lungs these processes are reversed since the carbon dioxide concentration of the plasma is higher than that in the alveoli.

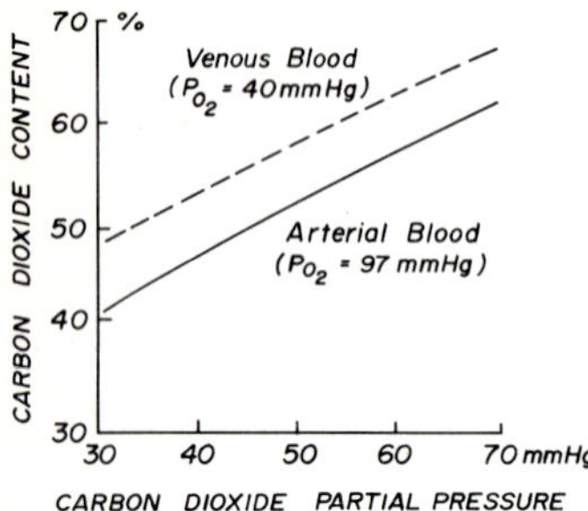

FIG. 2–3. Dependency of the binding properties of blood for carbon dioxide on the oxygen content. With increasing P_{CO_2} *(abscissa)* blood contains progressively more carbon dioxide *(ordinate)*. More carbon dioxide is transported when the oxygen content of the blood is low. Thus the loss of oxygen from arterial blood to the tissues facilitates the transport of carbon dioxide, whereas oxygenation of the blood in the lungs augments the release of carbon dioxide from the blood into the alveoli.

Hg. This is the P_{O_2} to which the blood is exposed as it passes through the lungs. The hemoglobin divests itself of oxygen to the body cells in proportion to the decrease in oxygen pressure in the tissues. The dissociation of the oxyhemoglobin is facilitated by the simultaneous increases in P_{CO_2}, H^+ concentration, and temperature which occur in active tissues (Fig. 2–1). When the amount of unsaturated hemoglobin exceeds 5 g/100 ml, the color of the blood changes from red to blue (cyanosis). As the oxygen diffuses from the hemoglobin to the tissues, carbon dioxide diffuses to the blood and partially binds to hemoglobin for transport to the lungs (Fig. 2–2). The amount of carbon dioxide transported by the blood at a given P_{CO_2} is greater when its oxygen content is lowered (Fig. 2–3).

The white blood cells are involved in the defense of the organism against infection and in immune responses.

The platelets (thrombocytes), named for their resemblance to tiny plates, are 2 to 4 microns in diameter. Their granules contain 5-hydroxytryptamine (serotonin; p. 101), adenosine diphosphate (ADP; p. 46), growth factors (p. 233), and enzymes. The platelets have mitochondria and a tubular system but are unable to synthesize proteins. Their membrane contains phospholipids. They play a major role in hemostasis by: (1) liberation of 5-hydroxytryptamine, which causes vasoconstriction (p. 22); (2) adhesion and aggregation to form a platelet thrombus, which temporarily prevents the blood loss; (3) initiation of blood clotting; and (4) initiation of the retraction of fibrin (p. 26).

The plasma is a solution of 90% water containing various salts, mainly sodium chloride, in concentrations similar to those of the fluid surrounding the body cells. It also contains glucose, free fatty acids, lipids, and proteins. The proteins, which are formed mainly in the liver, serve to transport molecules such as iron, hormones, and lipids. They also act as antibodies in immune responses, are operative in blood clotting (p. 23), and together with sodium bicarbonate, other salts, and hemoglobin help to buffer the changes in hydrogen ion concentration of the plasma. The total amount of proteins in solution determines the colloid osmotic pressure of the plasma (p. 83).

In relation to hemodynamics the physical properties of the blood merit special attention. These are described in the following sections.

Viscosity

The viscosity of a Newtonian fluid is independent of the dimensions of the tube through which it flows and of the rate of flow, provided the latter is laminar and not turbulent (Fig. 2–4). With a non-Newtonian fluid such as blood, which is a suspension of cells in liquid, the viscosity and hence the resistance to blood flow varies depending on the rate of flow, the hematocrit, the caliber of the small vessels, the axial orientation of the red cells, and their deformability. As a consequence, the term "apparent viscosity" is often applied to the value obtained for blood viscosity in the conditions under which it has been measured (p. 307).

When the number of cells per milliliter of plasma increases, so does the apparent viscosity of the blood. The normal value of the hematocrit provides for optimal oxygen transport capacity within the vascular system. If the hematocrit increases, as in polycythemia, the potential advantage for increased oxygen carriage is offset by the increase in blood viscosity, which reduces the flow to the tissues at the existing pressure. The converse is true in anemia, when the number of red cells is decreased. If blood is made to flow through a glass capillary tube, its apparent viscosity remains constant once the diameter of the tube exceeds 1 mm. With smaller diameters the apparent viscosity decreases markedly (Fahraeus–Lindqvist effect); the explanation of this is unknown. The influence of vessel diameter on the apparent viscosity is due in part to changes in the orientation of the red cells in the plasma as the blood passes through small vessels. Usually the red cells occupy the center position of the vessel

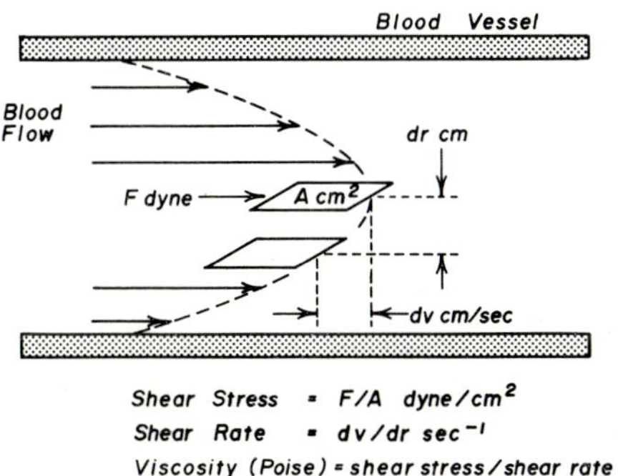

FIG. 2–4. The flow of a Newtonian fluid consists of a series of parallel laminae, moving over each other with different velocities. The frictional forces between adjacent laminae are responsible for the intrinsic resistance to flow and therefore determine the viscosity of the fluid. To move the fluid, a shearing force (F) is necessary to overcome the frictional force. This shearing force is proportional to the relative velocity of the fluid and to the contact area (A) between adjacent laminae; it is inversely proportional to the distance (dr) between the centers of the laminae. Hence $F/A \propto (dv/dr)$. The force per unit area (F/A, expressed in dynes/cm^2) is known as the shear stress; the ratio between the relative velocity and the distance between the centers of the laminae (dv/dr, expressed per second) is termed the shear rate. Viscosity (expressed in poise) equals shear stress divided by shear rate. (Courtesy of Dr. M. A. McGrath.)

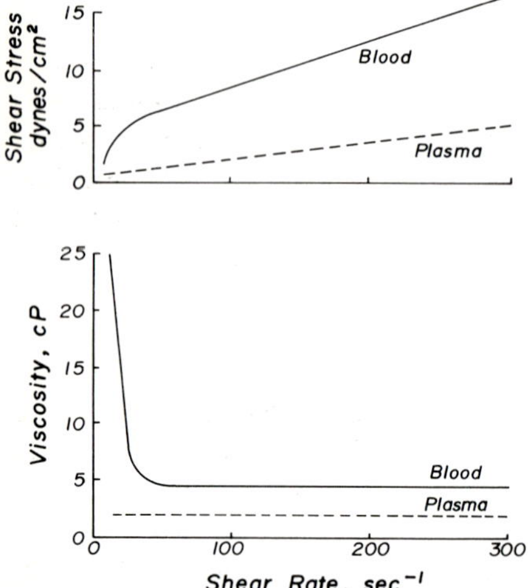

FIG. 2–5. Relations between shear stress and shear rate for blood and plasma **(top)** and dependence of blood viscosity on shear rate **(bottom).** An increase in viscosity at low shear rates is characteristic of non-Newtonian suspensions (e.g., blood). The viscosity of a Newtonian liquid (e.g., plasma) is independent of shear rate. (Courtesy of Dr. M. A. McGrath.)

where the linear flow rate is highest, whereas the majority of plasma flows in the slower-moving outer layers. The red cells move with their long axis parallel to the direction of flow. The axial migration, the constantly changing shape, and the membrane rotation of the red cells passing through the arteries and arterioles turns the blood into an emulsion of low apparent viscosity. Once this has occurred, the blood viscosity remains constant even with further increases in flow or driving pressure, provided turbulence does not occur (Fig. 2–5). At low rates of flow, the relative velocity of one layer of fluid decreases with respect to that of adjacent layers (low shear rate). This increases the tendency for the red cells to form aggregates (rouleaux formation), with a resultant increase in viscosity. Since the tendency for rouleaux formation is dependent on the concentration of large proteins in the plasma, particularly fibrinogen, the increase in viscosity when the shear rate is low is greater in any circumstance when the fibrinogen concentration is increased. The viscosity of the blood is inversely related to the deformability of the red cells. The red cell, when studied under the microscope, usually assumes the configuration of a biconcave disk with a diameter of 7 microns. As it progresses toward the capillaries, the ability of the red cell to undergo deformation becomes increasingly important, particularly in those circumstances where the diameter of the capillary becomes smaller (3 to 7 microns) than that of the cell. In these conditions the latter assumes a "bullet-like" or "parachute-like" configuration, which not only reduces the effective cell diameter but permits the presence of a lubricating plasma layer. The deformability of the red cell depends on the Ca^{2+} concentration in the plasma. If excess Ca^{2+} enters the red cell, as occurs when the blood contains less oxygen, the cell becomes stiffer and the viscosity of the blood increases. A similar increase in viscosity due to decreased deformability is characteristic of disorders such as sickle cell anemia.

Turbulence

Usually when fluid passes through a tube the flow velocity is not uniform from the periphery to the center of the tube. The central core moves faster than the immediately adjacent layer, whereas the fluid at the tube wall may be virtually stationary. Such a flow pattern is called laminar or streamline flow. If the flow velocity increases over a critical value, the layering is not maintained and irregular motions of the fluid elements develop (Fig. 2–6). Such a flow is called turbulent. When this occurs, a much greater pressure difference is required to achieve a given flow, and thus the apparent viscosity of the blood is increased. In normal circumstances turbulent flow occurs in the heart and occasionally in the aorta. In pathological conditions turbulence can develop in the cardiovascular system and is sufficient to cause resonance in adjacent structures; the resonance may be heard as a murmur. This occurs when there is obstruction to flow by narrowing of the mitral or aortic valve, since under these circumstances there is a great increase in the flow velocity across the smaller orifice. The most commonly used method for the indirect measurement of arterial blood pressure depends on creating turbulence resulting in a murmur (p. 307).

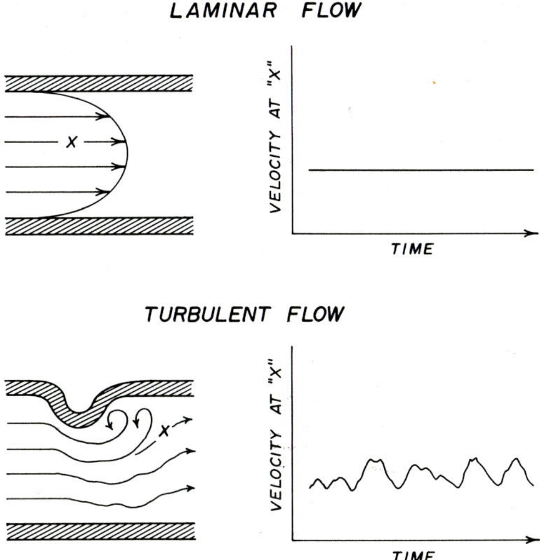

FIG. 2–6. Laminar **(top)** and turbulent **(bottom)** flow patterns. The factors determining whether flow is likely to be laminar or turbulent are related by the Reynolds number *(NR),* which is the ratio of inertial to viscous forces in a fluid. $NR = (\sigma/\eta)\ \bar{V}D$, where σ is the fluid density (g/ml), η the fluid viscosity (poise), $\bar{V}$ the average velocity of the fluid (cm/sec), and D the tube diameter (cm) (Reynolds, 1883). When the Reynolds number exceeds a critical value (about 2,000 in large, and 200 in small blood vessels), turbulence occurs. An increased flow velocity or a reduced blood viscosity (e.g., anemic murmur) predisposes to its development. It occurs normally in the ventricles, and in disease when a narrowed segment opens into a wider lumen (e.g., stenosis of one of the heart valves) or with narrowing of a large artery by an atherosclerotic plaque. When the turbulence results in vibration of the adjacent structures, a murmur is generated. (Courtesy of Dr. M. A. McGrath.)

THE LINING

Structure

All parts of the cardiovascular system are lined with a single continuous layer of thin cells (30 microns length, 10 microns width, 0.1 to 0.3 microns thick except in the nuclear region) called endocardial cells in the heart and endothelial cells in the blood vessels. In most parts of the system the adjacent cells are closely opposed; sometimes there are "tight junctions" when fusion occurs between adjoining cell membranes. In most capillaries, spaces (pores) exist between adjacent cells, the size of which varies but can approximate 0.02 micron.

At one extreme are most of the capillaries in the brain, which have no intercellular pores; this explains why certain molecules or drugs which pass easily through other capillary endothelial structures do not cross the "blood–brain barrier." At the other extreme are the capillaries in the kidney, certain glands, and the intestinal mucosa, where the endothelial cells form numerous large intracellular openings called fenestrations. Instead of capillaries, there are rela-

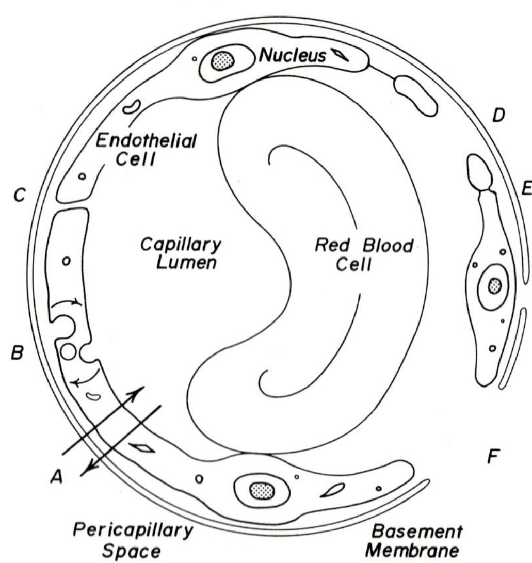

FIG. 2–7. Transport pathways in capillary endothelium. **A:** Transport through an endothelial cell of water, small nonpolar solutes, and lipid-soluble solutes. **B:** Pinocytosis. Cytoplasmic vesicles which shuttle between the cell membranes and exchange fluid and solutes. **C:** Intercellular junctions (pores). These provide a pathway for diffusion and ultrafiltration, and for the exchange of water and lipid-insoluble substances. If large enough, they may allow the passage of plasma proteins. **D:** Intracellular fenestrations, with or without a thin diaphragm, which permit the passage of large molecules. **E:** Tight junctions in the brain. Little exchange can occur through them. **F:** Large gaps seen in sinusoids of liver and spleen allow practically unlimited exchanges, including plasma proteins.

tively wide channels called sinusoids in the bone marrow, liver, and spleen. Here very large gaps occur between the endothelial cells, permitting the passage not only of macromolecules but also of blood cells (Fig. 2–7). In erectile tissues (e.g., corpora cavernosa of the penis) the arterioles open directly into venous sinuses, and no capillaries are present.

On the outer surface of the endothelial and endocardial cells, there is a basement membrane composed of fine connective strands which serve to bind these cells to the surrounding structures. In the capillary bed this basement membrane offers little hindrance to the movement of fluid and solutes. In the sinusoids the basement membrane is partially absent.

The capillaries, particularly at their venous side, may be embraced by long connective tissue cells called pericytes or Rouget cells, the function of which is unknown.

Function

Permeability

The endothelial membrane in normal conditions is permeable to water and solutes but not to most proteins (p. 83). However, a fraction of the plasma protein molecules gain access to the interstitial fluid around the tissue cells. This may be important in providing the latter with certain proteins and protein-bound substances. These proteins are returned to the plasma by the lymphatics in most tissues; in the kidney they are actively taken up by the proximal tubule of the nephron.

Metabolism

Certain endothelial cells, in addition to allowing exchanges between blood and tissues, have other functions. The endothelial cells of the lung capillaries are the best known examples. They not only provide an inert surface (estimated at 70 m^2 in man) for gas exchange but also can remove, produce, or modify bioactive materials. These cells have invaginations of the cell membrane (pinocytotic vesicles) and contain many enzymes. Besides their possible role in the transcapillary movement of lipid-insoluble macromolecules by the pinocytotic vesicles, the endothelial cells are the site of active transformation of plasma constituents such as angiotensin I, norepinephrine, 5-hydroxytryptamine, and prostaglandins. Each of these substances can affect the function of the cardiovascular system (Fig. 2–8).

Angiotensin and Bradykinin

When renin formed in the kidney is released into the blood, it transforms a plasma protein into an inactive decapeptide, angiotensin I. When the latter

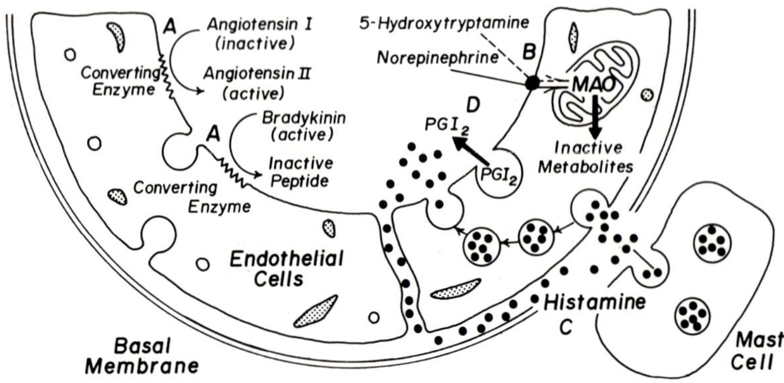

FIG. 2–8. The handling of bioactive substances by the pulmonary capillaries. **A:** Substances such as angiotensin I and bradykinin are transformed "on" the endothelium by converting enzymes, with resulting formation of active and inactive components, respectively. **B:** Substances such as norepinephrine and 5-hydroxytryptamine are actively taken up (●) and degraded enzymatically by monoamine oxidase (MAO). Other substances metabolically degraded by the lung capillaries include certain prostaglandins. **C:** During allergic and anaphylactic reactions substances such as histamine can overflow into the capillary lumen. **D:** It is likely that the lung capillaries can produce certain prostaglandin-like substances such as prostacyclin (PGI_2) and release them into the bloodstream.

passes through the lung capillaries it is transformed to an octapeptide, angiotensin II, by a converting enzyme on the surface of the endothelial cells. Angiotensin II is the most potent activator of the muscle cells of the arterioles (p. 120). The converting enzyme also degrades bradykinin if present in the blood (p. 102).

Norepinephrine

Some of the transmitter liberated by the sympathetic nerve endings may overflow into the blood and reach the lung capillaries; if so, it is taken up by the endothelial cells and is inactivated by the enzyme monoamine oxidase.

5-Hydroxytryptamine

5-Hydroxytryptamine is another potent vasoactive substance found in a variety of tissues but particularly in the platelets (p. 16). It is inactivated in the same way as norepinephrine.

Prostaglandins

The lung capillaries appear to play an important role in the metabolism (formation, transformation, and inactivation) of the prostaglandins; these are a group of ubiquitous lipids formed from arachidonic acid with a variety of biological effects (p. 103).

Other Substances

During allergic and anaphylactic reactions the lung produces a number of biologically active substances which can overflow into the blood. Among these are histamine (p. 101) and certain prostaglandins or their precursors.

The handling of bioactive material by the pulmonary capillaries is important because each minute an amount of blood equal to the total blood volume passes through them. However, this metabolic role is not confined to the lung endothelial cells. For example, converting enzyme is present in many blood vessels, as are the enzymes involved in the metabolism of prostaglandins.

Clotting

The entire lining of the cardiovascular system has the important function of inhibiting intravascular coagulation by preventing adherence of the platelets which continuously bombard it. To do so the endothelial cells synthesize prostacyclin, which, like the other prostaglandins (p. 103), is derived from arachidonic acid. Prostacyclin is a strong inhibitor of platelet aggregation (Fig. 2–9). Intravascular coagulation is further inhibited by the presence of natural anticoagulants. The most important are heparin, a polysaccharide formed in the liver and the pericapillary mast cells, and antithrombin III.

When a blood vessel is ruptured, the amount of bleeding depends on the pressure within the vessel, the nature of the interstitial space, the degree to which the injured blood vessel constricts, aggregation of the platelets, and formation of a blood clot. The vascular smooth muscle cells of the injured blood vessel contract because the aggregating platelets release vasoconstrictor substances, in particular 5-hydroxytryptamine (p. 16). When the interstitial space restricts the outflow of blood, the pressure within it rises quickly, the resultant hematoma counteracts the intravascular pressure, and the bleeding ceases. If the bleeding occurs from the skin surface or into the intestinal lumen or a body cavity, the intravascular pressure is unopposed.

The clotting process involves a complex interaction between the blood vessel wall, platelets, and coagulation factors (Fig. 2–10). The latter are plasma proteins synthesized in the liver; the synthesis of several of these factors (prothrombin and factors VII, IX, and X) requires vitamin K. Blood coagulation is initiated when the lining is injured and subendothelial elements are exposed to the blood. Von Willebrand factor is present as a subendothelial fibrillar network to which platelets adhere without aggregation or degranulation. The exposure to connective tissue, principally collagen, leads to platelet aggregation and release of the content of the platelet granules (p. 223). In addition to vasoactive substances (e.g., 5-hydroxytryptamine, prostaglandins) the platelets release a protein

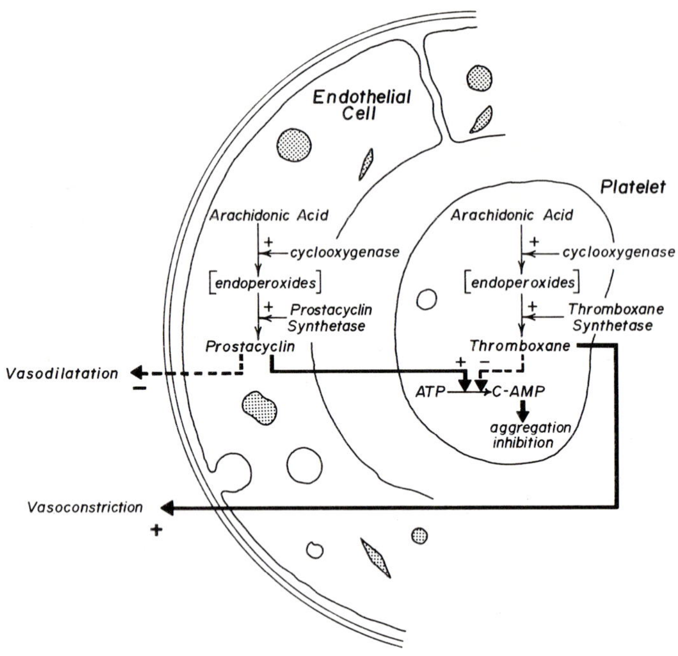

FIG. 2–9. Role of metabolites of arachidonic acid in platelet aggregation. The production of thromboxane by the platelets inhibits the formation of 3′5′ adenosine monophosphate (cyclic AMP, c-AMP) from adenosine triphosphate (ATP). By contrast, the vessel wall produces prostacyclin, which activates cyclic AMP formation and causes inhibition of platelet aggregation. When the endothelial cells do not produce prostacyclin because of trauma or disease, the production of thromboxane dominates and platelets adhere to the vessel wall. If the lining of the blood vessel is interrupted, the collagen fibers lying just outside the endothelium liberate an unknown substance which causes platelets to aggregate at the site of injury. Prostacyclin causes vasodilatation and thromboxane vasoconstriction. [Modified from Moncada and Vane (1978): In: *Mechanisms of Vasodilatation,* edited by Vanhoutte and Leusen, p. 107. Karger, Basel, 1978.]

(platelet factor 4) which neutralizes the inhibitory effect that circulating heparin has on the clotting process; platelet-factor-4-like activity may also originate from injured endothelial cells. The platelets also release adenosine diphosphate, which promotes further platelet aggregation.

The damaged endothelium and the platelets provide the phospholipid surface on which the activation of prothrombin ultimately occurs. This activation can be initiated directly by tissue factors (thromboplastin) stimulating the activity of the plasma enzyme proconvertin (factor VII), which in the presence of Ca^{2+} activates the prothrombin converting enzyme (factor X); this chain of reactions initiated by tissue damage is often referred to as the extrinsic pathway. Activation of prothrombin can also occur in the absence of tissue damage (intrinsic pathway), although subendothelial structures presented to the plasma by endothelial

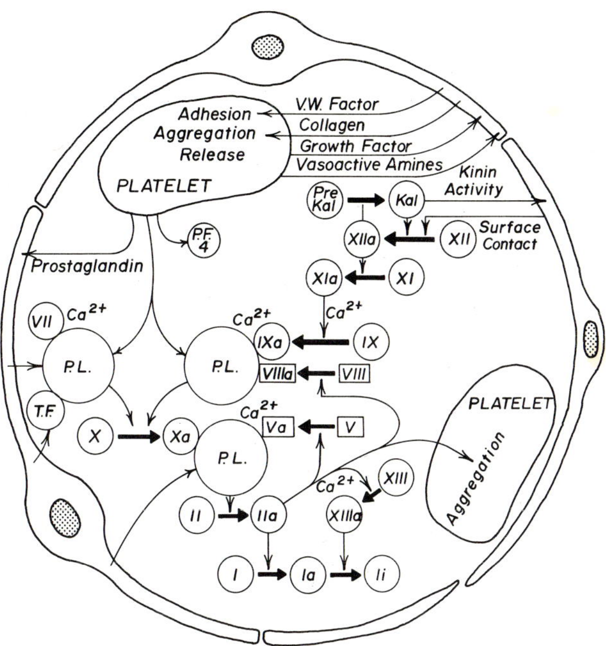

FIG. 2–10. Interaction between the blood vessel wall, platelets, and plasma coagulation factors. Factor X represents the crossover point between the "intrinsic" system (moderated by factors IX and VIII, Ca^{2+}, and phospholipids) and the "extrinsic" system of coagulation (moderated by factor VII, tissue factor, Ca^{2+}, and phospholipids). Factor X sets the conversion of thrombin in motion, which initiates the deposition of fibrin and accelerates the coagulation process at various levels (for details see text). a = activated form. I = fibrinogen. Ia = fibrin. Ii = cross-linked fibrin. II = prothrombin. IIa = thrombin. V = factor V, proaccelerine. VII = factor VII, proconvertine. VIII = cofactor VIII. IX = factor IX, plasma thromboplastin antecedent. X = factor X, prothrombin converting enzyme. XI = factor XI. XII = factor XII, Hageman factor. XIII = factor XIII, fibrin stabilizing factor. $P.F._4$ = platelet factor 4. P.L. = phospholipid. PreKal = prekallikrein. Kal = kallikrein. (Courtesy of Dr. K. Mann.)

damage facilitate the plasmatic blood coagulation cascade. In this cascade surface contact activates the Hageman factor (glass factor, factor XII). Once activated, factor XII in turn activates prekallikrein to kallikrein (p. 102); kallikrein serves as a feedback which accelerates the activation of factor XII. Activated factor XII initiates the formation of active factor XI, which in the presence of Ca^{2+} subsequently activates the plasma thromboplastic antecedent factor (factor IX). Activated factor IX is the intrinsic activator of factor X; its effective catalytic function requires Ca^{2+} ions, a phospholipid surface, and the cofactor protein factor VIII. As in the extrinsic pathways, the activated factor X in conjunction with phospholipid and Ca^{2+} (prothrombinase complex) sets in motion the conversion of prothrombin to thrombin. Once thrombin is formed it exerts a positive feedback on the coagulation process at different levels by promoting: (1) platelet aggregation; (2) proteolytic activation of the cofactor VIII, which favors the activation of factor X; and (3) activation of proaccelerin (factor V), which enhances the conversion of prothrombin. Thrombin is a proteolytic enzyme which converts fibrinogen into fibrin; it also activates fibrin stabilizing factor (factor XIII), which catalyzes the formation of cross links within the fibrin polymer deposition. The fibrin threads form an interlacing meshwork in which the blood cells are trapped and eventually seal off the damaged area of the endothelium (Fig. 2–10). Retraction of the fibrin threads is initiated by factors liberated by platelets adhering to the crossing points between these threads. The retraction results in expulsion of the remaining components of plasma (serum).

Tears of the endothelial or endocardial surface may precipitate the formation of an intravascular clot which may partially or completely occlude the lumen of the vessel (thrombosis). If the clot is dislodged by the bloodstream and wedged in a smaller, downstream vessel (embolus), it endangers the blood supply to the tissues. The resulting hypoxia, if prolonged, causes irreversible damage to the tissue cells (infarction; p. 227).

SUPPORTING STRUCTURES

In the heart and the blood vessel wall, the muscle cells are embedded in connective tissue consisting of elastin and collagen fibers. The relative distribution of these two types of fiber determines much of the passive behavior and the viscoelastic properties of the wall. In the heart, as well as in the peripheral veins, the connective tissue serves as the supporting skeleton for the endothelial and endocardial folds which form the valves.

Heart

The right and left heart each consist of two muscular chambers, an atrium and a ventricle (Figs. 2–11 through 2–13). The valves between the atria and ventricles are attached to fibrous rings which separate these chambers (Fig. 2–14). They consist of cusps composed of endocardium-covered collagen, which is characterized by its low distensibility; the left (mitral) valve has two cusps, and the right (tricuspid) valve has three. The free edges of these valves are connected by endocardium-covered strands of collagen (chordae tendinae) to finger-like processes of myocardium called the papillary muscles. These prevent valve eversion during systole and thus regurgitation of blood from the ventricle to the atrium.

The semilunar valves are placed at the origin of the aorta and the pulmonary artery, and have a composition similar to that of the mitral and tricuspid valves. Their function is to prevent reflux into the ventricles during diastole. The coronary arteries, which supply the heart muscle with blood, arise behind the aortic semilunar valves (sinuses of Valsalva).

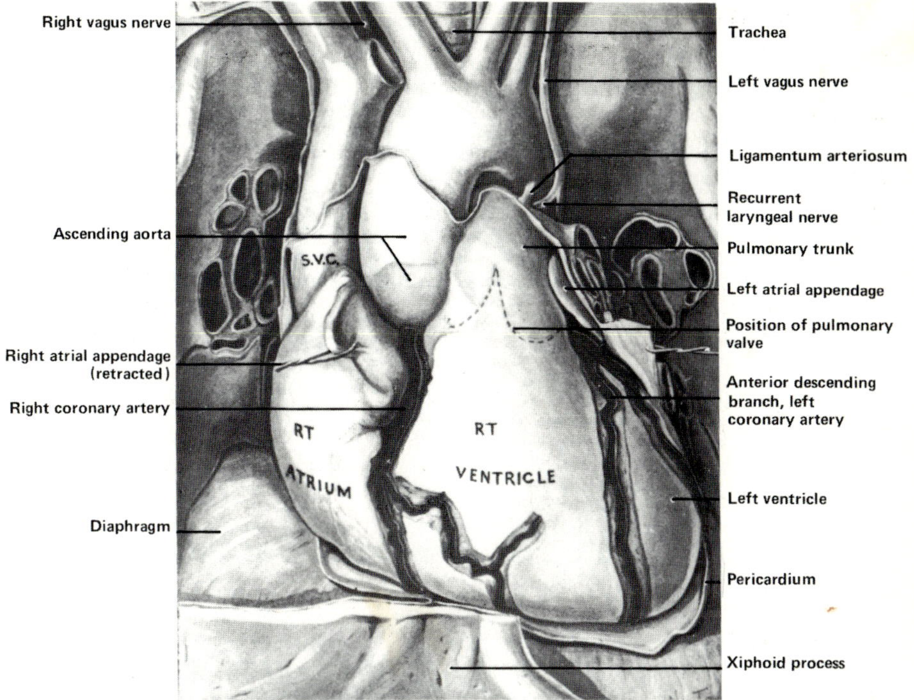

FIG. 2–11. The heart viewed from the front with the lungs retracted and the pericardium resected. S.V.C. = superior vena cava. (From Walmsley and Watson: *Clinical Anatomy of the Heart,* p. 61. Churchill Livingstone, Edinburgh, 1978.)

Arteries

The aorta is composed of an ascending part, an arch, and a descending part. It gives rise to the arteries supplying the tissues and organs of the body (Fig. 2–15).

Veins

In man, venous valves are more prominent in the veins of the leg than the arm, reflecting the adaptation to larger changes in hydrostatic pressure. Each valve possesses two cusps composed of endothelium-covered collagen. They are found in the superficial and deep venous systems of the leg, as well as in the branches connecting these two systems. In the latter they are designed to permit blood to flow from the superficial to the deep veins (Fig. 2–16). This arrangement of valves allows the massaging action of skeletal muscle contraction to propel blood toward the heart in the upright posture (muscle pump; p. 87).

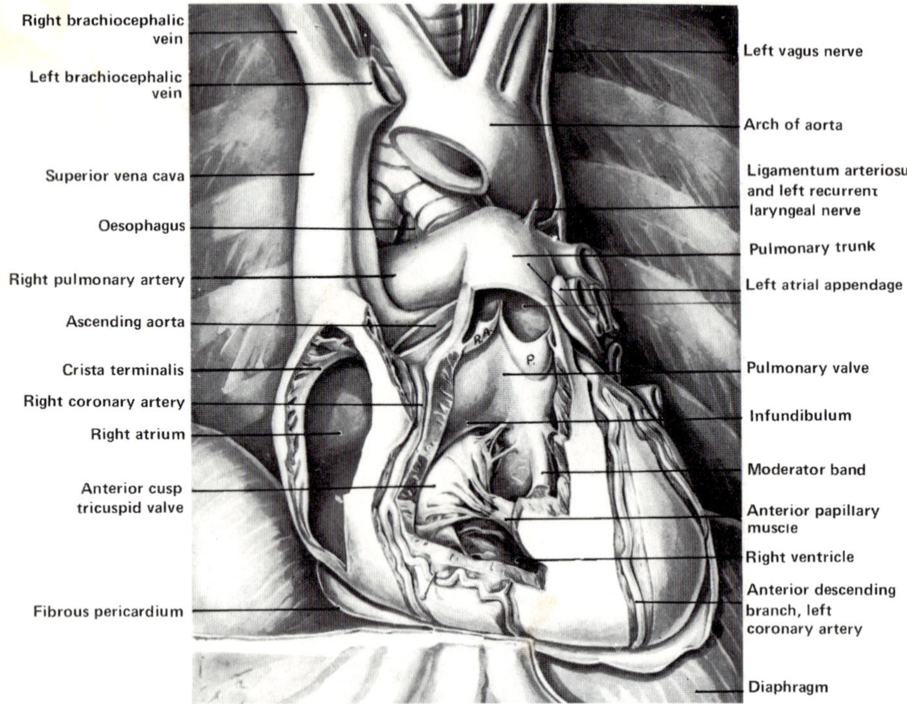

FIG. 2–12. The heart viewed from the front after removal of the lungs, the anterior wall of the right atrium and right ventricle, and most of the ascending aorta. The crista terminalis is a muscular ridge on the interior of the right atrium that extends downward from the front of the superior vena cava to the front of the opening of the inferior vena cava. Projecting forward from it are small muscle bundles which give the anterior part of the chamber a trabeculated appearance. The remainder of the right atrium is smooth-walled, and into this part the superior and inferior vena cava and coronary sinus open. The superior vena cava returns the blood from the upper part of the body and opens into the upper and posterior part of the atrium. There is no valve at the orifice. The inferior vena cava is larger than the superior, returns the blood from the lower part of the body, and opens into the lowest part of the atrium near the interatrial septum. The orifice is skirted anteriorly by a rudimentary semilunar valve. In the fetus this valve is large and serves to direct the flow from the inferior vena cava into the left atrium through an opening, the foramen ovale, in the interatrial septum (p. 270). The fossa ovalis and the limbus fossae ovalis mark the remains of the foramen ovale between the two atria. The coronary sinus returns the greater part of the blood from the heart muscle. Its opening is placed between the orifice of the inferior vena cava and the tricuspid valve. The valve of the coronary sinus covers the lower part of its orifice and serves to prevent regurgitation of blood into the sinus during contraction of the atrium.

The right ventricle has an inflow part and an outflow part. The inflow part has rough walls owing to the presence of irregular muscular columns (trabeculae carneae). It receives the blood from the right atrium through the tricuspid valve. The outflow part, infundibulum or pulmonary conus, has smooth walls and leads to the pulmonary orifice. The tricuspid valve has three somewhat triangular cusps: the anterior, the posterior, and the septal. The anterior, which is the largest, projects into the right ventricle and is interposed between the atrioventricular orifice and the infundibulum; the septal cusp is in relation to the ventricular septum. The moderator band is attached to the base of the anterior papillary muscle. Each cusp is formed by a duplication of the lining membrane of the heart strengthened by intervening layers of

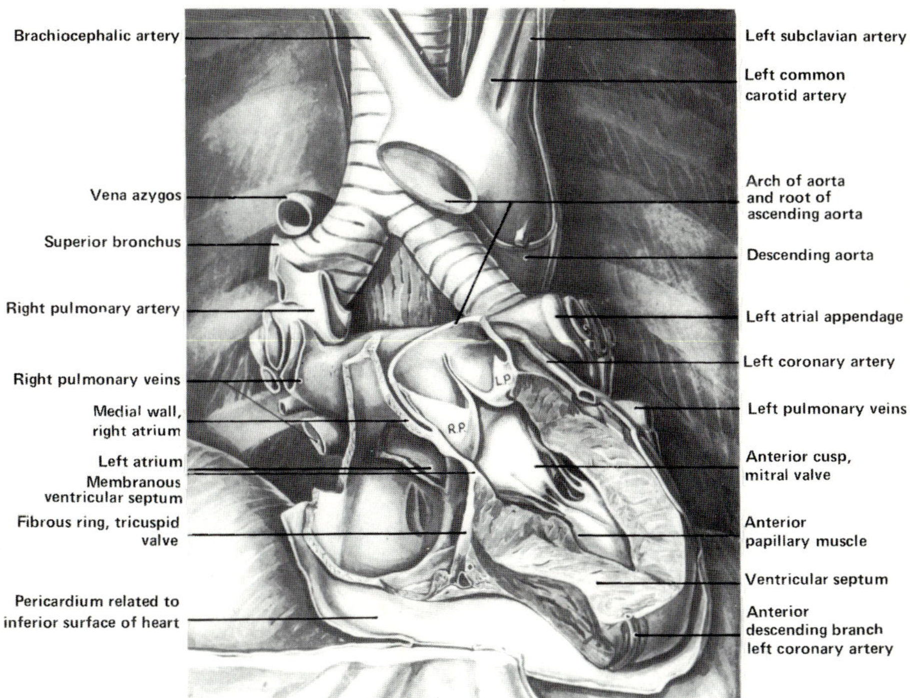

FIG. 2–13. The heart viewed from the front after removal of the right ventricle and much of the ventricular septum to expose the interior of the left ventricle and the root of the aorta. The left ventricle is longer and more conical than the right. The trabeculae carneae have a dense interlacement at the apex of the ventricle. The mitral valve has an anterior and a posterior cusp. The anterior cusp projects into the interior of the left ventricle; its smooth anterior surface forms the posterior wall of the left ventricular outflow tract. The chordae tendineae of two papillary muscles (anterior and posterior) are attached to both cusps of the mitral valve. At the upper part of the ventricular septum there is a thin oval membranous area called the membranous part of the ventricular septum. This is in continuity with the right side of the ascending aorta. Two of the three cusps of the aortic valve are shown. L.P. = left coronary cusp. R.P. = right coronary cusp. The left atrium is more posterior and to the right of the left ventricle. (From Walmsley and Watson: *Clinical Anatomy of the Heart,* p. 78. Churchill Livingstone, Edinburgh, 1978.)

←

fibrous tissue. Their bases are attached to the fibrous ring surrounding the atrioventricular orifice. Their atrial surfaces are smooth, and their ventricular surfaces give attachment to fine tendinous cords (chordae tendineae). These in turn are attached to two papillary muscles. The anterior is the larger, and its chordae tendineae are connected with the anterior and posterior cusps of the valve. The posterior is attached to the posterior and septal cusps.

The interior of the left ventricle is not seen, but its line of demarcation from the right ventricle is indicated by the anterior descending branch of the left coronary artery. (From Walmsley and Watson: *Clinical Anatomy of the Heart,* p. 68. Churchill Livingstone, Edinburgh, 1978.)

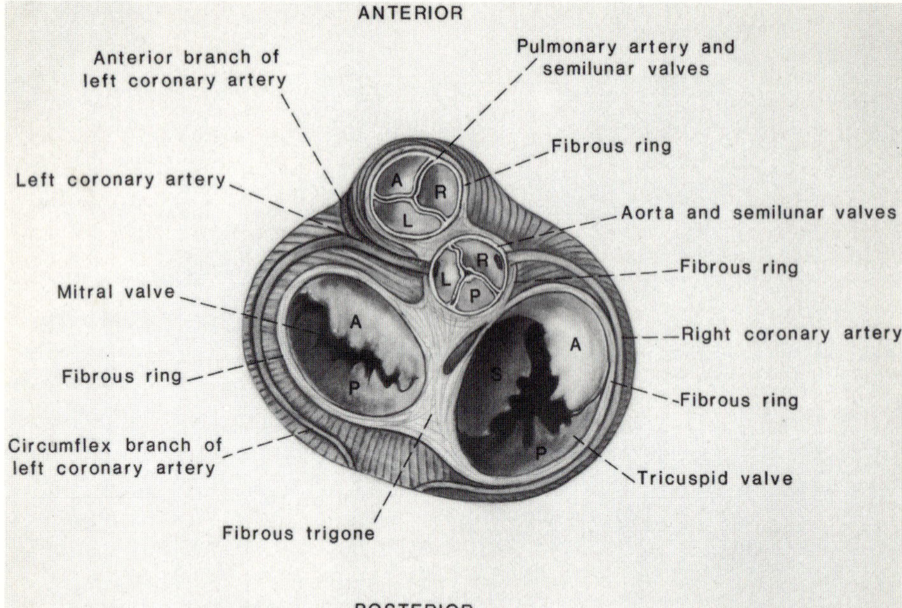

FIG. 2–14. Section through the base of the heart at the level of the fibrous ring supporting the cardiac valves. The coronary arteries arise from the sinuses of Valsalva behind the leaflets of the aortic valve. The right coronary artery arises from the anterior aortic sinus. The left coronary artery, larger than the right, arises from the left posterior aortic sinus. A = anterior. P = posterior. R = right. L = left. S = septal.

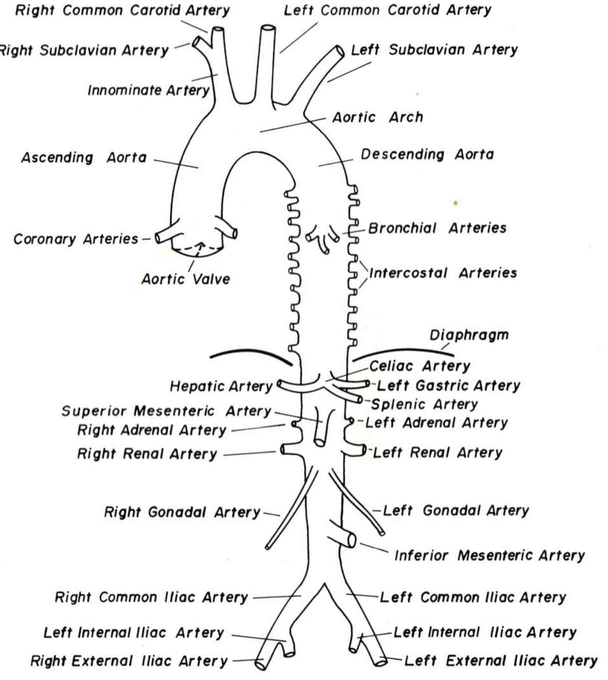

FIG. 2–15. Anatomy of the aorta and its branches.

SURROUNDING STRUCTURES

The external surface of the myocardium is covered with a thin layer of cells, the epicardium. The epicardium forms the inner surface of the pericardial sac, which invests the whole heart and the adjacent parts of the great vessels that enter or leave it. The pericardial sac contains 5 to 30 ml of clear fluid formed by the epicardium and is drained by the lymphatic system. The external layer (pericardium) consists mainly of collagenous tissue, which is highly resistant to distention and exerts a restraining influence on the left ventricle (Fig. 2–11). The double-layered membrane with the pericardial lymph lubricates the heart and minimizes the friction when it contracts and relaxes. If, in abnormal conditions, additional fluid accumulates in the pericardial sac, the heart is compressed, stroke volume decreases, and cardiac output is impaired (cardiac tamponade; p. 240).

The muscle layers of the blood vessel wall are surrounded by loose connective tissue, the adventitia.

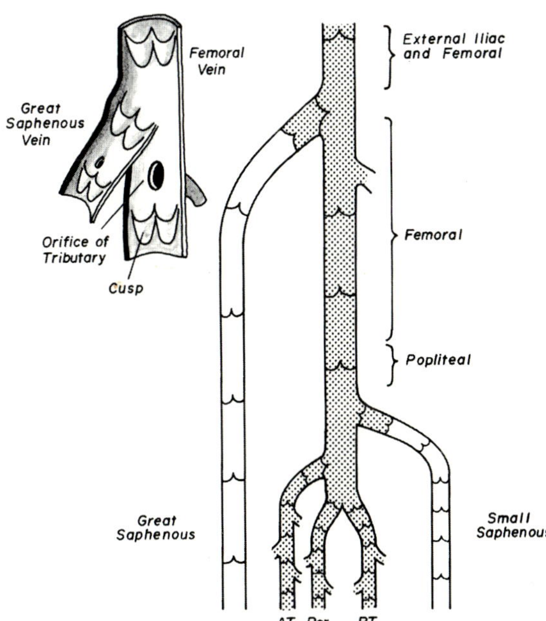

FIG. 2–16. Right: Valve frequency and distribution in the veins of the lower limb. Stippled = deep veins. Clear = superficial veins. AT = anterior tibial. Per = peroneal. PT = posterior tibial. (Modified from Ludbrook: *Aspects of Venous Function in the Lower Limbs.* Charles C Thomas, Springfield, Ill., 1966.) **Left:** Upper portions of the femoral and great (long) saphenous veins laid open to show valves.

MUSCLE OF CARDIAC AND VASCULAR WALLS

Morphology

Myocardial Cell

The fibrous rings surrounding the heart valves form the fibrous skeleton of the heart to which are attached the atrial and ventricular myocardium. The ventricular walls are composed of superimposed layers of muscle bundles running in a spiral from the base to the apex where they form the papillary muscle. Both atria are thin-walled muscular chambers (1 to 3 mm) separated from each other by the interatrial septum. In the adult the circumference of the orifice between the right atrium and ventricle (tricuspid) approximates 11 cm

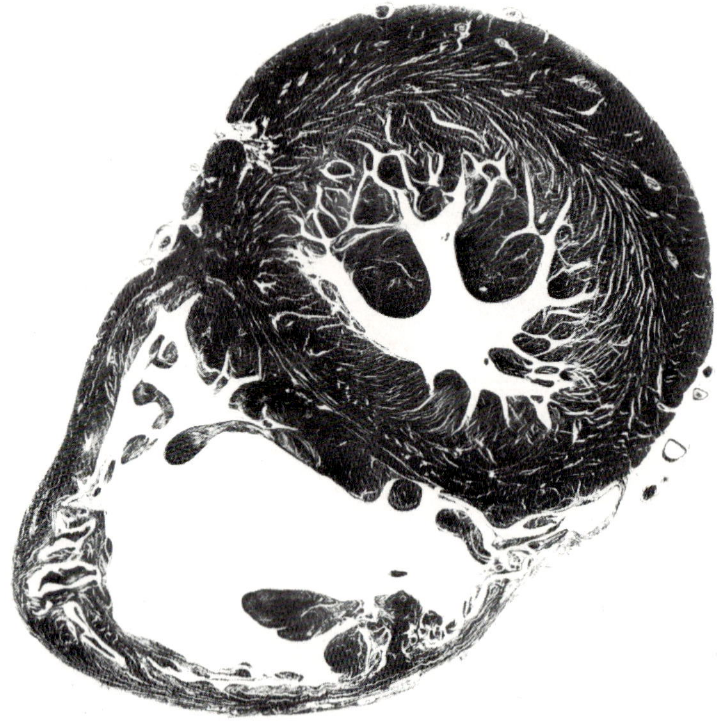

FIG. 2–17. A transverse section of the ventricles of an adult's heart about midway between the apex of the heart and the atrioventricular (coronary) sulcus. The specimen has been placed as nearly as possible in the position it occupied before removal from the thorax so that the right ventricle forms the greater part of the anterior surface and the left ventricle forms most of the inferior or diaphragmatic surface of the heart. Note, between the trabeculae carneae, the thick wall of the left ventricle as compared to that of the right ventricle. (From Walmsley and Watson: *Clinical Anatomy of the Heart,* p. 200. Churchill Livingstone, Edinburgh, 1978.)

and that between the left atrium and ventricle (mitral) 9.5 cm. The mass of the left ventricle (thickness 12 to 15 mm) is approximately three times that of the right. The two ventricles are separated by the intraventricular septum, whose muscle is as thick as that of the free wall of the left ventricle (Fig. 2–17). The cavity of the left ventricle is cone shaped; the inflow and the outflow tracts (mitral and aortic orifices, respectively) are adjacent at the base of the cone. The right ventricle is crescentic in cross section; the valves on the inflow and outflow tract (tricuspid and pulmonary valves) are separated so that the right ventricular cavity is U-shaped (Fig. 2–12 and 2–13; see Appendix, Table 3).

The myocardium consists of columns of large cylindrical muscle fibers (100

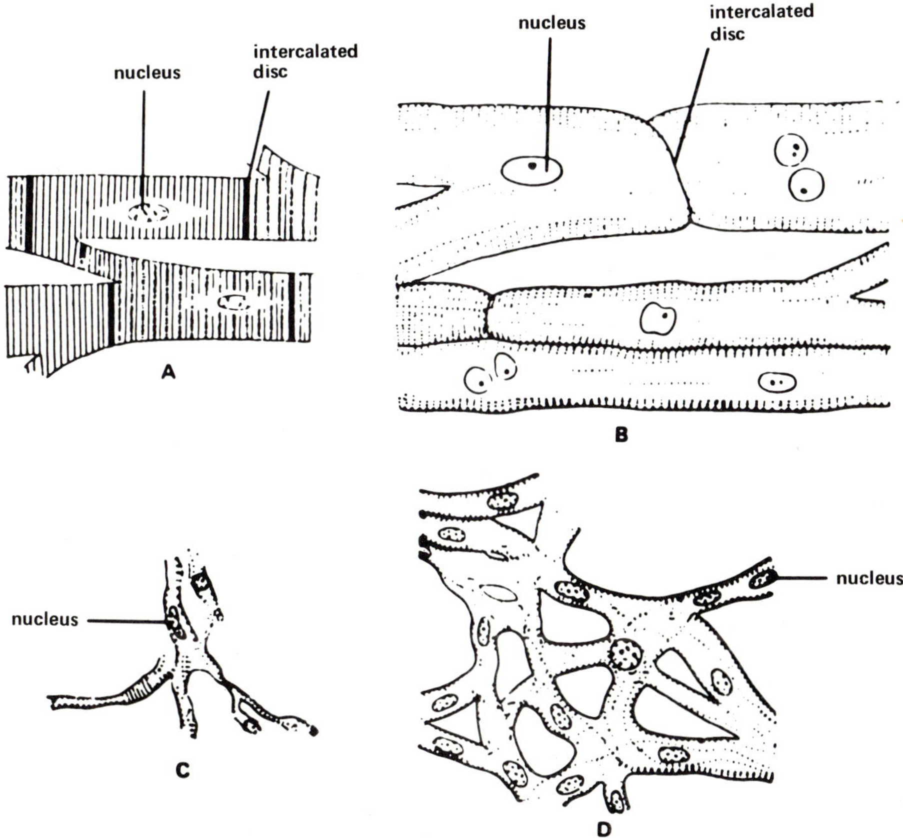

FIG. 2–18. Cells comprising the human heart. **A:** Working myocardial cell of the ventricle, showing intensely staining cross-striations, central nuclei, and intercalated discs. **B:** Purkinje fiber, showing large, faintly staining cells with sparse cross-striation. **C:** Sinus node. **D:** Atrioventricular node. Both nodes have a network of small, sparsely cross-striated cells. (Modified from Benninghoff: *Lehrbuch der Anatomie des Menschen,* 1944. Lehmanns Verlag, Munich. From Katz: *Physiology of the Heart.* Raven Press, New York, 1977.)

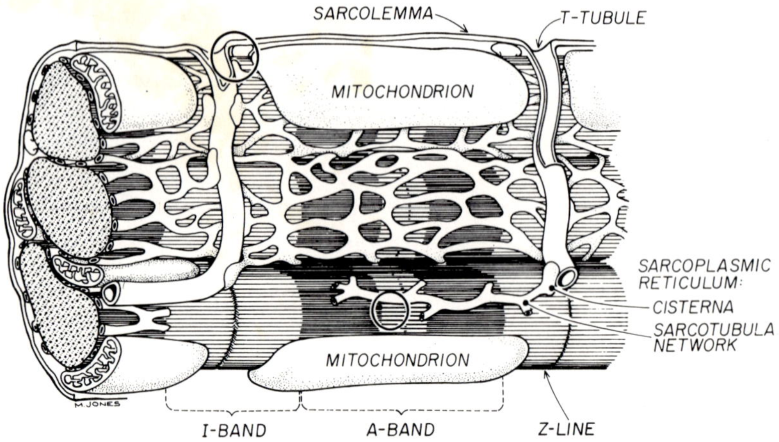

FIG. 2–19. Ultrastructure of the myocardial cell. Contractile proteins are arranged in a regular array of thick and thin filaments (seen in cross section at the left). The A-band represents the region of the sarcomere occupied by the thick filaments into which thin filaments extend from either side. The I-band is the region of the sarcomere occupied only by thin filaments; these extend toward the center of the sarcomere from the Z-lines, which bisect each I-band. The sarcomere, the functional unit of the contractile apparatus, is the region between each pair of Z-lines; it contains two half I-bands and one A-band. The transverse tubular system (t-tubule) is lined by a membrane that extends from the sarcolemma and carries the extracellular space into the myocardial cell. In contrast to the t-tubules of skeletal muscle, those of the myocardium can run in a longitudinal as well as a transverse direction. The sarcoplasmic reticulum, a membrane network that surrounds the contractile proteins, consists of the sarcotubular network at the center of the sarcomere and the cisternae, which abut on the t-tubules and the sarcolemma. Mitochondria are shown in the central sarcomere and in cross section at the left. (From Katz: *N. Engl. J. Med.,* 293:1184, 1975.)

microns length, 15 microns diameter) which branch to form a network (Fig. 2–18). Each cell consists of a cell membrane (sarcolemma) surrounding bundles of small fibers, the myofibrils, which are approximately 1 micron wide and 1.5 to 2.5 microns long and constitute about 50% of the cell volume. The cells contain numerous mitochondria (about 35% of the cell volume) and a centrally located nucleus (Fig. 2–19). Within the myofibrils the contractile proteins are arranged longitudinally into repeating units, the sarcomeres. These are composed of myofilaments, which are macromolecular complexes of contractile proteins. There are two types of myofilament. The thicker type, limited to the middle part of the sarcomere (A-band) consists of myosin. The thinner type consists of actin molecules, which are anchored at each end of the sarcomere to the anatomical and functional delineation of the contractile unit, the Z-line. Under the microscope the Z-line is recognized as a dark line crossing the myofibril. Where two cells merge, the terminal Z-lines together with the sarcolemma form a single membrane, the intercalated disc. Within the cardiac muscle cells the arrangement of Z-lines and A-bands from adjacent myofibrils is such that,

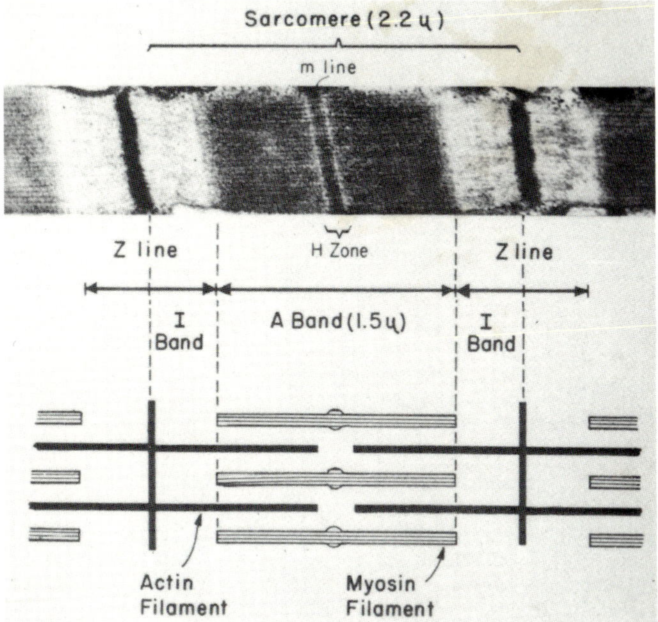

FIG. 2–20. Filamentous fine structure of the sarcomere *(below)* in relation to the sarcomere band pattern *(above).* (From Sonnenblick et al.: *Am. Heart J.,* 68:336, 1964.)

as in skeletal muscle, the cells present a cross-striated appearance (Fig. 2–20).

The sarcoplasmic reticulum forms a complex network of intracellular tubules which encircle the myofibrils and serve as the main source for release and reuptake of Ca^{2+} ions. The transverse tubules (t-system) are invaginations of the sarcolemma at the level of the Z-line which penetrate the cells and come in close contact, but are not continuous, with the terminal cisternae of the sarcoplasmic reticulum (Fig. 2–19).

Vascular Cells

Arteries, arterioles, and veins have muscle cells in the tissue layer (media) adjacent to the subendothelial connective fibers (intima). These cells usually are arranged in a circumferential manner, and their number varies with the function of the vessel (Fig. 2–21). Per unit of tissue mass, the cells are most numerous in the small arteries and arterioles, and in the splanchnic and cutaneous veins. The vascular muscle cells are 100 microns or less long and approximately 3 microns in diameter. They consist of a cell membrane and myofibrils arranged along the length of the muscle cells. These myofibrils show no cross striations, which prompted the name "smooth" muscle cells. They contain mitochondria

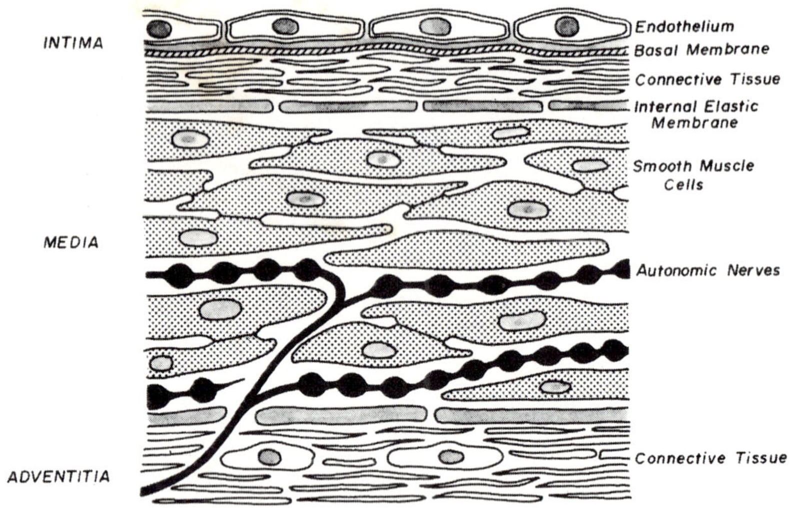

FIG. 2–21. Structure of the wall of a large artery showing the various layers (intima, internal elastic membrane, media, and adventitia). Depending on the type of vessel, only endothelium (capillaries), mainly smooth muscle (arterioles), or large quantities of elastic connective tissue (large arteries and veins) may be present. In arteries the autonomic nerves usually do not penetrate deep into the media; in veins the media usually is innervated throughout.

and a centrally located nucleus. In certain vascular tissues the cells are functionally connected by means of close apposition of the cell membranes of two neighboring cells (nexus, or tight junction). The filaments are attached to either the internal side of the cell membrane or to dark staining areas (dense bodies) in the cytoplasm. These dense bodies correspond to the Z-line of the cardiac muscle cells. As in cardiac muscle, the filaments consist of actin (thin filaments) and myosin (thick filaments). The absence of cross striations is explained by the fact that the actin and myosin are not lined up in a regular fashion within the cell. The sarcoplasmic reticulum of vascular smooth muscle is relatively sparse although present as a system of tubules running mainly longitudinally. The cell membrane shows invaginations (surface vesicles) which form close appositions with the sarcoplasmic reticulum and probably correspond to a primitive form of t-system (Fig. 2–22).

FIG. 2–22. Smooth muscle cells (SM) of the portal–anterior mesenteric vein. Scale = 0.1 μm. **A:** Transverse section showing the sarcoplasmic reticulum approaching the surface vesicles and cell membrane *(arrowheads)*. The surface vesicles are absent at the membrane areas occupied by dense bodies (DB), and the sarcoplasmic reticulum does not approach the cell membrane at these areas. Microtubules *(small arrows)* are present close to the sarcoplasmic

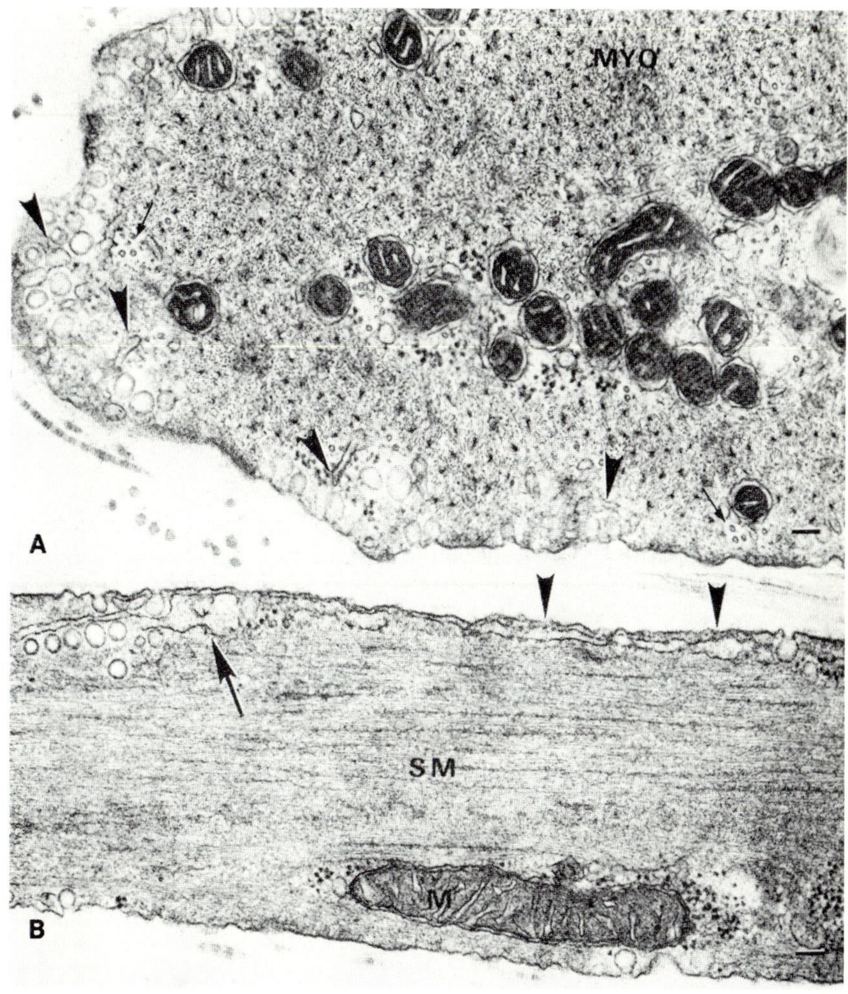

reticulum and mitochondria. Some mitochondria are in close apposition to surface vesicles (SV). Thick and thin filaments (MYO) are present, with a regular spacing of approximately 70 nm between the thick filaments. ×47,000. **B:** Longitudinal section showing an unusually long sarcoplasmic reticulum–tubule cell membrane relationship *(arrowheads)* and a dilated portion of the sarcoplasmic reticulum beside some surface vesicles *(large arrow).* Thick and thin filaments are present in the cytoplasm, and a mitochondrion (M) is in close association with a surface vesicle. ×47,000. (From Devine et al.: *J. Cell Biol.,* 52:690, 1972.)

The Contractile Process

The muscles of the heart and blood vessels are chemicomechanical transducers in that during contraction chemical energy is transformed into work.

Myocardial Cells

Changes in Membrane Characteristics

The cell membrane does not allow free movement of all the cell constituents to the extracellular space, permitting only certain extracellular molecules and ions to enter the cell. It thus is a semipermeable membrane which creates osmotic and chemical gradients between the inside and the outside of the cell; when ions are involved, electrical gradients ensue. The differences in permeability for various ions, together with the presence in the cell membrane of active carrier systems that can move ions against chemical or electrical gradients, result in the transmembrane potential difference at rest (resting membrane potential). During activation of the muscle cell there are profound changes in membrane behavior which are accompanied by electrical phenomena (action potential).

Resting membrane potential. The electrical potential which is necessary across the cell membrane to maintain equilibrium can be calculated from the knowledge of the intra- and extracellular concentration of a given ion at this equilibrium. In other words, the ionic flux resulting from the electrical force generated by the membrane potential must be equal and opposite to the ionic flux resulting from the diffusive force created by the concentration difference. This "equilibrium potential" (E_X), in millivolts (mv), is given by the Nernst equation:

$$E_X = \frac{RT}{Fz} \ln \frac{Xe}{Xi}$$

where R is the gas constant, T the absolute temperature, F the Faraday number, z the valence of the ion, Xe its extracellular concentration, and Xi its intracellular concentration. For example, in cardiac muscle, where the intracellular concentration of K^+ is high and that of Na^+ is low, the equilibrium potentials for these two ions are: $E_K = -90$ mV and $E_{Na} = +40$ mV. The situation in the intact cell is made complex by the fact that multiple ions determine the membrane potential. This is described by the Goldman equation, which relates the membrane potential *(E)* to the concentrations and permeability of the various ions involved:

$$E \log_{10} \frac{P_x X_e + P_y Y_e}{P_x X_i + P_y Y_i} \cdot \cdot \cdot \cdot$$

where P is the permeability and e the extracellular and i the intracellular concentration involved. From this equation it follows that the membrane potential tends to move toward the equilibrium potential for the ion with the greatest permeability. At rest the sarcolemma is very permeable to potassium (K^+) and relatively impermeable to other ions such as sodium (Na^+), chloride (Cl^-), and calcium (Ca^{2+}); hence the resting membrane potential is near the equilibrium potential for K^+. The cell membrane possesses an active carrier system, which in the resting state continuously pumps Na^+ from the inside to the outside against the existing high concentration gradient. Na^+ pumping is done in exchange for K^+, which is pumped from the outside to the inside of the cell. The Na^+,K^+ pump is an active process which requires energy derived from the enzymatic hydrolysis of adenosine triphosphate (ATP); the enzyme involved is activated by Na^+ and K^+ and has been named sodium-potassium-activated adenosine triphosphatase (Na^+,K^+-ATPase). As a result of the high intracellular K^+ concentration and the marked permeability of the resting membrane for the ion, part of the K^+ leaves the cell along the concentration gradient created by the Na^+,K^+ pump, so the myocardial cell at rest contains fewer positive ions than the extracellular fluid surrounding it. This then creates most of the electrical potential difference across the cell membrane (polarization). The normal value for the resting membrane potential is the highest in Purkinje fibers (around −95 mV) and the lowest in the atrioventricular node (around −65 mV).

Action potential. With the activation of a cardiac muscle cell, the permeability for Na^+ suddenly increases. As Na^+ pours into the cell the membrane potential decreases to zero and then becomes positive because Na^+ enters the cell faster than K^+ leaves it. The K^+ channels of the sarcolemma have strong rectifying properties, which means that they carry inward current more easily than outward current. The initial depolarization suddenly reduces the outward current, which is only slowly compensated for by an increase in the proportion of open K^+ channels. After the initial rapid depolarization (spike), the Na^+ permeability decreases but the increased influx of other positive charges, in particular Ca^{2+}, helps maintain a sustained depolarization (plateau) before repolarization occurs. The action potential of cardiac muscle cells is much longer than that of nerve and skeletal muscle cells, partly because of the presence of the slow inward Ca^{2+} current in the former (Fig. 2–23). These changes in membrane potential are necessary to initiate contraction of the myocardial cells (electromechanical coupling).

Excitation–Contraction Coupling

The sarcoplasmic reticulum, as the intracellular site for the release and the reuptake of Ca^{2+}, is the primary target for the changes in cell membrane potential. At rest, an energy-dependent process pumps Ca^{2+} from the cytoplasm into the sarcoplasmic reticulum to cause a high Ca^{2+} concentration in the latter; the Ca^{2+} carrier is linked to Mg^{2+}-ATPase, which provides the energy required by hydrolyzing ATP. The action potential spreads along the transverse tubules

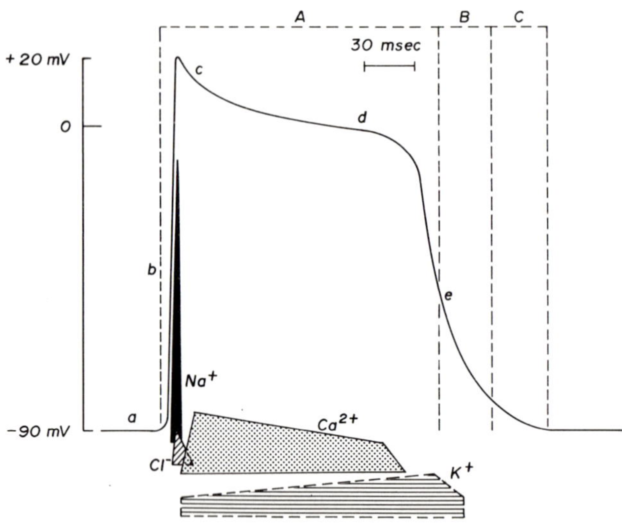

FIG. 2–23. Phases of the action potential and ion movements in a contracting myocardial cell. The transmembrane potential *(ordinate)* is recorded as a function of time *(abscissa).* (a) Resting potential. (b) Depolarization. Current flowing from a neighboring cell causes partial depolarization and increases the permeability for Na^+. The sudden influx of this ion (inward current) causes the interior of the cell to become positive with respect to the extracellular fluid (up to 20 to 30 mV). (c) Rapid repolarization. At the positive membrane potentials the permeability of the cell membrane for Na^+ decreases, but that for Cl^- increases; the inward movement of the negative ion combines with the leakage of K^+ to create an outward current, and the cell begins to repolarize. (d) Plateau phase. The action potential has initiated a slow inward movement of Ca^{2+} which results in a slow inward current; the latter neutralizes the outward movement of K^+, and as a result the membrane potential is relatively steady. (e) Restoration of resting potential. When the Ca^{2+} inward movement decreases, the increased leakage of K^+ restores the pre-excitation potential. A = effective refractory period. B = relative refractory period. C = supernormal period.

to cause instantaneous inhibition of the Ca^{2+} carrier and an increase in permeability of the sarcoplasmic reticulum. Since the Ca^{2+} concentration is highest in the latter, the sudden increase in permeability causes the discharge of Ca^{2+} into the cytoplasm in the vicinity of the myofibrils, where the Ca^{2+} concentration increases by a factor of 10 and becomes greater than 10^{-6} M. The increase in Ca^{2+} concentration then initiates the final sequences of the contractile process (Fig. 2–24). The amount of Ca^{2+} available for release by the sarcoplasmic reticulum is determined in part by the amount of the ion which enters the cell during the preceding action potential (slow inward current).

Contractile Proteins

During contraction the thin actin filaments slide between the thicker myosin filaments so that the sarcomere shortens. The thin and thick filaments remain constant in length during this process and interact (actomyosin interaction)

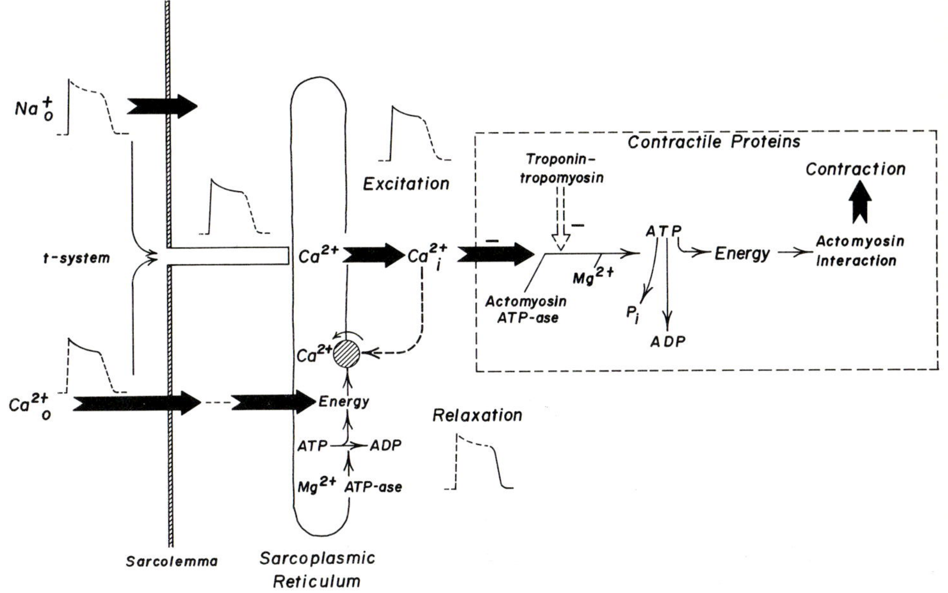

FIG. 2–24. Major steps in the excitation and contraction processes in cardiac muscle cells. ATP = adenosine triphosphate. ADP = adenosine diphosphate. o = extracellular. i = intracellular. − = inhibition. + = activation. ● = active carrier.

by virtue of cross-bridges formed between them (Fig. 2–25). The cross-bridges, which are the projecting parts of the myosin filaments, become attached to specific sites on the actin filaments. As force develops between the filaments, the actin is pulled toward the center of the sarcomere. In order to shorten further, cross-bridges must detach and reattach to a new binding site.

The velocity of shortening depends on the speed at which the cross-bridge can attach, pull, detach, and resume the original configuration. The force development by the muscle depends on the number of cross-bridges attached at a given time. Hence it is not surprising that an inverse relationship exists between force and velocity (force–velocity relationship) (Fig. 2–26). Theoretically the maximal velocity of shortening (V_{max}) is reached when no load is imposed on the muscle. Such condition can be obtained in the laboratory with isolated fragments of myocardium but not in the intact organism (p. 293).

The force a muscle can generate depends on the degree of overlap of the actin and myosin molecules at the time the muscle is activated (active length–tension relationship). If the passive stretch on the muscle is such that no overlap occurs, the cross-bridges cannot attach and no mechanical response is possible. If the sarcomere length is reduced, the cross-bridges are facing the attachment sites on the actin, and shortening (or tension development) can occur. When all cross-bridges are adjacent to their attachment sites, optimal interaction is possible, and the mechanical response is maximal. This occurs at sarcomere

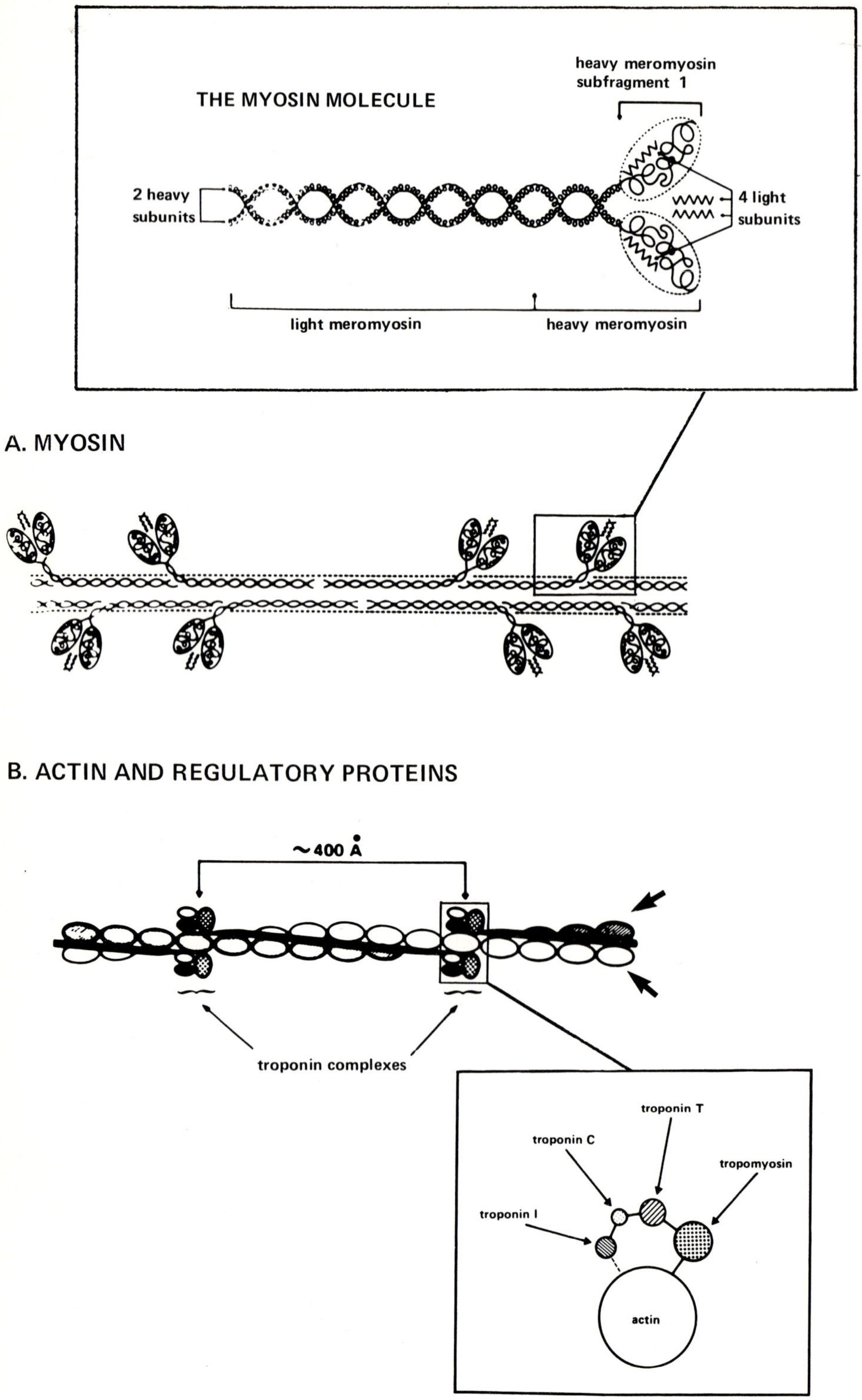

THE MYOSIN MOLECULE

heavy meromyosin subfragment 1

2 heavy subunits

4 light subunits

light meromyosin

heavy meromyosin

A. MYOSIN

B. ACTIN AND REGULATORY PROTEINS

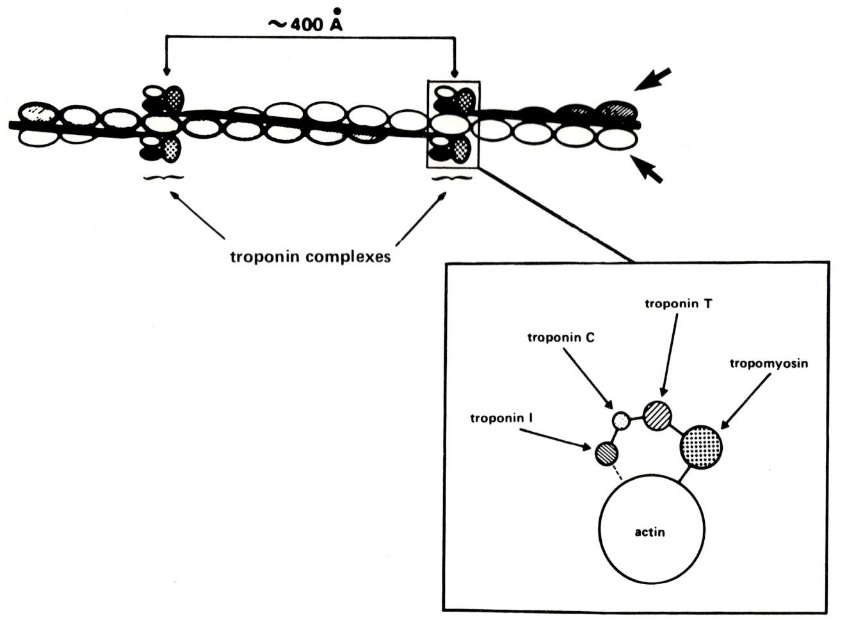

lengths of about 2.2 microns. When little stretch is imposed on the muscle the sarcomere becomes too short, and the mechanical efficiency is reduced.

In the relaxed state the actin molecule is not accessible for the cross-bridges because it is embraced by another protein complex, troponin and tropomyosin. When Ca^{2+} binds to the troponin–tropomyosin complex, the actin molecules become accessible for the cross-bridges, and the actomyosin interaction starts. The hydrolysis of ATP by the ATPase contained in myosin (actomyosin ATPase) yields the energy for the cycling of the cross-bridges.

Relaxation

Relaxation occurs when the transverse tubules and the cell membrane repolarize and when the Ca^{2+} concentration in the vicinity of the troponin–tropomyosin complex decreases below 10^{-6} M. This is caused by: (1) active reuptake of Ca^{2+} by the sarcoplasmic reticulum: (2) uptake in mitochondria by an active process, linked to oxidative metabolism, which moves Ca^{2+} in exchange for H^+; and (3) extrusion of Ca^{2+} at the cell membrane by a Na^+,Ca^{2+} carrier which allows extracellular Na^+ to flow into the cell down its concentration gradient and provides the necessary energy for the transport of Ca^{2+} against its concentration gradient. The Na^+ is then removed by the Na^+,K^+-ATPase.

←

FIG. 2–25. Organization of the contractile and regulatory proteins in the sarcomere. **A:** Organization of individual myosin molecules in the thick filament. The backbone of the thick filament is delineated by dashed lines. Individual myosin molecules have opposite polarities in the two halves of the sarcomere *(right* and *left).* The bare area in the center of the thick filament is a region devoid of cross-bridges, which can be seen to arise from the tail-to-tail organization of myosin molecules unique to the center of the thick filament. The cross-bridges represent the heads of the individual myosin molecules, which project at right angles to the long axis of the thick filament. **Inset:** Myosin molecules. Myosin is an elongated molecule consisting of a tail *(left)* and a head *(right).* The tail is composed of two α-helical chains wound around each other that extend into the paired globular head of the molecule. The head contains, in addition, four light subunits. Enzymatic cleavage at the point indicated by the arrow produces heavy and light meromyosins. The approximate molecular weight of myosin is 480,000 (two heavy chains of 200,000, two light chains of 19,000 and two light chains of 24,000). **B:** Actin exists in the sarcomere as the F-actin polymer, which provides the backbone of the thin filaments. It is composed of two strands of G-actin monomers *(ovals)* wound around each other. The G-actin monomers in the two strands *(arrows)* are identical. Each half turn of the F-actin filament contains approximately seven pairs of monomers and has a length of approximately 350 Å. The molecular weight of actin is 42,000. Tropomyosin is composed of two helical peptide chains wound around each other and joined by a single disulfide bond. It has a molecular weight of 68,000 and is found along with actin in the thin filament where it is located in the groove between the two strands of G-actin monomers. Troponin complexes are bound to tropomyosin at approximately 400-Å intervals along the thin filament and consist of three proteins (troponin T, I, and C with molecular weights of 41,000, 28,000, and 18,000, respectively). **Inset:** Cross section of half of the thin filament at the level where the troponin complexes are located. This shows proposed relationships between actin, tropomyosin, and the three components of the troponin complex. The dashed line between troponin I and actin represents a bond postulated to vary in strength depending on the binding of calcium to troponin C. (From Katz: *Physiology of the Heart.* Raven Press, New York, 1977.)

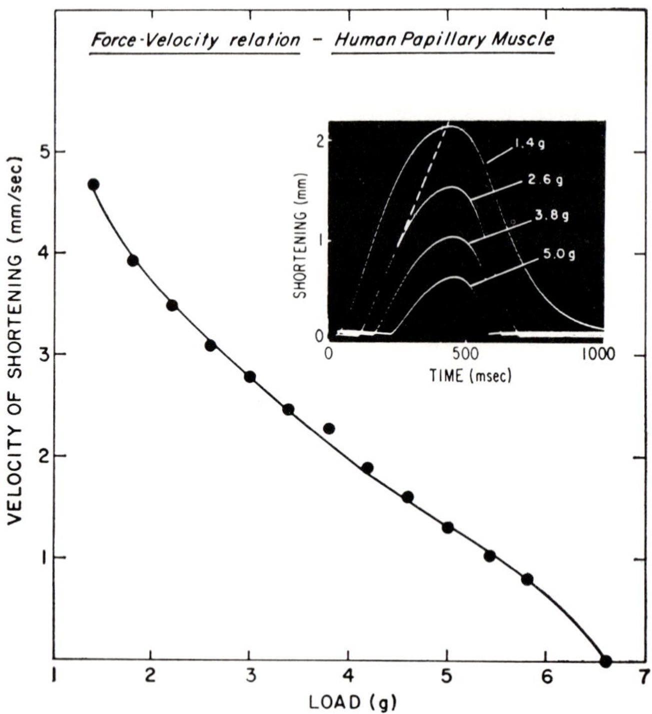

FIG. 2–26. Relationship between velocity of isotonic shortening *(ordinate)* and force, or load *(abscissa),* in a human papillary muscle stimulated at a frequency of 12 per minute. **Inset:** Original recordings of the actual contractions at four loads. (From Sonnenblick et al.: *J. Clin. Invest.,* 44:966, 1965.)

Vascular Smooth Muscle Cells

The main concepts outlined for cardiac muscle, particularly the role of Ca^{2+} as an activation coupling agent and the sliding filament mechanism of contraction, also apply for vascular smooth muscle (Fig. 2–27). However, vascular smooth muscle cells have certain pecularities:

1. Although contraction of these cells can be induced by membrane depolarization (electromechanical coupling), such changes in membrane potential either are an intrinsic property of the smooth muscle cell (automaticity, spontaneous rhythmicity) or are induced by vasoactive substances. Certain hormones and drugs can cause contraction of vascular smooth muscle without altering the membrane potential (pharmacomechanical coupling) (Fig. 2–28).

2. The sarcoplasmic reticulum plays a smaller role in the supply of Ca^{2+} for activation, since the penetration of Ca^{2+} from the outside can increase the cytoplasmic concentration of the ion to the level required to activate the contractile process. Mobilization of Ca^{2+} from intracellular stores occurs with certain

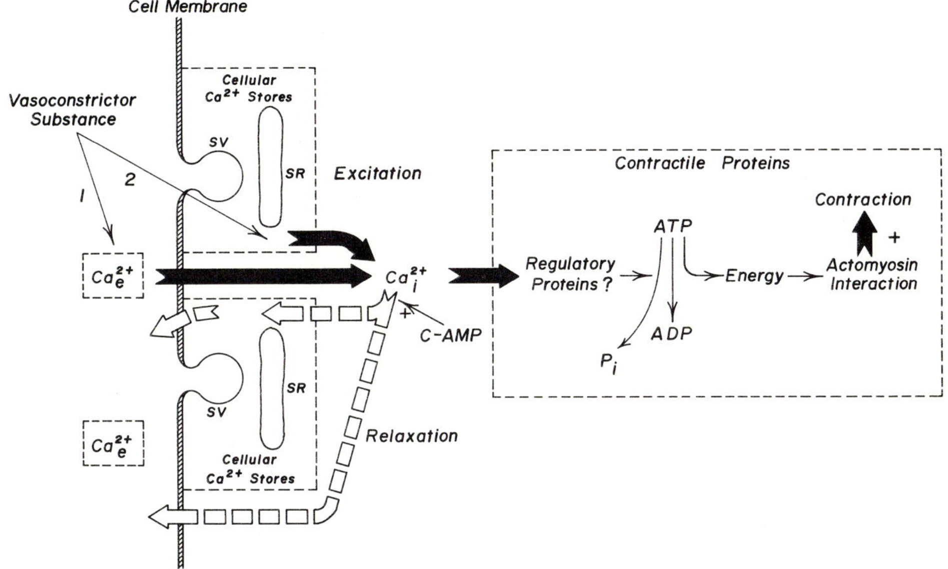

FIG. 2–27. Major steps in the excitation and contraction processes in vascular smooth muscle cells. ADP = adenosine diphosphate. ATP = adenosine triphosphate. c-AMP = 3′,5′ adenosine monophosphate. e = extracellular. i = free intracellular. Pi = inorganic phosphate. SR = sarcoplasmic reticulum. SV = surface vesicles.

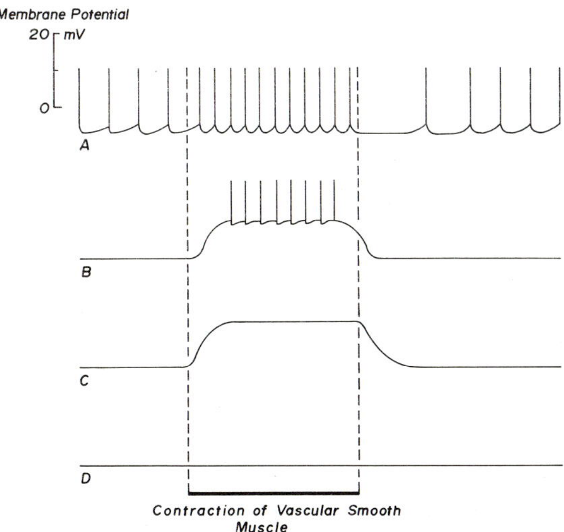

FIG. 2–28. Patterns of changes in membrane potential in vascular smooth muscle during contraction. **A:** The intrinsic spontaneous activity of the cell is augmented. **B:** Depolarization with superimposed action potentials. **C:** A sustained depolarization. **D:** No changes in membrane potential.

vasoactive substances, in particular norepinephrine and other alpha-adrenergic drugs (p. 184).

3. The role of the troponin–tropomyosin complex or of other regulatory proteins has not been established.

Metabolism

ATP Production

The contractile process itself does not require oxygen since the energy is provided by the hydrolysis of ATP. However, to maintain contractile activity, the cells must regenerate ATP. The muscle cells contain phosphocreatine, which, in the presence of the enzyme creatine phosphotransferase, can rapidly regenerate ATP according to the equation: phosphocreatine + ADP → creatine + ATP. Since the amount of ATP is less than that of phosphocreatine, and since the enzyme creatine phosphotransferase is abundant, phosphocreatine plays a major role in the instantaneous regeneration of ATP. Although phosphocreatine provides an immediate reserve of energy, it is not sufficient to sustain prolonged activity. Ultimately regeneration of the energy-rich phosphate compounds involves the breakdown of metabolic substrates such as fatty acids, glucose, and lactate. This can occur aerobically or anaerobically. The former results not only in the production of more ATP per molecule of substrate but also in the formation of carbon dioxide and water as end-products, which diffuse easily from the contracting cell. By contrast, the anaerobic consumption of substrates terminates with the production of fixed acids. When the concentration of the latter rises, intracellular acidosis becomes unavoidable since these acids are not freely diffusible. The various end-products of metabolism exert a positive feedback on the intracellular enzymatic processes as well as on the oxygen delivery to the working cells, which continuously adjusts energy production to its utilization (Fig. 2–29).

The mitochondria in close vicinity to the myofibrils are the sites of oxidative phosphorylation. Of all muscles, the myocardium contains the greatest number

FIG. 2–29. Major steps in the production of energy in muscle cells and of the factors modulating it. Myocardial cells preferentially use free fatty acids (FFA) as substrate for oxidative metabolism; the fatty acids have to be combined with coenzyme A (CoA) before they can enter the mitochondria and be transformed to acetyl coenzyme A (acetyl CoA). The vascular smooth muscle cells preferentially use carbohydrates as substrate and degrade them aerobically and anaerobically. The aerobic metabolism of a fatty acid with 11 C-atoms yields the net production of 95 molecules of adenosine triphosphate (ATP); that of glucose yields 38 molecules of ATP. The breakdown products of ATP have a positive feedback on the metabolism chain, which continuously adjusts energy production to the needs of the cell. AMP = adenosine monophosphate. ADP = adenosine diphosphate. c-AMP = cyclic AMP. P_i = inorganic phosphate. C = creatine. PC = phosphocreatine. PFK = phosphofructokinase. CPT = creatine phosphotransferase. β = beta-adrenergic receptor.

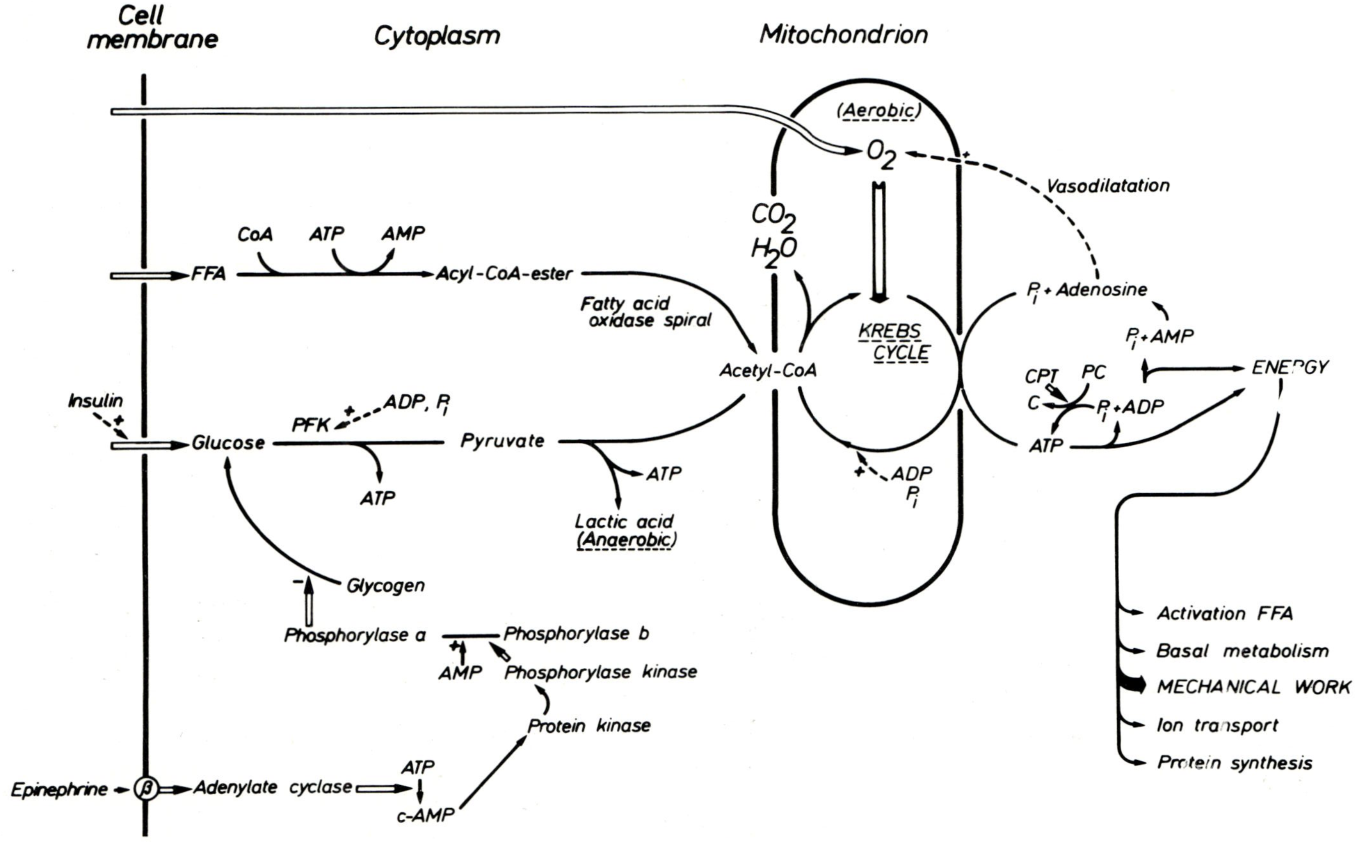
Cell membrane
Cytoplasm
Mitochondrion
(Aerobic)
O_2
Vasodilatation
CO_2
H_2O
CoA
ATP
AMP
FFA
Acyl-CoA-ester
Fatty acid oxidase spiral
KREBS CYCLE
P_i + Adenosine
P_i + AMP
Acetyl-CoA
ENERGY
CPT
PC
C
P_i + ADP
Insulin
ADP, P_i
PFK
Glucose
Pyruvate
ATP
ATP
ATP
ADP
P_i
Lactic acid
(Anaerobic)
Glycogen
Phosphorylase a
Phosphorylase b
AMP
Phosphorylase kinase
Protein kinase
ATP
Epinephrine
β
Adenylate cyclase
c-AMP
Activation FFA
Basal metabolism
MECHANICAL WORK
Ion transport
Protein synthesis

of mitochondria. This illustrates the fact that, in order for the heart to be able to function continuously, such large amounts of ATP are required that only aerobic metabolism can provide them. Thus myocardial oxygen consumption is a measurement of the total energy consumption of the heart; it augments when the heart has to perform more work and, in particular, when cardiac contractility is increased. By contrast, most vascular smooth muscle can function for relatively long periods anaerobically. This is particularly true for the veins, which are exposed to relative hypoxia throughout life.

The efficiency (work divided by energy production) of muscular contraction is relatively low. Only 5 to 20% of the total energy utilized during muscle activity is converted into external work; most of the energy is dissipated as heat. With increasing loads the efficiency decreases and even more heat is produced relative to the external work performed (Fenn effect); as a consequence the total energy consumption augments. In the heart, particularly the left ventricle, the initial load depends on the wall tension. According to Laplace's law the wall tension of the left ventricle is directly proportional to its radius and the intraventricular pressure, and inversely related to wall thickness (p. 72). Thus in disease, when the left ventricle dilates, its oxygen consumption augments for a given amount of external work to be performed (p. 258).

Whereas large amounts of ATP are required to sustain contraction (about 70% of the total energy expenditure), much smaller quantities (about 30%) are necessary for the synthesis of cellular constituents, for the ion transport systems (e.g., Na^+,K^+-ATPase), and in the case of vascular smooth muscle for the synthesis of connective fibers.

Cyclic Nucleotides

After a neurohumoral mediator binds with a specific receptor on the cell membrane (p. 181), the combination of hormone and receptor can activate the enzyme adenylate cyclase (adenyl cyclase) located in the cell membrane. The adenyl cyclase converts cytoplasmic ATP to cyclic 3′,5′-adenosine monophosphate (cyclic AMP), which brings about the specific response within the cell. One example of such responses is the positive inotropic effect of catecholamines on cardiac muscle cells. How it occurs is unknown. The cyclic AMP activates protein kinases, which catalyze the transfer of phosphate from ATP to other cell enzymes or to proteins which initiate the physiological response (activation or inhibition). Cyclic AMP is often called the "second messenger" for hormonal-mediated responses of cells, the "first messenger" being the hormone itself, which binds to the membrane receptor site (p. 181). Cyclic AMP is inactivated by conversion to 5′-AMP by the enzyme phosphodiesterase (Fig. 2–30).

The cyclic derivative of guanosine, guanosine 3′,5′monophosphate (cyclic GMP), is also present in the cells (Fig. 2–30). It too can mediate a variety of cellular responses. In some cells cyclic AMP and cyclic GMP appear to interact, one causing stimulation and the other inhibition.

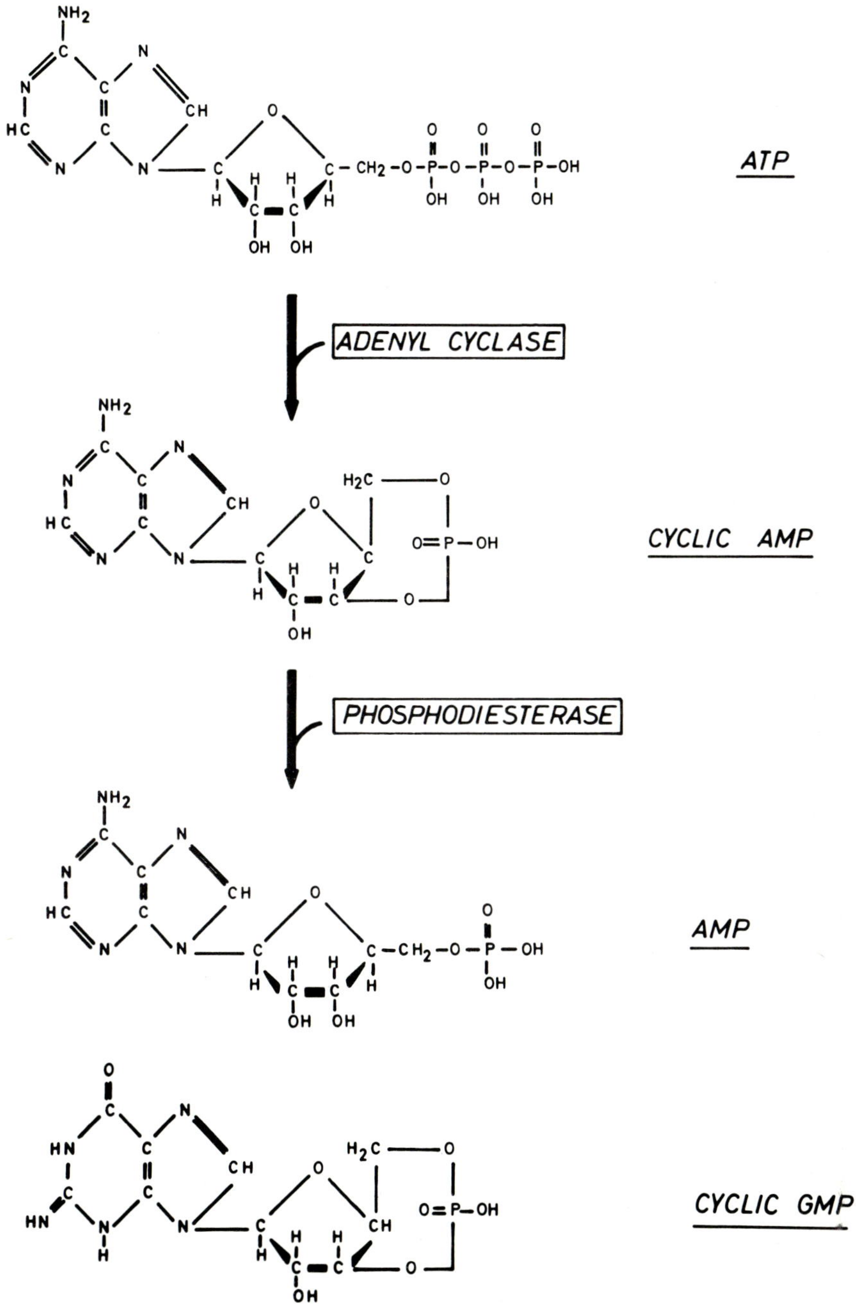

FIG. 2–30. Formation and deactivation of 3′,5′-adenosine monophosphate (cyclic AMP) and structure of guanosine 3′,5′-monophosphate (cyclic GMP). AMP = adenosine monophosphate. ATP = adenosine triphosphate.

Functional Characteristics

Passive Properties

When a muscle is stretched, there is a progressive increase in tension with increasing length. The relationship obtained is not a linear one because the muscle is composed of various constituents with different moduli of elasticity (Figs. 2–31 and 2–32). When stiffer components predominate, the curve shifts toward the tension axis. For example, the arterial wall is less distensible than

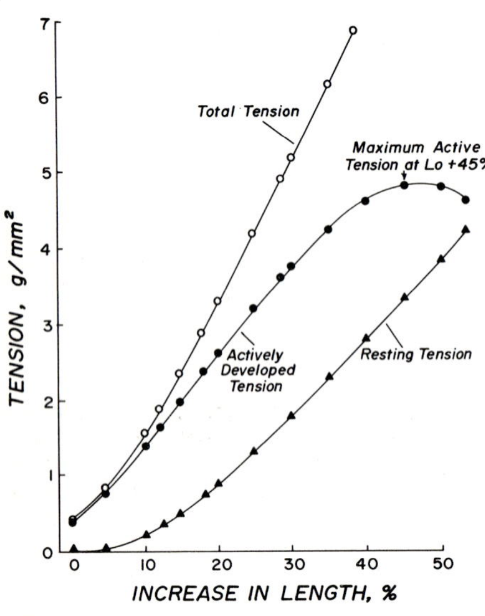

FIG. 2–31. Length–tension relationships of excised human papillary muscle. When the length is progressively increased *(abscissa)* the resting tension augments *(ordinate)*. If at each length the muscle is stimulated, the amount of isometric force the muscle can develop augments progressively to reach a maximum at a length which is 45% greater than the initial length Lo = length at which resting and active tensions approach zero. (From Sonnenblick et al.: *J. Clin. Invest.*, 44:966,1965.)

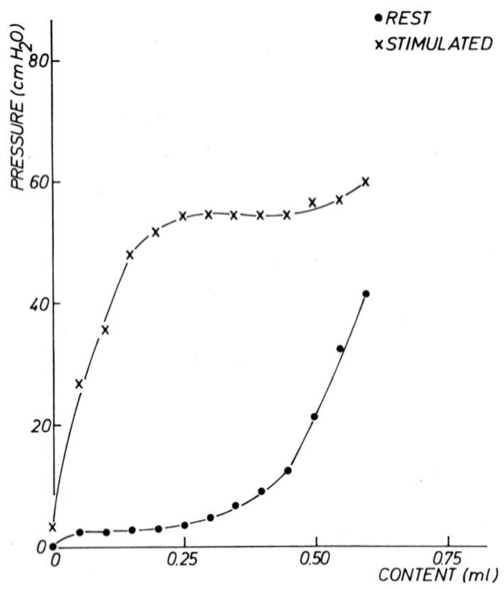

FIG. 2–32. Venous reactions depend on the degree of distention, as demonstrated in an isolated segment of cutaneous vein. The intraluminal pressure is recorded, and the content is increased by infusing known amounts of physiological solution. The plot shows the intraluminal pressure at rest and at the maximum of a contraction induced by nerve stimulation. (From Vanhoutte and Leusen: *Pfluegers Arch.*, 306:341, 1969.)

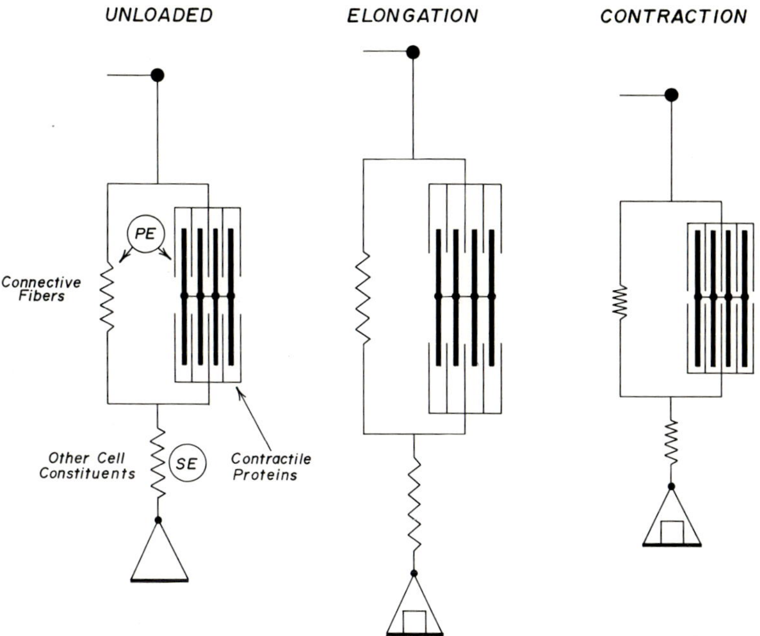

Fig. 2–33. Alterations in the elastic components of a muscle cell with elongation and contraction. When the muscle carries no load, the connective fibers within it are unstretched and the contractile proteins overlap without attachment of cross-bridges. When a load is carried by a resting muscle, these elements (parallel elastic elements; PE) are stretched until their elastic resistance offsets the load imposed. When the muscle contracts, the parallel connective fibers are unstretched when the contractile proteins actively take over the load, but shortening can occur only by compression of the other constituents of the cells, which resist this compression (series elastic components; SE).

the venous wall, which is in keeping with the role of the latter in the control of vascular capacity.

The elastic components within the muscle are of two kinds. Some resist elongation and thus are responsible for the passive length–tension relationship outlined above. In the resting state they carry the load imposed on the muscle. These elements (parallel elastic elements) consist mainly of connective tissue and contractile proteins. On the other hand, when the muscle cell shortens, the contractile elements unload the parallel elastic components, actively taking over the load attached to the muscle. However, to shorten they have to overcome the inertia and the internal resistance of the cell, which are termed the series elastic components (Fig. 2–33).

Interaction of Passive and Active Properties

If the muscle is stretched progressively and its response to an identical stimulus recorded at each length, the initial response is small. With additional stretching, it increases to a maximum (optimal length) and then decreases when further stretch is imposed. Such "active length–tension relationships" exist in cardiac (Fig. 2–31) and vascular (Fig. 2–32) muscle, and they are fundamental for understanding the functioning of the intact heart (p. 70) and the blood vessels (p. 97). The active length–tension relationship is usually explained by the fact that changes in length within the sarcomere changed the number of cross-bridges which can interact (p. 41). However, alterations in length also affect the rate at which the cross-bridges attach and detach by influencing Ca^{2+} movements within the cells.

If the load imposed on a muscle is small or moderate the muscle can shorten, and during the shortening the tension it develops remains constant (isotonic response). If the load imposed on the muscle is too large, even at maximal activation it is unable to shorten but does develop tension (isometric response). In fact, all muscular responses are a combination of isometric and isotonic components. In isometrically contracting muscles the contractile elements shorten by distending the series elastic elements (internal shortening) even if the ends of the muscle fibers are fixed. In isotonic contractions the muscle cells have to unload the parallel elastic components and carry the external load before shortening can occur (Fig. 2–33). In most cases this load corresponds to the amount of stretch imposed (preload) prior to activation. In other circumstances the load is not encountered by the muscle until actual shortening begins (afterload). The total load carried by the muscle is the sum of preload and afterload. In the beating heart a succession of isotonic and isometric phases occur whereby the filling pressure of the chambers of the heart constitute the preload, and the pressure in the aorta and the pulmonary artery the afterload (p. 71). Likewise, venous responses are a combination of isometric and isotonic components, the former to resist changes in hydrostatic pressures and the latter to mobilize blood.

Excitability

Muscle cells are "excitable" and can react to a stimulus coming from the outside of the cell or generated within the cell membrane. The latter is the case for specialized cells in the heart and certain blood vessels. The excitability of a cell refers to its ability to generate an action potential and thus to trigger the sudden increase in Na^+ permeability (Fig. 2–23). This occurs at a certain level of membrane depolarization (threshold potential). The effectiveness of a stimulus depends on its intensity and its duration. Once a stimulus is higher than threshold it is fully effective, and further increases in intensity or duration evoke no greater responses of the activated sarcomere or vascular smooth muscle cell (all-or-none phenomenon). Further increases in response can be obtained only by adjusting the degree of stretch, augmenting the contractility of the activated units, or recruiting more muscle cells.

An effective stimulus can activate the cell only when the membrane potential is below the threshold. After the cell depolarizes there is an effective refractory period, during which stimuli of any strength are unable to elicit a propagated action potential. When the membrane potential is returning toward the resting value, there is a time when a very strong stimulus may elicit a new depolarization. This relative refractory period is followed by the supernormal, or vulnerable, period when the resting values for Na^+ permeability are restored but the membrane is not yet fully repolarized; at this time stimuli less than the threshold can evoke action potentials (Fig. 2–23).

Action potentials are propagated normally only if they occur after the full recovery period, which ends a few milliseconds after the membrane potential returns to its resting value. Action potentials generated in the relative refractory and the supernormal periods are propagated at a slower speed. The duration of the refractory period depends on the duration of the action potential. Hence it is much longer in cardiac muscle than in other excitable cells.

Contractility

For a muscle cell in a given condition, effective stimuli always evoke the same degree of interaction between the actin and myosin molecules, which cease to be freely extensible and either develop tension or cause the sarcomere to shorten (active state). The intensity of the interaction (i.e., the number of cross-bridges involved in the response) depends on the amount of activated proteins and thus on the amount of liberated Ca^{2+}. The duration of the interaction is determined by the length of time the cytoplasmic concentration of Ca^{2+} is increased. Increasing either the amount of Ca^{2+} liberated or the liberation period augments the intensity or prolongs the duration of the active state, respectively. The intensity of the active state determines the "contractility" of the muscle or its potential to shorten and/or to develop tension. This means that changes in contractility can be caused only by interventions that either augment or reduce that intensity and thus augment or reduce the amount of Ca^{2+} liberated per stimulus.

When comparing skeletal, cardiac, and smooth muscle cells, it appears that in skeletal muscle the amounts of Ca^{2+} released upon stimulation in normal conditions is so overwhelming that a maximal intensity of active state is reached in the stimulated sarcomeres. This is not true for cardiac or vascular smooth muscle. For example, in cardiac cells the intensity of the active state can be either increased (positive inotropic effect) or decreased (negative inotropic effect). Such changes are caused mainly by external signals reaching the cell, the most important example being the positive inotropic effect of catecholamines (p. 86).

Although it is relatively easy to define and assess changes in contractility, it is more difficult to do so for contractility itself, since the latter is a consequence of the integration of the biochemical and biophysical events resulting in the actomyosin interaction and can be described only by a complex relationship between the force exerted by the muscle, its velocity of shortening, its length,

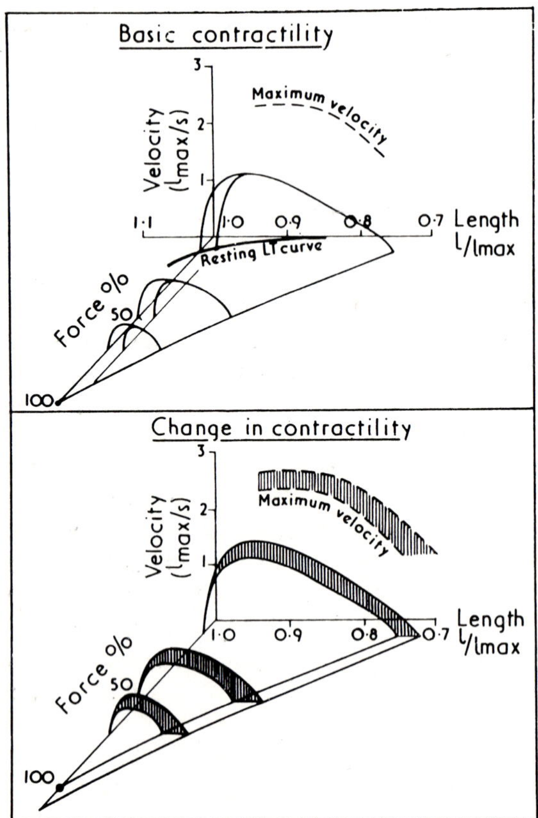

FIG. 2–34. Relationships between force, velocity of shortening, and length in an isolated papillary muscle during isotonic shortening at various loads. The three-dimensional construction shows: the force–velocity plane to the left, the velocity–length plane to the right, and the isotonic force–length relation on the base. The resting length–tension (LT) curve is indicated on the basal plane. The maximum shortening velocity, obtained at zero load, is shown in the velocity–length plane *(dashed line).* In this representation basic contractility is viewed as the time-independent interrelationship between force, velocity, and length **(top).** It is described by the force–velocity–length surface during external shortening and is independent of the initial muscle length from which the muscle starts to shorten. A change in contractility **(bottom)**—in the example a positive inotropic effect—moves the entire surface to a new position. (From Brutsaert and Paulus: *Cardiovasc. Res.,* 11:1, 1977.)

and the time of the contractile cycle at which these parameters are measured (Fig. 2–34). Changes in contractility are evidenced, at a given preload, by changes in the maximal velocity of shortening, increases in the maximal isometric tension reached, or the rate of tension development. Any change in the work performed by an isolated strip of muscle that is not caused by the physical rearrangement of the contractile filaments due to alteration in initial fiber length is due to a change in contractility. In the intact heart, changes in contractility of the ventricles can be identified when the work performed per beat changes without a change in end-diastolic volume (p. 75).

Interaction of Contractility and Excitability

When a muscle contracts with a single twitch, the actomyosin interaction reaches its maximum rapidly. However, the mechanical response of the muscle is slower because the inertia and the internal resistance must be overcome. Thus the actomyosin interaction decays (decay of active state) at a time when the contractile response still augments. In the case of skeletal muscle, since the action potential and thus the refractory period is short, a second stimulus can reach the cell and cause a new action potential at a time when it is still actively contracting. The renewed actomyosin interaction therefore causes a greater contractile response (summation). If a train of impulses reaches the cells, a prolonged activation can be obtained (tetanic contraction). Summated and tetanic contractions also are possible in vascular smooth muscle, which explains how vasoconstrictions can be sustained. However, in the heart the refractory period outlasts the mechanical response, and summation and tetanic contractions are impossible, which ensures proper functioning of the pump.

The heart rate by itself can affect myocardial contractility. If the heart is beating slowly and its frequency is suddenly increased, subsequent systoles become progressively stronger and reach a new steady state within a few beats. This phenomenon (positive staircase, Treppe, or Bowditch effect) may be accounted for by a larger inflow of extracellular Ca^{2+} with the increasing frequency of action potentials, combined with the decreased time for extrusion of Ca^{2+} between beats. Postextrasystolic potentiation, in which contractions following premature beats are markedly augmented, probably has the same explanation. By contrast, in the rapidly beating heart a further increase in frequency decreases the force of the subsequent contractions (negative staircase), presumably because there is insufficient time for the storage of Ca^{2+} in sites from which it can be recycled.

GENERATORS AND CONDUCTORS OF IMPULSES

Heart

The cells of the heart have the intrinsic ability to generate the impulse that causes their own contraction as well as the ability to conduct impulses passed on by neighboring cells. Hence cardiac muscle acts as a functional syncytium. The cell-to-cell conduction is possible because the intercalated discs offer a low electrical resistance. The action potential in an active cell causes current flow, which depolarizes the adjacent cells; if these reach threshold depolarization, they generate their own action potential.

For the intact heart to function as a pump, it is necessary for the chambers

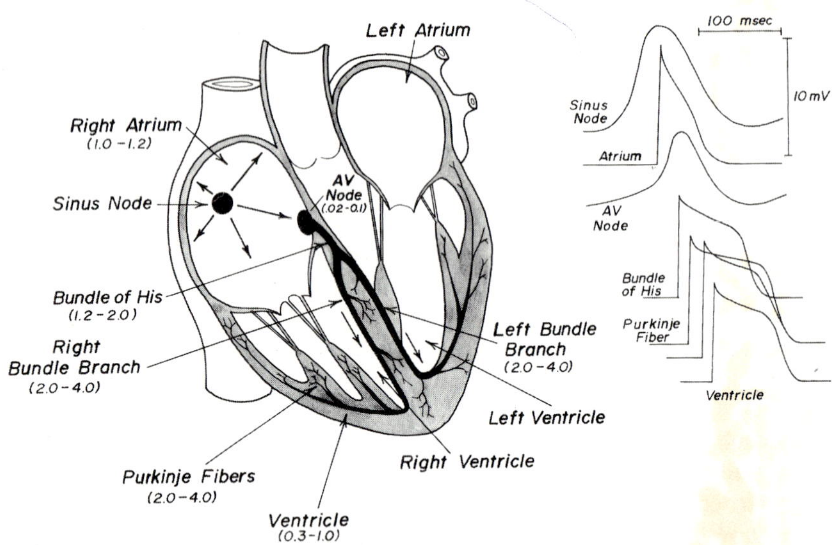

FIG. 2–35. Left: Conducting system of the human heart. The electrical impulse which causes rhythmic contraction of the muscle of the heart originates in the sinus node. The impulse spreads across both atria and is conducted to the ventricles via the atrioventricular node, the bundle of His, the right and left bundle branches, and the Purkinje fibers. The numbers in the circles indicate the conduction velocity (meters/second). **Right:** Transmembrane action potentials recorded from single fibers of the sinus node, atrial muscle, atrioventricular node (AV node), bundle of His, proximal and terminal Purkinje fibers, and ventricular muscle. Note the sequence of activation and the differences in amplitude, configuration, and duration of the action potentials. The sinus and atrioventricular nodes exhibit a relatively slow depolarization. The slow depolarization of the sinus node triggers the action potential when it reaches a threshold value. (Data from Hoffman and Cranefield: *Electrophysiology of the Heart,* p. 261. McGraw-Hill, New York, 1960.)

to contract sequentially, with appropriate time for filling, and to achieve coordination of the contractions of the different chambers. This is accomplished by specialized types of muscle fibers, which in the process of evolution have altered their ability to generate or conduct impulses and have lost their property to contract (Fig. 2–35). This is consistent with the smaller number of mitochondria and myofibrils in these cells (Fig. 2–18).

The initiation of the heart beat occurs in the sinus node, which is situated in the sulcus terminalis in the wall of the right atrium near its junction with the superior vena cava. The sinus node is about 10 to 20 mm long, 3 mm wide, and 1 mm thick. The cells that comprise it set the heart rate because they have the greatest ability to spontaneously initiate an action potential. This property is due to an inherent instability of the cell membrane, which, presumably because of a decreased permeability for K^+, does not succeed in maintaining the resting potential. As a result a spontaneous depolarization (pacemaker potential) commences and at about −55 mV (threshold potential) initiates an action potential (Fig. 2–35). The generated action potential is transmitted in all directions to the atrial cells and spreads across the functional syncytium at a speed of 1.0 to 1.2 m/sec. Because the sinus node determines the heart rate, it is often referred to as the natural "pacemaker" of the heart.

The impulse cannot be conducted from the atria to the ventricles on a cell-to-cell basis because it is halted by the connective attachment of the atrioventricular valves. Another group of cells specialized in conduction are located just above this fibrous barrier in the vicinity of the opening of the coronary sinus, in the posterior wall of the right atrium. This atrioventricular node is 7 mm long, 3 mm wide, and 1 mm thick. It is normally the major conducting pathway connecting the atria to the ventricles and is a region of slow conductance (0.02 to 0.1 m/sec). This ensures the necessary delay between the contractions of atria and ventricles, thus allowing time for ventricular filling. The slow conduction by the atrioventricular node reflects mainly the membrane properties of the cells in its middle part. In these cells the action potential rises much slower and is of lower amplitude than in other myocardial cells because these cells are less permeable to Na^+ (Fig. 2–35 and 2–36).

Although no anatomically defined link exists between the sinus and the atrio-

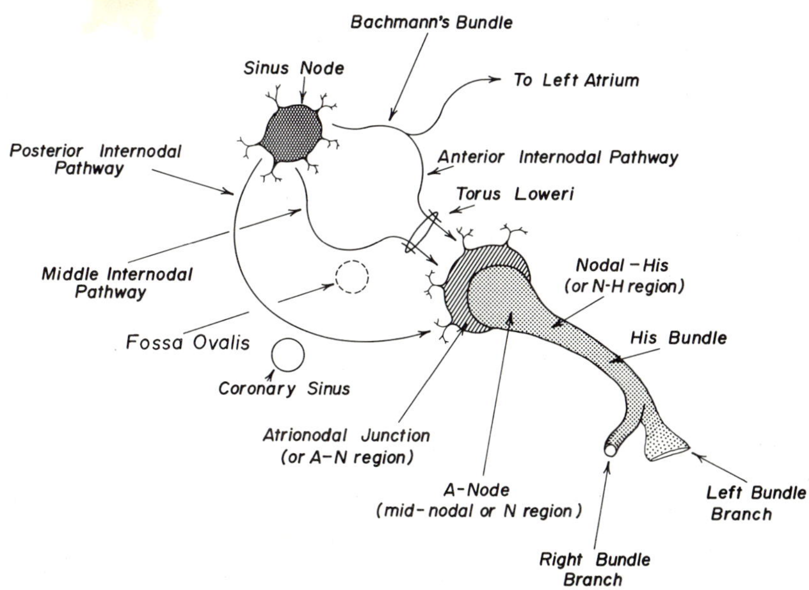

FIG. 2–36. Three interatrial pathways connect the sinus node to the atrioventricular (AV) node. The anterior and middle of these merge in the torus Loweri, a thick muscle bundle in the interatrial septum running anterior to the fossa ovalis. Part of the anterior pathway forms the major interatrial pathway. Three parts of the atrioventricular node have been identified based on characteristic electrophysiological responses, including features of the action potential. The slowest rate of depolarization and the lowest action potential are found in the middle region. The two bundle branches should be visualized with the right bundle branch coming toward, and the left going away, from the viewer. (Courtesy of Dr. T. N. James.)

ventricular nodes, the internodal cell-to-cell conduction occurs more rapidly along three functional interatrial pathways. One of these, the anterior pathway, continues on through the atrial septum as the anterior interatrial band (Bachmann's bundle) and aids in synchronizing the two atria. The internodal pathways consist of a mixture of ordinary myocardial cells and cells more specialized in conduction (Fig. 2–36).

Besides the atrioventricular node, additional strands of conducting tissue that link atria and ventricles are sometimes found in normal human hearts and in abnormal circumstances may become involved (p. 252).

The atrioventricular bundle (bundle of His) arises from the lower part of the atrioventricular node and conducts the impulses at a velocity of 1.2 to 2.0 m/sec. It crosses the atrioventricular fibrous barrier and travels toward the intraventricular septum. At the top of the latter, it gives rise to the left bundle branch, which fans out under the endocardium of the left ventricle. The right bundle branch is the continuation of the bundle of His. It runs beneath the endocardium on the right side of the interventricular septum, toward the anterior papillary muscle, and forms a ridge known as the "moderator band" (Fig. 2–12 and 2–35).

The end-branches of the bundles form a network consisting of large specialized cells (Purkinje cells) that form a subendocardial plexus and conduct at the same high velocity as the bundle branches (2.0 to 4.0 m/sec). The Purkinje cells form close apposition with the less-differentiated subendocardial cells in which cell-to-cell conduction occurs (0.3 to 1.0 m/sec). This eventually causes the synchronous contraction of the whole ventricular wall.

When an impulse generated by the sinus node spreads over the bundle branch system, the interventricular septum and the papillary muscles contract first. The contraction of the septum makes it stiffer, allowing it to act as a platform for contraction of the remaining parts of the ventricles. Contraction of the papillary muscle prevents eversion of the atrioventricular valves during ventricular contraction. Since the left ventricle is thicker than the right, its outer parts (epicardial surface) are activated later. Further, the ventricles are activated in sequence from the apex to the base, which facilitates their emptying.

Vascular Muscle

Although certain blood vessels possess inherent rhythmicity and intrinsic tone, there is no evidence of specialized structures conducting the impulses generated or recognized by certain cells to other parts of the blood vessel wall. When conduction of impulses occurs, it happens on a cell-to-cell basis. The tight junctions, or nexuses, provide a low-resistance channel for transfer of membrane potential changes.

As with the myocardial cells, the property of a vascular smooth muscle cell to trigger its own contraction (automaticity) rests on the instability of the cell membrane. The loss of stability results in the occurrence of spontaneous spike potentials, which can spread to the neighboring cells. The consequence of spontaneous activity of vascular smooth muscle is either rhythmic changes in wall tension or sustained reduction of the caliber of the vessel. The former is seen in the large splanchnic veins, where this phenomenon helps propel the blood from the intestine into the portal circulation ("portal venous heart"; p. 97). The latter occurs mainly in the arterioles, where the presence of high myogenic tone is one of the determinants of the resistance to flow (Fig. 2–28).

METABOLIC SUPPORT

In the hearts of cold-blooded animals, where the metabolic rate is low, diffusion to and from the blood flowing through the chambers is sufficient to ensure adequate nutrition. With the large muscle mass of the myocardium in vertebrates and its higher metabolic requirements, simple diffusion from the chambers becomes insufficient and contributes only to the nourishment of the subendocardial muscle cells. A complex system of nutritional vessels, the coronary arteries, subserve the myocardium (Figs. 2–37 and 2–38). The large coronary vessels (left and right coronary arteries and their branches) lie on the surface of the

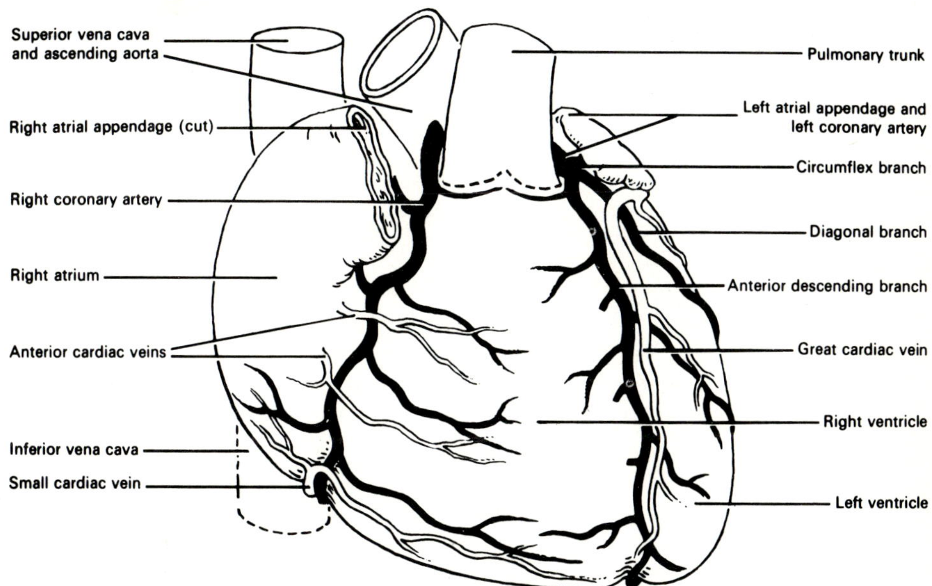

FIG. 2–37. Principal arteries and veins on the anterior surface of the heart. Part of the right atrial appendage has been resected to expose the origin of the right coronary artery from the right (anterior) coronary aortic sinus. The left coronary artery arises from the left (left posterior) coronary aortic sinus and appears on the anterior surface between the root of the pulmonary trunk and the left atrial appendage. In this case it terminates in three branches: the anterior descending (interventricular) and circumflex branches, which are constant, and one diagonal branch. (From Walmsley and Watson: *Clinical Anatomy of the Heart,* p. 203. Churchill Livingstone, Edinburgh, 1978.)

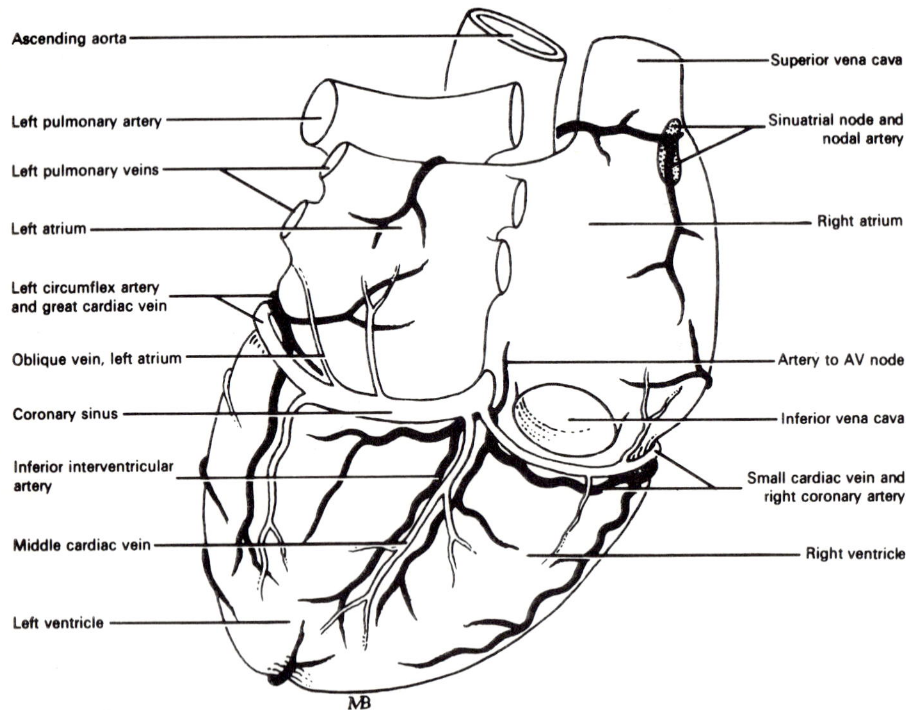

FIG. 2–38. Principal arteries and veins on the posterior and inferior surface of the heart. The large coronary sinus with its tributaries lies immediately above the terminal parts of the left circumflex and right coronary arteries. The artery to the sinus node arises from one of these arteries. The artery to the atrioventricular (AV) node arises from the right coronary artery or rarely from the left circumflex artery. (From Walmsley and Watson: *Clinical Anatomy of the Heart,* p. 205. Churchill Livingstone, Edinburgh, 1978.)

heart underneath the epicardium. From these large vessels, smaller arteries pass at right angles into the myocardium and branch to form arterioles and capillaries. Most of the venous blood returning from the coronary capillaries, and particularly that from the left atrium and ventricle, drains into the right atrium through the coronary sinus whose orifice lies just above the tricuspid valve. The venous blood derived from the right ventricle enters the right atrium by the anterior cardiac vein. A small fraction of the coronary blood flow returns directly into any of the four chambers through small channels (Thebesian veins).

Larger arteries are supplied with nourishment from the arterial tree by small vessels called the vasa vasorum. In smaller vessels nutrition is ensured by exchanges with the blood in the lumen and with the surrounding interstitial fluid.

SELECTED REFERENCES

Bakhle, Y. S., and Vane, J. R. (1974): Pharmacokinetic function of the pulmonary circulation. *Physiol. Rev.,* 54:1007.

Bayliss, L. E. (1962): The rheology of blood. In: *Handbook of Physiology, Sect. 2: Circulation,* Vol. 1, p. 137. American Physiological Society, Washington, D.C.

Bohr, D. F. (1978): Vascular smooth muscle. In: *Peripheral Circulation,* edited by P. C. Johnson, p. 13. Wiley, New York.

Brutsaert, D. L., and Paulus, W. J. (1979): Contraction and relaxation of the heart as muscle and pump. In: *International Review of Physiology, Cardiovascular Physiology III,* Vol. 18, edited by A. C. Guyton and D. B. Young, p. 1. University Park Press, Baltimore.

Carmeliet, E. (1978): Cardiac transmembrane potentials and metabolism. *Circ. Res.,* 42:577.

Ebashi, S. (1976): Excitation-contraction coupling. *Annu. Rev. Physiol.,* 38:293.

Endo, M. (1977): Calcium release from the sarcoplasmic reticulum. *Physiol. Rev.,* 57:71.

Huxley, A. F. (1974): Muscular contraction. *J. Physiol. (Lond),* 243:1.

James, T. N. (1973): The sinus node as a servomechanism. *Circ. Res.,* 32:370.

James, T. N., and Sherf, L. (1971): Specialized tissues and preferential conduction in the atria of the heart. *Am. J. Cardiol.,* 28:414.

Jewell, B. R. (1977): A reexamination of the influence of muscle length on myocardial performance. *Circ. Res.,* 40:221.

Katz, A. M. (1970): Contractile proteins of the heart. *Physiol. Rev.,* 50:63.

Korner, P. I. (1974): Present concepts about the myocardium. *Adv. Cardiol.,* 12:1.

Langer, G. A., Frank, J. S., and Brady, A. J. (1976): The myocardium. In: *International Review of Physiology, Cardiovascular Physiology II,* Vol. 9, edited by A. C. Guyton and A. W. Cowley Jr., p. 191. University Park Press, Baltimore.

Mann, K. G. (1976): Prothrombin. *Methods in Enzymology, Proteolytic Enzymes (Part B),* edited by L. Lorand, p. 123. Academic Press, New York.

Mann, K. G., and Downing, M. R. (1977): Thrombin generation. In: *The Chemistry and Biology of Thrombin,* edited by R. L. Lundblad, J. W. Fenton, and K. G. Mann, p. 11. Ann Arbor Press, Ann Arbor, Michigan.

Massing, G. K., and James, T. N. (1976): Anatomical configuration of the His bundle and bundle branches in the human heart. *Circulation,* 53:609.

Michel, C. C. (1972): Flows across the capillary wall. In: *Cardiovascular Fluid Dynamics,* edited by D. H. Bergel, Vol. 2, p. 241. Academic Press, New York.

Noble, M. I. M., and Pollack, G. H. (1977): Controversies in cardiovascular research: Molecular mechanisms of contraction. *Circ. Res.,* 40:333.

Renkin, E. M. (1977): Multiple pathways of capillary permeability. *Circ. Res.,* 41:735.

Reuter, H. (1974): Exchange of calcium ions in the mammalian myocardium: Mechanisms and physiological significance. *Circ. Res.,* 34:599.

Schmid-Schönbein, H. (1976): Microrheology of erythrocytes, blood viscosity, and the distribution of blood flow in the microcirculation. In: *International Review of Physiology, Cardiovascular Physiology II,* Vol. 9, edited by A. C. Guyton and A. W. Cowley Jr., p. 1. University Park Press, Baltimore.

Somlyo, A. P., and Somlyo, A. V. (1968): Vascular smooth muscle. I. Normal structure, pathology, biochemistry and biophysics. *Pharmacol. Rev.,* 20:197.

Suttie, J. W., and Jackson, C. M. (1977): Prothrombin structure, activation and biosynthesis. *Physiol. Rev.,* 57:1.

Tada, M., Yamamoto, T., and Tonomura, Y. (1978): Molecular mechanism of active calcium transport by sarcoplasmic reticulum. *Physiol. Rev.,* 58:1.

3

Dynamic Behavior

This chapter puts the individual units of the cardiovascular system together and demonstrates how the behavior of each component is influenced by events occurring both upstream and downstream from it.

OXYGEN DELIVERY

The blood carries oxygen to the tissues. At the normal arterial partial pressure of oxygen (Po_2 = 95 mm Hg), it contains 19.7 ml of oxygen per 100 ml of blood, of which 0.3 ml is in physical solution and 19.4 ml is combined with hemoglobin. The arterial blood is distributed to all tissues, where oxygen extraction occurs as a function of the metabolic needs. As a consequence, there are differences in the oxygen saturation of the streams of venous blood entering the right atrium. In the normal resting subject the blood in the superior vena cava has an oxygen saturation of about 80%, in the inferior vena cava of about 85%, and in the coronary sinus of 30 to 45%. The streams of venous blood do not mix adequately in the right atrium but have done so by the time the blood reaches the pulmonary artery. Here the mixed venous blood is about 80% saturated and has a total oxygen content of about 16 ml/100 ml of blood. The body as a whole extracts about 4 ml of oxygen per 100 ml of blood passing through the tissues.

After passage through the pulmonary capillaries the blood has equilibrated with the alveolar air (Po_2 = 100 mm Hg) and has an oxygen saturation of 97 to 99%. In the left heart its saturation decreases through admixture with cardiac venous blood entering the cavities of the left atrium and ventricle via the Thebesian veins. This explains why oxygen saturation of the arterial blood (94 to 98%) is slightly below that of the blood in the pulmonary veins (p. 327).

The oxygen consumption of the whole body is the sum of that consumed by the individual tissues. It reflects the overall metabolic needs of the organism without providing information on the specific needs of its individual parts. The requirements of the latter are the basic determinants of their blood supply. In many tissues there is a strict correlation between the metabolic activity and blood flow; the most typical examples are the heart and skeletal muscle. However, in other tissues the blood supply fulfills other functions not related to their metabolism. The prime examples are the glomerular blood vessels in the kidney, whose main concern is filtration, and the skin blood vessels, which play a key role in body temperature regulation. These various functions of the blood are reflected in the ratio between blood flow through the tissue and the amount of oxygen the latter extracts. For example, in resting conditions the coronary flow is 250 ml/min, and 10.8 ml of oxygen is extracted per 100 ml of blood, whereas in the kidneys the blood flow averages 1,100 ml/min and only 1.5 ml of oxygen per 100 ml of blood is extracted (Fig. 3–1); (p. 325).

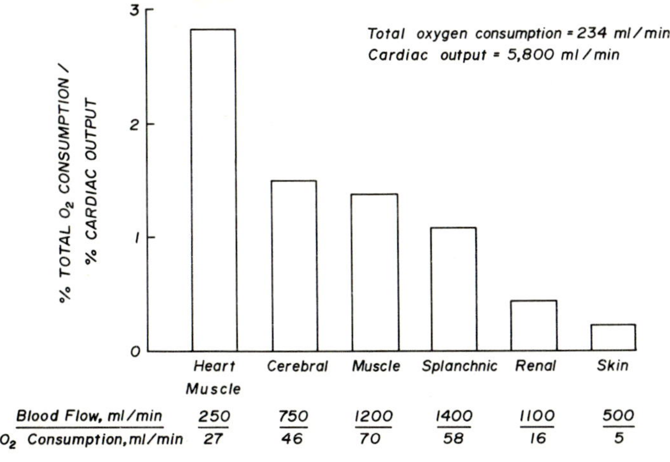

FIG. 3–1. Relation of oxygen requirements to blood supply for various vascular beds. Values are for a normal subject at rest in a comfortable environment. Note that the heart muscle extracts large amounts of oxygen relative to the blood flow compared to the kidney and skin, where flow is greatly in excess of metabolic requirements.

CARDIAC PERFORMANCE

The development of techniques for placing radiopaque catheters in all chambers of the heart and in the great vessels, the attachment of these to manometers for precise measurement of pressures, and the use of oximeters for measuring oxygen saturation of the blood has provided vital information on cardiovascular function. The injection of dye and radiopaque substances through these catheters permits the measurement of cardiac output, stroke volume, end-systolic and end-diastolic volumes of the ventricles, the volume of blood in the heart and lungs, and visualization of the heart chambers and the coronary vessels. Together with noninvasive procedures such as the electrocardiogram for the analysis of the electrical behavior of the heart, the phonocardiogram for the analysis of heart sounds, and the use of ultrasound to portray the movements of heart valves and the contraction of the myocardial wall, these various procedures permit the study of human cardiac function in normal and abnormal circumstances (Chapter 12).

The driving force for the flow of blood is the total energy imparted to it. This total fluid energy is determined by the sum of the potential energy stored as pressure, the kinetic energy, and the gravitational potential energy. If a system is perfused at constant flow and does not change in configuration, the total energy at each level of the circuit remains the same. Thus when the velocity of flow is higher in a given part of the circuit (e.g., narrowing of a vessel) more of the total fluid energy is converted to kinetic energy at the expense of the potential energy or pressure (Bernouilli's principle) (Fig. 3–2). Transformation from potential (pressure) into kinetic (velocity) energy occurs throughout the vascular system when the cross-sectional area decreases (Fig. 1–4) and vice-versa.

When the blood flows through the consecutive sections of the vascular tree,

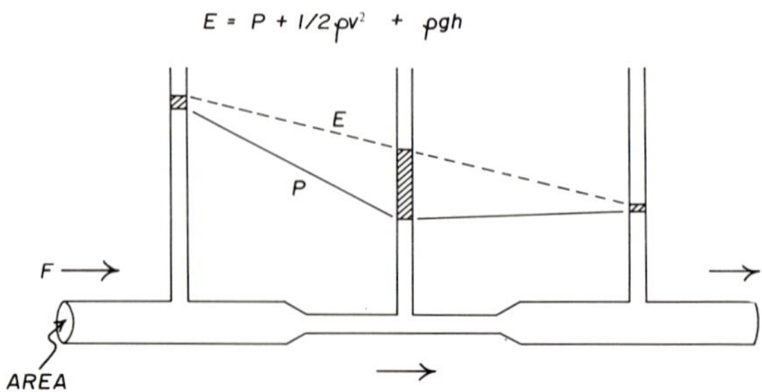

FIG. 3–2. Illustration of Bernouilli's principle at the narrowing of a tube demonstrating how flow (F) occurs down the gradient of total fluid energy (E; *dotted line*) rather than down the pressure gradient (P; *solid line*). When the area of the tube decreases, the kinetic energy *(hatched area)* augments and thus so does the velocity, at the expense of the potential energy stored as pressure. Along the tube the total fluid energy decreases because of dissipation due to frictional forces. ϕ = density. v = velocity. g = gravitational acceleration. h = height above reference level.

it progressively loses part of its total fluid energy because of the frictional forces between the blood and the vessel walls. The energy lost is dissipated in heat. The main function of the cardiac pump is to restore the total fluid energy in order to maintain the forward movement of blood.

The Heart as a Pump

Ventricular ejection is caused by a reduction in circumference and a decrease in the longitudinal axis as the base of the heart (atrioventricular rings) is pulled toward the apex. The contraction of the muscle around the valve orifice assists in valve closure. During systole the heart rotates to the right, which brings it in contact with the chest wall in the region of the fifth left intercostal space (apex beat).

Most of the understanding of the basic characteristics of myocardial muscle has been derived from studies performed on isolated fragments of the heart, shortening longitudinally while carrying a fixed load (e.g., Fig. 2–34). However, the conditions of loading of the intact ventricle are different from those obtained in isolated muscles since the ventricle must eject a viscous content, the blood, into a viscoelastic container, the vasculature. The ability of the heart to function properly as a pump depends on the interrelation between: (a) synchronous activation of the different cardiac chambers; (b) potential of the ventricular wall to perform muscular work; (c) total load imposed on the myocardial fibers; (d) ventricular dimensions; and (e) appropriate filling between systoles.

The Cardiac Cycle

To describe the complex sequence of events during the cardiac cycle, it is convenient to discuss the electrical changes and their interpretation before the mechanical events.

Electrical Events

Cellular basis. The changes from resting potential to action potential described in Chapter 2 can be determined only by intracellular recording. This is not possible in the intact human heart. However, since the myocardium is a large muscle mass, its electrical activity can be recorded by extracellular electrodes, either placed within the cavities of the heart (intracardiac recording) or, more commonly, applied to the body surface (electrocardiogram; p. 281). The principle of such extracellular recording is that when a muscle bundle is at rest, with the inside of the cell negative to the outside, two electrodes placed at the outside of the cell show no difference in potential. As soon as one end of the bundle depolarizes as the action potential spreads, the extracellular recording indicates that the depolarized part now is negative when compared to the part of the bundle which is still polarized. When the whole bundle is depolarized, the extra-

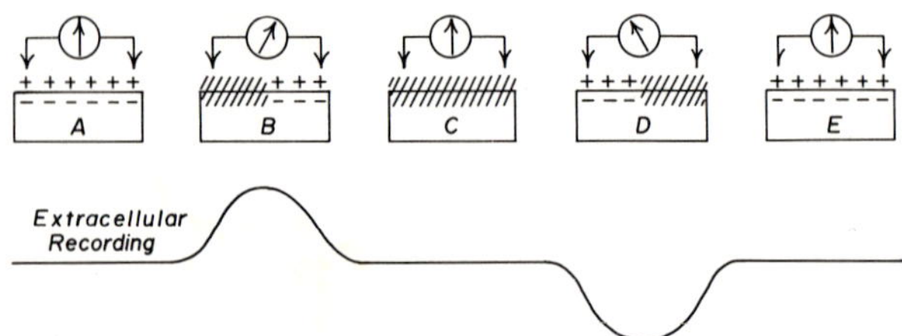

FIG. 3–3. Changes in extracellular electrical potential in a bundle of cardiac muscle cells; the bundle depolarizes and repolarizes from left to right. Potential changes are shown as right versus left part of the bundle. At rest (**A** and **E**) the whole bundle is polarized, and no extracellular potential is recorded. When the bundle starts to depolarize **(B)** the outer surface of the right part remains positive and an upward deflection of the potential recording is noted. When the whole bundle is depolarized, the recording indicates no potential difference **(C)**. On repolarization **(D)** the reverse occurs.

cellular recording returns toward the zero line. When the part of the bundle which depolarized first now repolarizes, it becomes positive relative to the other end, which is still depolarized. When the latter repolarizes in turn, the original resting state is recovered. Thus the extracellular recording is biphasic (Fig. 3–3).

The electrocardiogram. The electrocardiogram is the extracellular recording of the summation of the spread of action potentials over all the cells of the heart. Its appearance is complex and varies with the site of recording (limb leads, precordial leads, intracardiac recording; p. 281). Taking the peripheral leads as an example, the first deflection is the P wave, which corresponds to the depolarization of the atria. Its duration reflects the time needed for the wave of depolarization to spread over the latter. After atrial depolarization the extracellular recording returns to zero and stays there until the ventricles are activated. The interval between atrial and ventricular depolarization, from

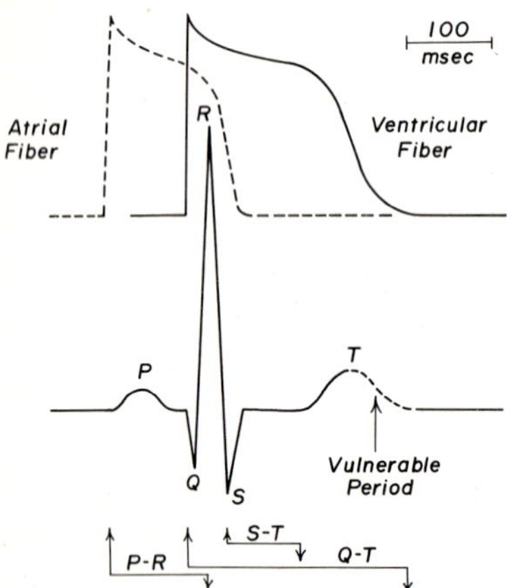

FIG. 3–4. The PQRST complex of the normal electrocardiogram as recorded in peripheral lead II (p. 281). Note the commonly used intervals (P–R, Q–T, and S–T). For comparison the superimposed action potentials of atrial and ventricular fibers are shown to indicate the temporal relationship between the transmembrane potential changes and the extracellular recording. The complexity of the electrocardiogram is due to the fact that it represents the summation of the extracellular potentials of all parts of the heart.

the beginning of the P wave to the first deflection of the QRS complex, indicates the time necessary for the impulse to be propagated from the atria to the ventricles. During this interval the atrioventricular node, the bundle of His and its branches, and the Purkinje network are activated, but the small amount of tissue involved does not generate a signal of sufficient magnitude to be detected by recording from surface leads. The QRS complex reflects the spread of depolarization through the ventricular mass. Its amplitude is much greater than that of the P wave because the tissue mass involved is larger. During the QRS complex the atria repolarize. After the QRS complex, the recording returns to or toward the electrical zero. This phase, where the whole ventricular mass is depolarized, is called the S–T segment. When the ventricles repolarize, this generates the T wave. Since the repolarization is a relatively slow process, the T wave is longer than the QRS complex (Fig. 3–4).

Mechanical Events

During the cardiac cycle there are rapid changes in pressure and volume in the cardiac chambers, as each chamber alternately connects and disconnects from its neighbors to provide for the efficient propulsion of blood through the pulmonary and systemic circulation (Fig. 3–5). At the end of diastole (diastasis) the atrioventricular valves are open, the aortic and pulmonary valves are closed, and the atrial and ventricular muscles are relaxed. The atria and the ventricles are in free communication. Blood returns from the caval veins and from the coronary sinus to the right atrium and from the pulmonary veins to the left atrium because of the pressure difference (Fig. 1–3). This returning blood distends the atria, causing an increase in atrial pressure. As a consequence, blood flows from the atria into the ventricles, causing the pressure in the latter to increase slightly. At the end of diastasis the sinus node generates an impulse causing the P wave, which is followed by atrial contraction. The atrial contraction is responsible for approximately 20% of total ventricular filling at rest and increases the pressure in the ventricles. When the active contraction of the atrial wall stops, the pressure in the atrium drops. As soon as this pressure is lower than that in the ventricle, backflow of blood closes the tricuspid and mitral valves, giving rise to the first heart sound. After atrioventricular valve closure, the pressures in the atria and the ventricles change independently.

The QRS complex announces the contraction of the ventricular wall. At the time this occurs, the atrioventricular and semilunar valves are closed. The myocardium contracts isovolumetrically (isometric phase) until the pressure within the ventricular chambers exceeds that in the great vessels. However, the contraction of the ventricles is not completely isometric since the sudden increase in intraventricular pressure causes the atrioventricular and semilunar valves to bulge toward the atria and the aorta and pulmonary artery, respectively.

When the pressure in the ventricle exceeds that in the aorta and the pulmonary artery, the semilunar valves open and a continuous chamber is established be-

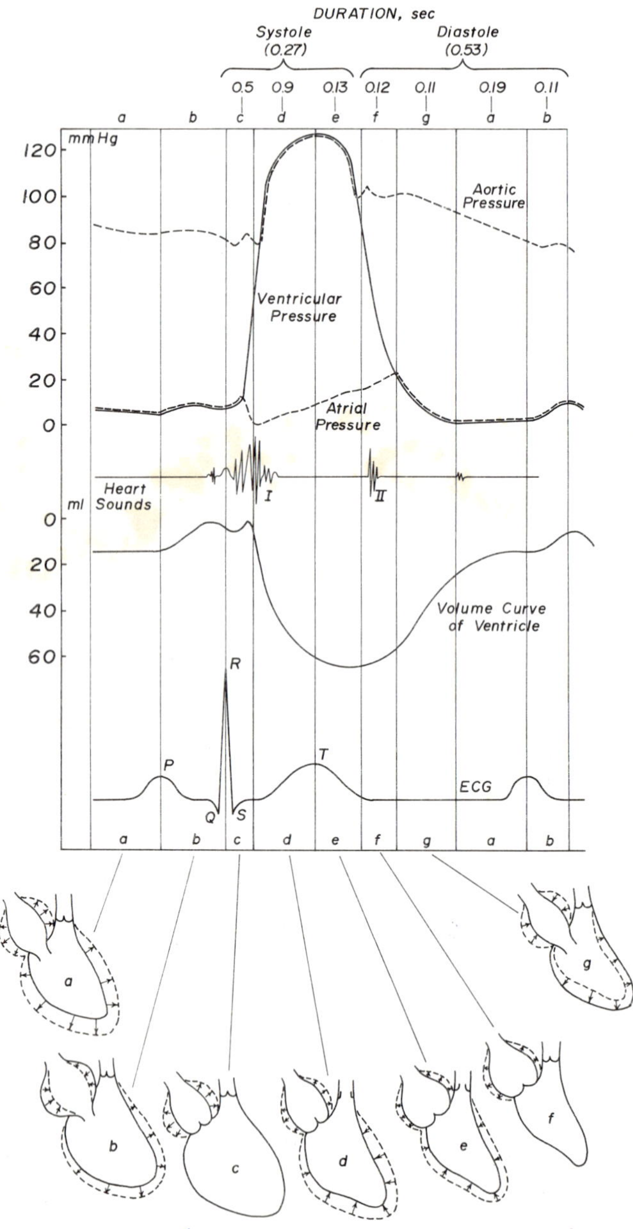

FIG. 3–5. The changes in aortic, left ventricular, and left atrial pressures, and in left ventricular volume, in relation to the phonocardiogram and the electrocardiogram during the cardiac cycle. **Insets:** Changes in configuration of left atrium, mitral valve, left ventricle, and aortic valve in the various phases of the cycle. The duration of each phase is indicated at the top of the figure. I = first heart sound; II = second heart sound. a = diastasis. b = atrial contraction. c = isovolumetric ventricular contraction. d = rapid ejection. e = slow ejection. f = isovolumetric relaxation. g = rapid filling. (Modified from Wiggers: *Circulatory Dynamics.* Grune & Stratton, New York, 1952.)

tween the ventricles and the great vessels. The myocardium now shortens isotonically (ejection phase), and blood is rapidly expelled into the aorta and the pulmonary artery. The ventricular and great vessel pressures follow the same pattern. In the first, or rapid, ejection phase, the amount of blood pumped by the heart exceeds the amount which can leave the great vessels through their peripheral branches. The ventricular as well as the aortic and pulmonary pressures increase further, and by virtue of their elastic properties the aorta and the pulmonary artery accumulate the excess blood. Next follows the reduced ejection phase, during which the outflow from the ventricles becomes less than the runoff through the small systemic and pulmonary vessels, the pressure in the ventricles and in the great vessels decreases slightly, and the T wave announces ventricular repolarization.

When the ventricles relax, the ventricular pressure falls rapidly. The great vessels, which have been distended, recoil passively but at a slower rate than the relaxing myocardium. The pressure in the aorta and the pulmonary artery decreases more slowly than that in the ventricles. The backflow of blood closes the semilunar valves, giving rise to the second heart sound. As long as the pressure in the ventricles is higher than that in the atria, which in the meantime have become filled with blood, the atrioventricular valves remain closed. This is the isovolumetric relaxation phase.

With the opening of the atrioventricular valves, there is an abrupt fall in atrial pressure and rapid filling of the ventricles. Normal cardiac valves offer little resistance to the forward flow of blood. Since the flow traverses the atrioventricular valves only during diastole, the flow rate through the valves is about twice the value of the cardiac output; the same holds for the semilunar valves during systole.

The ability of the heart to ensure the forward movement of blood depends on activation of its various parts in the sequence just described. Thus disorderly activation of the heart chambers endangers the function of the heart as a pump (arrhythmias; p. 245). Too strong contraction of part of the ventricular wall also interferes with the normal ejection of blood (hypertrophic cardiomyopathy; p. 244). Conversely, if segments of the ventricular wall do not function properly because of organic disease, cardiac performance is impaired (cardiomyopathies, p. 245; myocardial infarction, p. 247).

Heart Muscle

The ability of the heart muscle to expel blood against a given load is determined by the number of muscle cells activated and by the force of contraction of the individual cells. The mass of the ventricular wall depends on the chronic load with which it is confronted. Normal heart muscle grows to match the work load imposed on it. Since stroke work is the product of stroke volume and systolic pressure (p. 75), the myocardium grows when either its stroke volume or its systolic pressure is chronically augmented. The physiological example of the former is the increase in ventricular mass in athletes; that of the

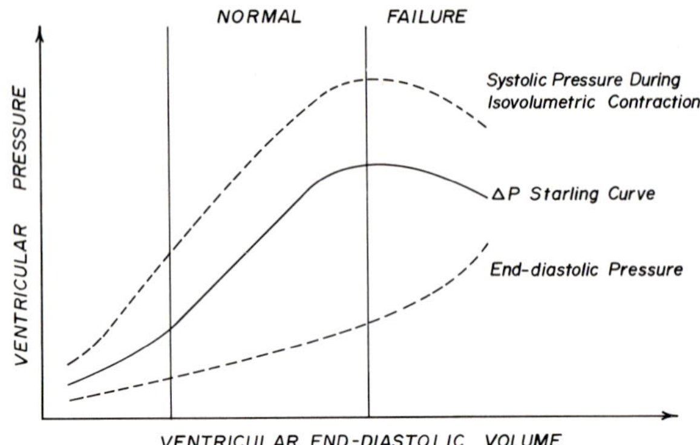

FIG. 3–6. Starling's law of the heart. This states that if the ventricles are filled to a greater extent than normal, the subsequent contraction is more vigorous than normal and a greater stroke volume is ejected. The figure shows the relationship between the amount of pressure developed during isovolumetric contraction of a ventricle and its end-diastolic volume. As end-diastolic pressure (ventricular filling pressure) increases in the normal heart, so does the end-diastolic volume and the pressure generated during the isometric phase of ventricular contraction. In the failing heart the filling pressure is abnormally high, and less pressure is generated during the contraction. The difference between the end-diastolic and systolic pressure (Δp) describes a curve with an ascending limb, a maximum, and a descending limb (Starling curve). In health this local myogenic mechanism permits the output of each ventricle to be adjusted on a beat-to-beat basis to meet the continuously changing demands on the circulatory system.

latter is the difference in wall thickness between left and right ventricles. Pathological examples are the hypertrophy occurring in conditions where the cardiac output or the systolic pressure are chronically augmented.

Two factors influence the force of contraction of the myocardial cells in normal conditions. The filling pressure of the ventricles (end-diastolic ventricular pressure) adjusts the degree of stretch of the muscle cells prior to their activation and thus determines the point on the active length–tension curve at which the myocardium operates. This in turn determines the force of the subsequent systole. This relationship was recognized by Starling (1914), who stated that if the filling of the heart is increased it contracts more forcefully (Starling's law of the heart, Frank-Starling mechanism) (Fig. 3–6). The dependency of the stroke volume on the degree of filling is the major factor in ensuring that the two sides of the heart remain in balance. The second factor determining the force of contraction is the contractility of the myocardial fibers (p. 53). Positive inotropic interventions increase the contractility of the myocardium at each fiber length; negative inotropic interventions have the opposite effect (Fig. 3–7). Such changes in contractility usually are due to variations in the levels of norepinephrine (sympathetic nerves), epinephrine (adrenal medulla), or other hormones (e.g., thyroxine) in the vicinity of the cardiac muscle cells. They also can be induced by the rate of contraction of the heart (e.g., staircase effect; p. 55). It is likely that changes in length and inotropism ultimately influence

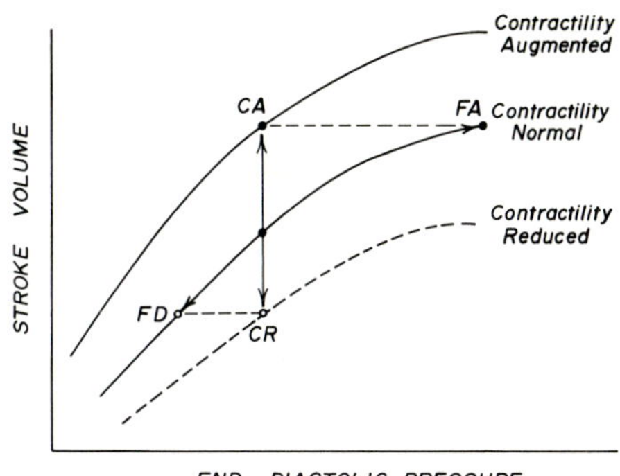

FIG. 3–7. Effect of alterations in myocardial contractility on the relationship between ventricular stroke volume and end-diastolic pressure. When contractility is increased [e.g., by norepinephrine or *cardiac glycosides* (positive inotropic effect)], more work is performed at the same end-diastolic pressure and less when contractility is decreased [e.g., by heart failure (negative inotropic effect)]. FD = ventricular fiber length decreased. FA = fiber length augmented. CA = contractility augmented. CR = contractility reduced. In normal circumstances there is a continuous adjustment of fiber length (Frank-Starling mechanism) and of contractility so the stroke output and cardiac output meet the requirements of the body tissues.

cardiac responses by altering the major controller of the actomyosin interaction, the intracellular Ca^{2+} concentration (p. 53). Increases in force of contraction of the ventricular wall augment stroke volume or help maintain it despite an increase in resistance to the ejection of blood from the ventricles.

The proper functioning of the ventricular muscle depends on the appropriate supply of oxygen and substrate (p. 91). Any restriction in coronary flow endangers the function of the cardiac pump (p. 227).

Ventricular Load

The muscle fibers in the ventricular wall sense a continuously changing load which is the instantaneous resultant of the preload and the afterload to which they are exposed. The preload is determined by the end-diastolic ventricular pressure and thus by the filling of the ventricle. The latter depends mainly on the venous return and on compliance of the cardiac chambers (p. 72). The pressures in the aorta and the pulmonary artery at the end of diastole dictate the energy that must be generated by the ventricles before the semilunar valves open. The afterload of the ventricle is determined by the factors that oppose shortening of the myocardial cells. The resistance offered by the vascular tree imposes an additional force on the myocardial fibers that is proportional to the velocity of shortening. The compliance of the large arteries creates an elastic feedback when they are filled by the ejected blood, which is proportional to cardiac fiber shortening. The mean ejection pressure, at a given ejection rate, reflects the average afterload encountered; moment-to-moment changes in resistance and compliance of the vascular tree are determined by the physical properties of the aorta and its branches, and represent the impedance of the vascular system. In the normal circulation preload and afterload are in dynamic equilibrium. For example, the injection of angiotensin II (p. 193) causes an acute increase in systemic vascular resistance and thus in afterload of the left ventricle. However, the widespread arteriolar constriction results in passive mobilization of blood toward the heart (p. 85); it increases venous filling of the right heart and, through the Frank–Starling mechanism, augments stroke volume. In congestive heart failure (p. 255) the venous filling pressure, and thus the preload, is high; drugs such as sodium nitroprusside (p. 198) shift blood from the central circulation to the peripheral veins and help compensate for the mismatch between preload and afterload. The preloading by the venous return and the afterloading by the arterial system illustrate the interdependence of the various segments of the vascular system.

For a given viscoelasticity of the arterial tree, if the ventricle is to eject blood more rapidly it must develop higher pressures and higher active wall tensions. To maintain the same flow in a less compliant vascular tree, the systolic pressure must be higher; the physiological illustration of this is provided by the increase in systolic aortic pressure seen with aging (p. 209).

Ventricular Dimensions and Wall Tension

The relationships between ventricular dimensions, ventricular wall tension, and intraventricular pressure can be approximated from Laplace's law for spherical or cylindrical structures (Fig. 3–8): (1) For a given pressure the passive wall tension is inversely related to the diameter. This means that at each end-diastolic pressure the wall stress is greater in a larger ventricle. The muscle must develop a force equal to the wall tension (preload) before it can generate pressure and shorten against the vascular resistance (afterload). Thus in a large ventricle overcoming the passive wall tension demands a large contribution to the total energy developed. (2) During ejection the changes in dimension of the ventricle depend on the extent of myocardial fiber shortening. A given degree of ventricular fiber shortening causes a greater increase in stroke volume in a large than in a small ventricle. (3) A small ventricle requires less force to generate the same pressure, and during the ejection phase the force developed by the ventricular wall is progressively reduced even if the intraventricular pressure still increases. These relationships are of particular importance for the failing heart (p. 258).

Ventricular Filling

Ventricular filling is determined by the active relaxation of the myocardium, the ventricular compliance, the atrial contraction, and the return of blood from the systemic vascular beds and the pulmonary circulation.

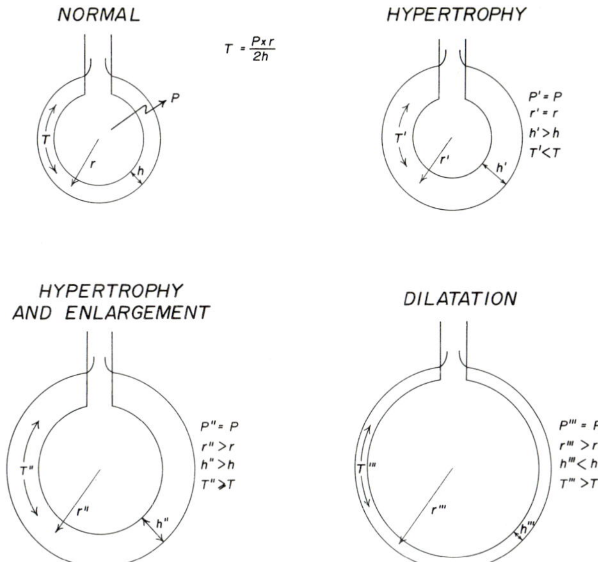

FIG. 3–8. On the assumption that the left ventricle is a sphere with uniform wall thickness, Laplace's law predicts that the load on the muscle fibers (wall tension; *T*) is determined by the product of the pressure *(P)* and the radius *(r),* divided by twice the wall thickness *(h).* In the normal ventricle the end-diastolic pressure determines the preload and the systolic pressure the afterload. If the latter augments, the wall tension increases and the myocardium has to develop greater force to eject the same stroke volume *(upper left).* If the ventricle hypertrophies, the thickening of the wall reduces the wall tension. In athletes the cardiac wall hypertrophies but the systolic pressure is normal; hence a greater reduction of diameter is obtained when the myocardial fibers are activated, and the stroke volume augments. In patients with arterial hypertension the systolic pressure is increased. The hypertrophy compensates for the increase in wall tension due to the high pressure, and the stroke volume is maintained *(upper right).* If the ventricle is enlarged, the wall tension is greater during diastole and systole, although the circumferential shortening required to eject a given stroke volume is reduced; if hypertrophy has occurred, it partially reduces the increase in wall tension *(lower left).* In the failing ventricle (p. 258) the pressure and the end-diastolic volume are augmented and the heart dilates. The resulting increase in radius and decrease in wall thickness markedly augment wall tension and thus the energy required to eject the blood; the stroke volume cannot then be maintained *(lower right).*

Relaxation of the ventricle is due to the active removal of Ca^{2+} from the cytoplasm surrounding the myofibrils. The relaxation rate is greatest when the load is smallest because at lower loads the sarcoplasmic reticulum is more effective in Ca^{2+} pumping. Increases in load augment the total number of cross-bridges that are activated during the contraction so that more time is needed for their detachment. When the atrioventricular valves open, the ventricular wall is still actively relaxing and during the first phase of the rapid filling aspirates part of the blood contained in the atria (Fig. 3–5).

The compliance of the ventricle determines how much blood it can store during diastole. When the ventricular wall becomes stiffer, it accommodates

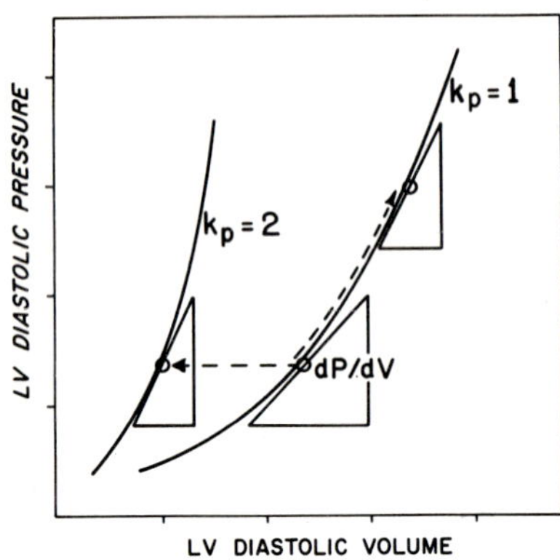

FIG. 3–9. Determination of the compliance of the left ventricle (LV) by plotting changes in diastolic pressure (P) versus changes in diastolic volume (V). The slope of a tangent to the pressure–volume curve *(dP/dV)* represents the modulus of stiffness of the ventricular chamber at a given filling pressure *(k_p)*. Thus any ventricle will become progressively stiffer with progressive filling *(curve on the right)*. An increase in the modulus of chamber stiffness (an increase in k_p from 1 to 2) likewise may result in an increase in the tangent slope *(dP/dV)*. (From Levine and Gaasch: *Mod. Concepts Cardiovasc. Dis.*, 47:95, 1978, by permission of The American Heart Association.)

less blood for each increase in distending pressure. To obtain satisfactory filling of a stiffer ventricle, higher end-diastolic ventricular pressures are needed (Fig. 3–9). This in turn augments the wall tension and thus the load and work of the ventricle. The compliance of the ventricles depends on: (1) *dimensions:* smaller ventricles are stiffer than larger ones; (2) *wall thickness:* hypertrophic walls are less compliant, and the left ventricle is stiffer than the right; (3) *muscle activity:* incomplete relaxation, as seen in the hypoxic heart, augments the stiffness of the ventricular wall; (4) *composition:* the presence of fibrous tissue, as in the scars resulting from myocardial infarction (p. 227) and infiltration of abnormal components (myxedema, amyloid) decrease the compliance of the ventricular wall; and (5) *external compression:* when the pericardium loses its elasticity (constrictive pericarditis, p. 240) or when the pericardial content augments abnormally (cardiac tamponade, p. 240), the expansion of the ventricles during diastole is limited; likewise, increases in right ventricular end-diastolic pressure and volume restrict the diastolic filling of the left ventricle. Increases in ventricular stiffness interfere with the proper pump function of the heart and precipitate its failure (p. 260).

Besides distensibility, the end-diastolic pressure in the ventricle, and thus its filling, also depends on the duration of ventricular diastole, the force of atrial systole, and the venous return. In resting conditions ventricular systole occupies about one-third of the total cardiac cycle, there is ample time for filling, and atrial contraction contributes relatively little to the filling of the ventricles. If the heart were to quicken without a change in myocardial contractility, the duration of systole would remain relatively constant, and at a maximal heart rate of 180 to 190 beats/min it is likely that the filling of the heart would be endangered and the stroke volume decreased. However, in normal circumstances the increase in heart rate is accompanied by an increase in contractility of both atria and ventricles. This, together with the increased surge of blood from the peripheral veins, combines to shorten mechanical systole, increase the atrial contribution, and accelerate the filling of the heart.

Cardiac Output

Cardiac output is determined by the product of stroke volume and heart rate. In the normal resting adult each ventricle discharges approximately 80 to 90 ml of blood per beat. The ventricle does not empty completely, and the volume remaining at the end of systole, after the stroke volume is expelled, is called the end-systolic, or residual, volume. The stroke volume at rest approximates 65% of the total ventricular content at the end of diastole. In heart failure, when the chambers of the heart dilate, the residual volume becomes larger and the stroke volume relatively smaller (p. 258). The normal adult, when lying or sitting quietly, has a heart rate of around 60 to 70 beats/min. This value does not reflect the intrinsic rate of the sinus node since the rate of discharge of this pacemaker is greatly influenced by the sympathetic and vagal nerves (p. 117 and p. 126). At rest the vagal nerves predominate, and in healthy young subjects the heart rate decreases only slightly if the sympathetic nerves are blocked. By contrast, if the vagal control is interrupted, the heart rate augments markedly. Simultaneous abolition of sympathetic and vagal control augments heart rate from about 70 to 110 beats/min. The latter rate reflects the intrinsic rate of discharge of the sinus node.

Since the cardiac output under resting conditions depends on the size of the individual, it has been customary to relate it to the body surface area, which is a function of height and weight. In the resting supine, sitting, or lying subject, normal values range from 2.8 to 4.2 liters/min/m^2 of body surface area. Increases in cardiac output are obtained by increasing the heart rate (up to 210 beats/min), stroke volume (up to 120 ml in nonathletes and 150 ml in athletes), or both. Thus the cardiac output can increase up to about 12.5 to 15 liters/min/m^2.

Cardiac Work

The total external work of the heart depends on the amount of pressure (pressure–volume work) and kinetic energy it has to generate. The pressure–volume work is defined as that performed when ejecting a given volume of blood from each ventricle into the great arteries at a given pressure. The stroke work can be calculated as the stroke volume times the pressure at which the blood is ejected (Fig. 3–10). Strictly speaking, the calculation of stroke work should account for the rates of change of pressure and volume during each systole. The aortic pressure is about five times greater than the pulmonary artery pressure. Both ventricles eject the same amount of blood. Hence the pressure–volume work of the left ventricle is about five times more than that of the right. Additional work is performed by each ventricle to generate the kinetic energy necessary to accelerate the blood; the amount of work involved approximates 5% of the total external work of the heart. The amount of external work per minute (minute work) is given by the product of the stroke work

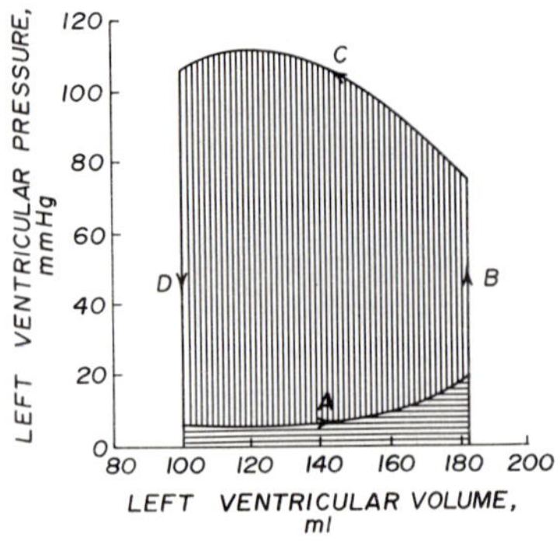

FIG. 3–10. Work diagram of the human left ventricle. **A:** Filling phase. During diastole, as blood flows from the left atrium into the left ventricle, the pressure in the latter increases slightly and the volume increases markedly. Toward the end of diastole, atrial contraction causes a further increase in pressure and volume (end-diastolic pressure). The area under this pressure curve *(horizontally hatched area)* represents the work done by the blood on the ventricle. **B:** Isometric contraction. The mitral and aortic valves are closed and the myocardium contracts isovolumetrically. No external work is done, but elastic energy is stored in the heart muscle. **C:** Ejection phase. The pressure in the ventricle exceeds that in the aorta; the aortic valves open; and the myocardium shortens isotonically. The shaded area *(vertical hatching)* represents work done by the ventricle on the blood during a single cardiac cycle. **D:** Isovolumetric relaxation phase. The ventricle relaxes, and the pressure falls rapidly. The aortic and mitral valves are closed, so the volume of the ventricle is unchanged. No work is done, but stored elastic energy is given back.

and heart rate. Any change in ejection pressure, heart rate, or stroke volume affects the minute work and hence the metabolic requirements of the heart muscle (Fig. 3–11).

Besides the external work, the heart muscle expends energy to overcome the inertia of the series–elastic components of its wall (internal work); this internal work is wasted in heat and has not been quantified.

The amount of work performed correlates with the oxygen requirements of the heart (p. 46), which are different during "volume loading" and "pressure loading." An example of the former is rhythmic muscular exercise in which the cardiac output increases markedly and compensates for the fall in peripheral resistance caused by the vasodilatation in the working muscles, whereas the aortic blood pressure changes little. By contrast, in chronic hypertension the cardiac output is normal but the blood pressure is high because of the increased systemic vascular resistance due to the decrease in diameter of the peripheral vessels (p. 209). For the same amount of calculated external work, a lower oxygen consumption by the myocardium is required for volume loading than for pressure loading. Hence the efficiency (external work/oxygen utilization; p. 48) of the heart increases during volume loading. In other words, if the heart performs a given amount of external work to generate pressure, this costs more energy and thus more oxygen than to perform the same amount of external work to eject blood.

DISTRIBUTING VESSELS

Pulse Pressure

The intermittent ejection of blood from the left ventricle into the aorta causes a pressure pulse in the arterial system. In the normal young adult the pressure

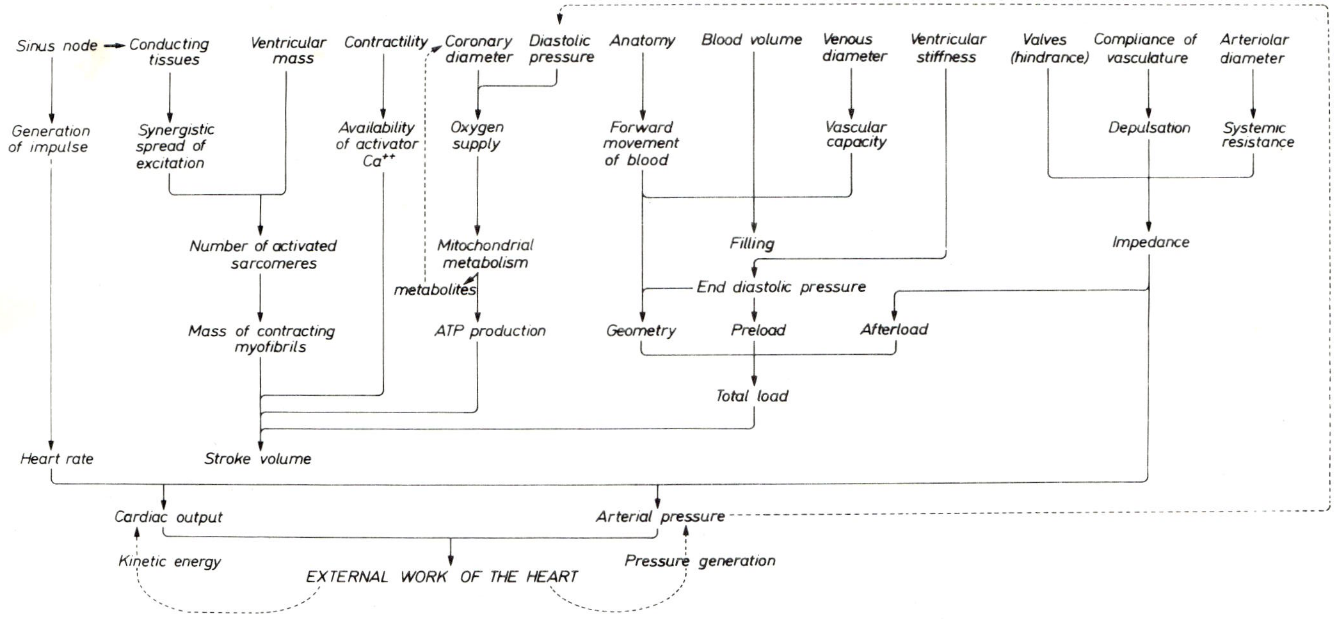

FIG. 3–11. Factors which influence the external work of the heart. Geometry refers to ventricular dimensions, and to Laplace's law. The hindrance offered by the valves becomes important only in valvular disease (p. 236). For details see text.

at the height of the pulse (systolic blood pressure) is about 120 to 125 mm Hg, and the lowest pressure (diastolic blood pressure) is about 80 mm Hg. The reason the pressure in the main arteries remains relatively high during ventricular diastole, when the pressure in the ventricle drops almost to zero, is the combination of the elastic recoil of the arterial wall and the peripheral resistance. There is a temporary imbalance between the volume of blood ejected by the ventricle and the amount allowed to flow through the narrow arterioles and the capillaries. The excess blood pumped by the heart is accommodated during systole by distention of the aorta and the large arteries. After closure of the aortic valve, the great vessels recoil further to resume their original configuration. This recoil imparts energy to the blood, maintaining its flow throughout diastole. The difference between the systolic and diastolic pressures is called the pulse pressure, which is mainly a function of the stroke volume and the elasticity (compliance) of the arterial tree.

The pulse contour in the aorta shows a rapid upstroke during left ventricular

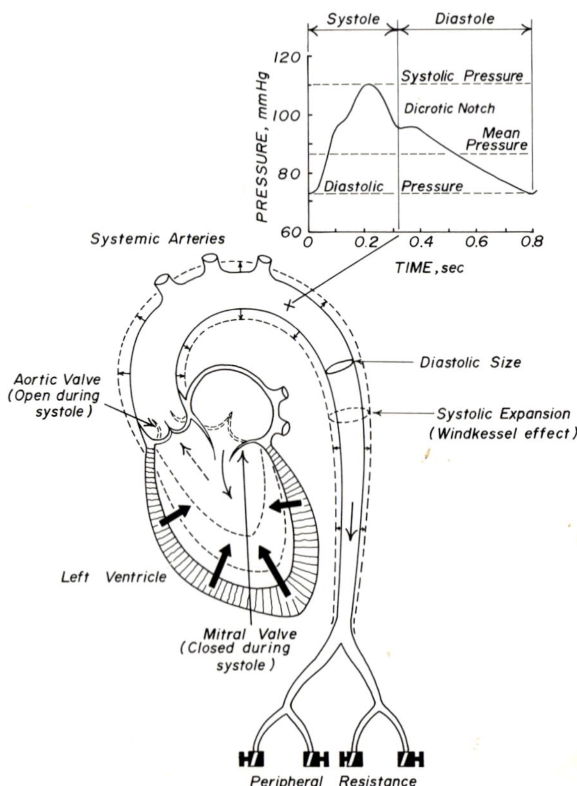

FIG. 3–12. The dampening role of the aorta and the large arteries on the pulsatile flow from the heart during systole (Windkessel effect). **Inset:** Changes in aortic pressure during the cardiac cycle.

systole followed by a slower rise to the peak pressure. The end of ventricular systole is indicated by a brief downward deflection (notch or incisura) of the pressure contour due to the reversal of flow when the ventricular pressure decreases below that in the aorta. The sudden closure of the aortic valve and the subsequent rebound of blood from it give a brief rise in pressure immediately following the notch. As blood flows out of the aorta into the peripheral vessels during diastole the pressure decreases rapidly at first and then more slowly as the driving force declines (Fig. 3–12).

Transmission of Pulse Pressure

The pulse pressure which develops in the proximal aorta as the blood is ejected into it is transmitted down the aorta and to the periphery where it can be detected easily by palpation in the larger vessels. The pressure pulse is transmitted with a greater velocity than that of the blood because of the latter's inertia. The velocity of transmission of the pulse wave approximates 4 m/sec in the aorta, 8 m/sec in the large arteries, and 16 m/sec in the smaller arteries. This is 15 and 100 times faster than blood velocity in the aorta and the arteries, respectively. As the pressure wave is transmitted to the periphery, it undergoes a gradual transformation of contour. This is due to a summation of the incident pulse waves with reflected waves from the periphery and resonance effects in the peripheral arteries. The summation of incident and reflected waves explains

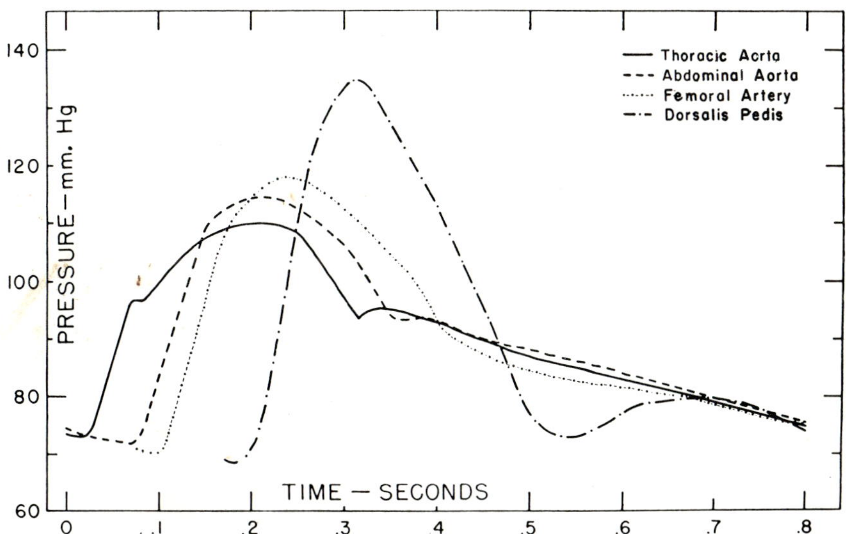

FIG. 3–13. Pressure pulses in a normal subject recorded from thoracic aorta, abdominal aorta, femoral artery, and dorsalis pedis artery. (From Remington and Wood: *J. Appl. Physiol.,* 9:433, 1956.)

why the systolic pressure is higher in the medium-sized arteries than in the aorta, although the diastolic pressure is lower (Fig. 1–3). As a consequence, in a vessel such as the radial artery the pulse pressure is about 40 to 45% greater, whereas the mean pressure is about 5% less, than in the central aorta (Fig. 3–13). The small arteries and arterioles act to dampen the pressure wave, which becomes almost absent in the capillaries, except when the former vessels are dilated.

The Pulmonary Circuit

The pressure in the pulmonary artery of the normal adult averages 23 mm Hg during systole and 16 mm Hg during diastole. The pulsatile pattern is maintained throughout the pulmonary bed including the capillaries (Fig. 1–3).

RESISTANCE VESSELS

The smallest arteries and the arterioles are characterized by a small diameter and a large wall-to-lumen ratio; the major components of the wall are the smooth muscle cells, which are arranged circumferentially. The arterioles offer the major resistance to blood flow. Because of their smooth muscle layers, they can actively vary their wall tension and their diameter, and thus the resistance they offer (Fig. 3–14). These changes in resistance not only provide for perfusion of the individual vascular beds in accordance to their metabolic needs but also have a primary role in the regulation of the systemic arterial blood pressure.

Provided the arterial blood pressure remains constant, the degree of opening of the arterioles determines the amount of blood flowing through them and thus the capillary perfusion. Alteration in the diameter of the arterioles affects not only the flow but also the pressure within the capillaries and veins, which has important implications for capillary exchanges and venous function (Fig. 3–15).

The arterial blood pressure, which governs perfusion of the tissues, is determined by the cardiac output and the total systemic vascular resistance. The

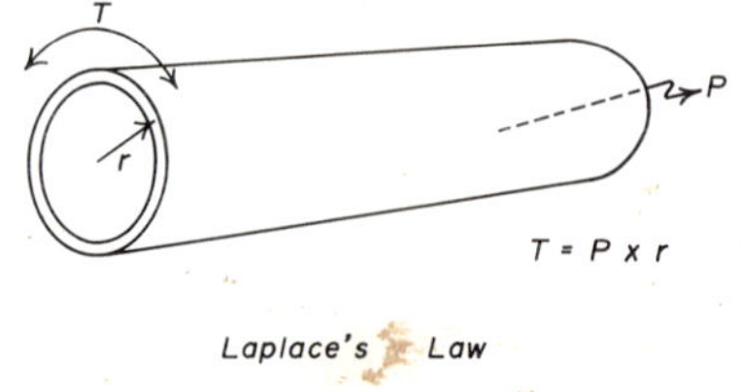

FIG. 3–14. In blood vessels the degree of opening (radius, *r*) is determined by the distending pressure *(P)* and the wall tension *(T)*, as predicted by Laplace's law for thin-walled cylindrical structures. The vascular smooth muscle in the wall can actively augment wall tension, which either opposes distention and maintains the diameter, or reduces the radius of the vessel. If the smooth muscle relaxes, the vessel is distended by the intraluminal pressure to the extent determined by its elasticity, which is greatest in the veins and lowest in the capillaries. Laplace's law also implies that large reductions in diameter, which result in active mobilization of blood, require less generation of active wall tension in the venous side of the circulation.

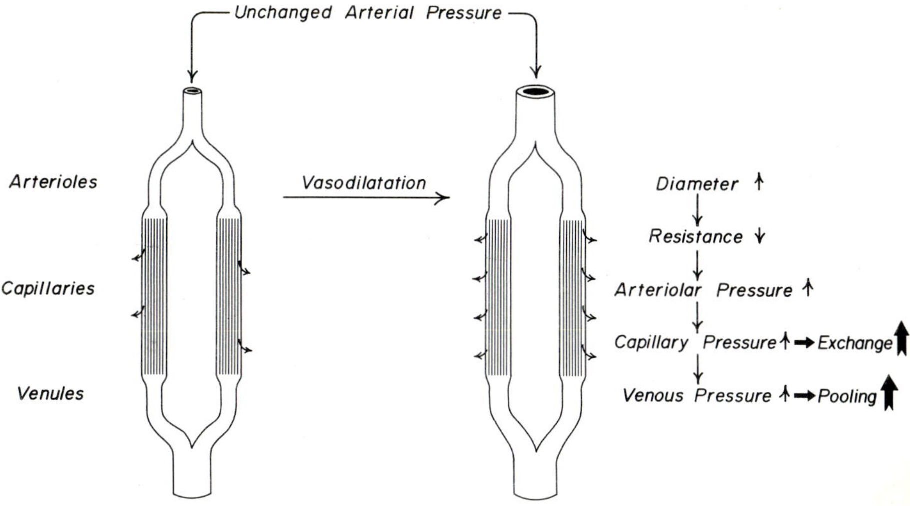

FIG. 3–15. Effects of arteriolar dilation on the capillaries and venules. When the arteriole dilates, its resistance decreases and the pressure drop across it is reduced. Thus the pressure in the capillaries and in the veins augments. This causes a greater filtration of fluid in the former and passive accumulation of blood in the latter.

latter depends on the totality of the individual resistances, each one of which is inversely proportional to the diameter of the arterioles involved (Fig. 1–8). Important increases or decreases in vascular resistance in given beds (e.g., skeletal muscle, kidney) affect the total systemic vascular resistance and arterial blood pressure unless compensatory changes in resistance of other beds and/or cardiac output take place.

EXCHANGE VESSELS

The ultimate goal of the cardiovascular system is fulfilled at the capillary level. Here oxygen and other essential substances leave the bloodstream to feed the tissue cells, and carbon dioxide and other metabolites are drained away. This is made possible by a combination of fluid exchanges (filtration/reabsorption) and diffusion. A small fraction of the total exchange, in particular the transport of macromolecules, occurs by pinocytosis (Fig. 2–7).

Diffusion

Diffusion along concentration gradients is the way by which oxygen reaches the cells and carbon dioxide is removed. These gases are lipid-soluble and therefore pass freely through the entire lining of the cardiovascular system. Other lipid-soluble substances also can cross the endothelial cells, whereas lipid-insoluble substances must traverse pores through or between them (Fig. 2–7). The bulk of water flowing across water-filled pores has been calculated by Poiseuille;

$$(1) \quad Jv = \frac{\pi r^4 n}{8 \eta \Delta x} \Delta P \quad \textit{(Poiseuille)}$$

$$(2) \quad Js = -Ds \frac{As}{\Delta x} Cs \quad \textit{(Fick)}$$

FIG. 3–16. Equations governing the flow of water (1) and the diffusion of solutes (2) across water-filled pores. J_v = total flow. r = pore radius. n = number of pores per unit area of membrane. n = viscosity of the fluid in the pores. P = pressure. Δx = thickness of the membrane = length of pores. J_s = solute diffusion. D_s = free diffusion coefficient of the solute in water. C_s = concentration of solute within the membrane. A_s = the apparent area available for diffusion of the solute in the water-filled channels of the membrane. The area is apparent because of additional frictional forces between the solute molecules and the walls of the pore, and of steric factors operating at the entrance of the pore.

the rate of diffusion of solute may be calculated from the application of Fick's law of diffusion to the pore channels (Fig. 3–16).

When the size of the lipid-insoluble substances increases and approaches that of the pore, the diffusion becomes limited. For smaller molecules (e.g., water, salts, urea, and glucose) the hindrance offered by the pores is minimal, and equilibration occurs readily throughout the cardiovascular system including the cerebral vessels; the total diffusion is limited only by the amount of blood flowing through the tissue (Fig. 3–17).

Fluid Movements

The filtration–reabsorption process, and thus the direction and the amount of fluid movement across the capillary membrane, depends on capillary permeability and the equilibrium between four forces. These are (Fig. 3–18): (1) The pressure of the blood within the capillary (hydrostatic pressure), which tends to force fluid through the pores. (2) The counterpressure exerted by the tissues

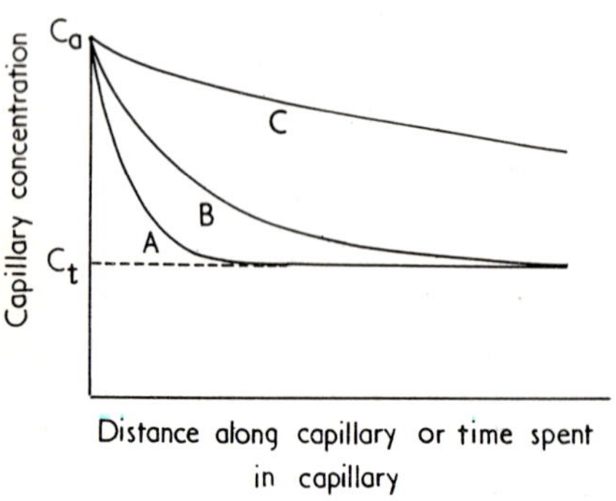

FIG. 3–17. The fall in blood concentration of three substances as they equilibrate with the tissues during their passage through a capillary. The capillary wall is more permeable to A than B, and more permeable to B than C. Because equilibrium is achieved for A and B before the blood leaves the capillary, net movement of these substances from the blood into the tissues can be increased only by increasing the blood flow, and the exchange of A and B is said to be flow-limited. Substance C does not equilibrate completely during a single transit, and its exchange is said to be diffusion-limited. (From Michel: In: *Cardiovascular Fluid Dynamics,* Vol. 2, edited by Bergel, p. 241. Academic Press, New York, 1972.)

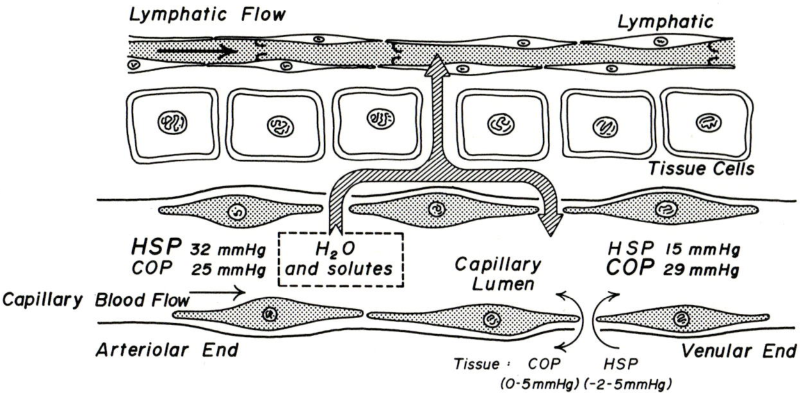

FIG. 3–18. Fluid exchanges at the capillary level. HSP = hydrostatic pressure. COP = colloid osmotic pressure.

(interstitial fluid hydrostatic pressure). The exact values for the hydrostatic pressure of the interstitial fluid are still debated. Assumptions that it was equal to or slightly greater than atmospheric pressure have been challenged by measurements from an implanted capsule or wick, which suggest that it is several millimeters of mercury less than atmosphere. (3) The attraction exerted by the plasma proteins on the interstitial fluid (plasma colloid osmotic pressure), which favors reabsorption. The colloid osmotic pressure of the plasma is more than 200 times smaller than the total osmotic pressure of the blood; this is because the proteins are the only components that do not pass freely back and forth across the capillary wall as do the crystalloids, which are the major determinants of plasma osmotic pressure. Of the plasma proteins (see Appendix, Table 8), the most numerous are the albumins and hence they are the major determinants of the colloid osmotic pressure. (4) The presence of some proteins in the interstitial fluid determines the interstitial colloid osmotic pressure, which resists reabsorption.

The amount of fluid filtered through the capillaries can increase in two ways. One is if the number of open capillaries is increased, thereby increasing the surface area available for diffusion. Since the capillaries have no smooth muscle, they are not capable of active changes in caliber. The number of open capillaries in each vascular bed is determined either by the degree of opening of the arterioles, which function as precapillary sphincters, or by the postcapillary pressure; these two factors are the determinants of the distending pressure in the capillaries. The other possibility is an increase in capillary permeability. How this occurs is uncertain, but it may involve altered activity of contractile proteins in the endothelial cell. An increased capillary permeability implies widening of the existing pores so that substances larger than normal leave the capillary bed, leading to an excessive loss of proteins to the tissues. This may be caused by substances such as histamine, 5-hydroxytryptamine, and bradykinin or by severe anoxia.

The hydrostatic pressure approximates 32 mm Hg at the arteriolar end of most capillaries (Fig. 1–3); in arterial blood the plasma colloid osmotic pressure averages 25 mm Hg. In normal conditions the interstitial fluid hydrostatic pressure and the interstitial colloid osmotic pressure are small and balance each other, and the movement of fluid is determined mainly by the equilibrium between the hydrostatic and the colloid osmotic pressure of the plasma. At the arteriolar side of the capillary the hydrostatic pressure dominates and fluid is filtered to the interstitial space. Along the capillary the hydrostatic pressure decreases, to reach approximately 15 mm Hg at the venous end. As fluid is filtered into the interstitial space, the concentration of the plasma proteins and thus the colloid osmotic pressure in the capillaries increases steadily. As soon as this pressure becomes greater than the hydrostatic pressure, the movement of fluid is reversed and reabsorption occurs.

In normal conditions the colloid osmotic pressure of the plasma and of the interstitial fluid, as well as the pressure of the latter, remain remarkably constant. Within the same capillary, variations in filtration and reabsorption are brought about mainly by altering the level of hydrostatic pressure. The most common example is the human who sits for a long time with the legs in a dependent position. The feet swell because the hydrostatic pressure in the dependent parts is increased. Another example is the exercising muscle, where local metabolic changes cause widening of the arterioles and a decrease of the arteriolar resistance; the small pressure drop across the arteriole results in high capillary hydrostatic pressure (Fig. 3–15). As a consequence, the fluid exchanges are proportional to the metabolic needs of the tissue.

The hydrostatic pressure is not the same in all capillaries. Hence the importance of the filtration process varies considerably among different tissues. At the two extremes are the kidney and the lung. In the glomeruli of the kidney the hydrostatic pressure is more than double that in the other systemic capillaries because the preglomerular arterioles are relatively short and wide. The increased hydrostatic pressure leads to a large filtration volume from the glomerular capillaries into the nephrons (approximately 170 liters/24 hr). Of that filtrate, most is reabsorbed by the renal tubule, and only about 2 liters is expelled as urine. The large glomerular filtration followed by selective tubular reabsorption permits the total plasma volume to be cleared repeatedly of toxic substances with a minimal loss of water and essential ions. By contrast, in the lungs it is vital that no fluid passes from the capillaries to the alveoli since this would interfere seriously with the exchange of gases. Here a constant predominance of the reabsorption process is ensured by the fact that the colloid osmotic pressure (25 mm Hg) greatly exceeds the hydrostatic pressure (8 to 10 mm Hg). The necessity of avoiding filtration to the alveoli, which could result in pulmonary edema (p. 257), explains why the pressure must be lower in the pulmonary circuit than in the systemic circulation.

LYMPHATICS

All the fluid filtered at the arteriolar side of the systemic capillaries is not reabsorbed at the venous end; the amount not reabsorbed is returned to the systemic circulation by the lymphatics. These originate as thin-walled, capillary-like, closed-ended channels and are present in all tissues (Fig. 3–18). Their walls are permeable even to macromolecules. The total amount of protein they carry per day approximates one-fourth to one-half of the plasma proteins. The lymphatics, which have valves, pass through the lymph glands and eventually unite to form larger vessels, the most important of which is the thoracic duct, which enters the left internal jugular vein. Besides draining the fluid and proteins from the tissues and returning them to the general circulation, they form, with their associated lymphatic glands, the first line of defense against infection. In addition, in the intestinal mucosa the lymphatics play an important role in the absorption process by carrying tiny droplets of fat (chylomicrons) to the circulating blood. The lymphatic flow is due to: (1) suction exerted by the high-velocity flow in the large veins; (2) contraction of the smooth muscle cells in the wall of the large lymphatic ducts; and (3) pressure exerted by the tissues (e.g., contracting skeletal muscle). The total lymphatic flow averages 4 liters/24 hr.

CAPACITANCE VESSELS

The major components of the vein wall are collagen, elastin, and smooth muscle. Leg veins contain more muscle than do arm veins, and in both the arm and the leg superficial veins contain more muscle than do deep veins. These differences are in keeping with the higher hydrostatic pressure in the lower extremities and the more active role played by the cutaneous veins. The venous wall is very distensible. This means that minimal changes in distending pressure cause either a passive displacement of blood toward the heart (decreased distending pressure) or a venous pooling (increased distending pressure). The distensibility of the normal venous wall is limited by its collagen structure and by the contraction of its venous smooth muscle (Fig. 2–32). The latter also permits active adjustments of the peripheral vascular capacity.

Transmural Pressure

The effective venous distending pressure (transmural pressure) is determined by the pressure of the blood within the vein minus the counterpressure exerted by the surrounding tissues. The venous blood pressure depends on: (1) The arterial pressure and the diameter of the arterioles. When the arterioles dilate, the venous pressure is augmented, leading to an increase in venous capacity; when the arterioles constrict, the venous distending pressure decreases, resulting in passive emptying of the system. (2) The hydrostatic load, which is dependent on gravitational forces. (3) The pressure in the downstream part of the low-pressure system.

Influence of Gravity

The most common gravitational stress for the human occurs when he/she changes from the supine to the standing position. When lying, the hydrostatic load is nearly the same for all parts of the body, and the pressures within the blood vessels depend on the force generated by the heart. Large hydrostatic gradients occur on standing (Fig. 3–19). The veins above heart level become increasingly elliptical as the pressure within them approaches tissue pressure. As long as the volume of the cerebrospinal fluid remains constant, the transmural pressure of the intracranial veins and of those in the spinal column remains about the same because the cerebrospinal fluid and these veins are exposed to an identical hydrostatic load. Thus the venous flow from the central nervous system is little affected by gravitational forces. The same is true in the abdomen where the increase in venous hydrostatic pressure is balanced by the increased tissue pressure exerted by the abdominal viscera. This places the splanchnic veins in an ideal position for modulation of vascular capacity. In the dependent extremities the arterial and venous pressures are increased to the same extent by the hydrostatic load, so there are no changes in the driving force to flow.

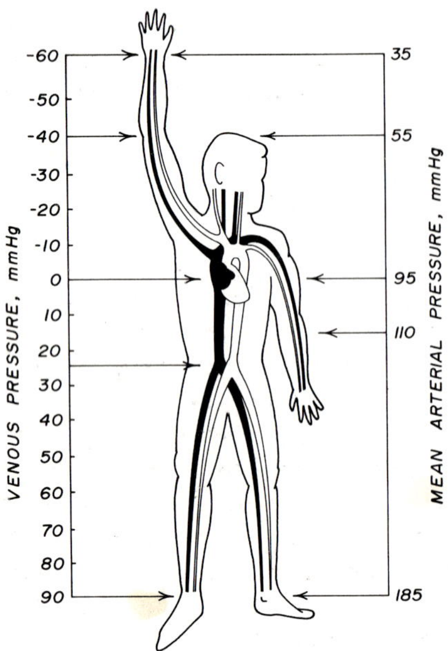

FIG. 3–19. Arterial and venous pressures in the motionless, standing subject. Influence of hydrostatic pressure on the columns of blood in the arteries *(open vessels)* and veins *(solid vessels).*

The increased pressure, however, has two consequences. One is to increase capillary pressure, causing increased filtration. The other is to cause pooling of blood at the venous side. The accumulation of blood in the limb veins is limited by the collagen fibers of the venous wall and by the presence of venous valves, which subdivide the venous blood column into segments (Fig. 2–16). The pressure inside these segments is less than would occur if the valves were absent. If the standing is prolonged, the maintained hydrostatic load above the proximal venous valves causes their insufficiency, and this process continues until the most distal valves become insufficient. At this time the venous pressure in the foot approximates the pressure of a column of blood extending vertically from the foot to the heart and hence may approach 90 mm Hg. As a consequence several hundred milliliters of blood accumulate in the lower extremities.

Muscle Pump

The peripheral pooling of blood on standing may bc counteracted effectively by the massaging action of the leg muscles during their contractions (skeletal muscle pump). During the latter the veins within the muscles are compressed, the pressure distending them decreases, and blood is mobilized toward the heart; the competency of the valves is restored, and the long hydrostatic column again is broken into shorter segments. The decrease in pressure in deep veins allows blood to flow into them from the superficial veins through communicating branches; hence the pressure in the cutaneous veins also decreases (Fig. 3–20). The resulting translocation of blood from the legs increases the amount of blood in the central vascular reservoir, improves the filling of the heart, and augments the stroke volume. In addition, the decrease in venous pressure increases the pressure difference between the arteries and the veins, and thus augments blood flow through the lower limbs.

Influence of Respiration and Heart Beat

As the veins traverse the abdomen and enter the thorax, the respiratory variations in pressure in the thoracic and abdominal cavities induce fluctuations in the venous return to the right heart. During deep inspiration the intra-abdominal pressure increases and forces blood into the thorax because retrograde flow into the legs is prevented by the valves in the iliac and femoral veins. Since the venous pressure inside the thorax decreases below atmospheric pressure during inspiration, this increases the pressure difference between the periphery and the right atrium, thus increasing venous return through both caval veins.

The pressure in the great veins reflects the pressure changes seen within the atria. Of importance is that the downward movement of the ventricles during their contraction increases the atrial size and causes an abrupt decrease in atrial and central venous pressure with a sudden rush of blood into the atria.

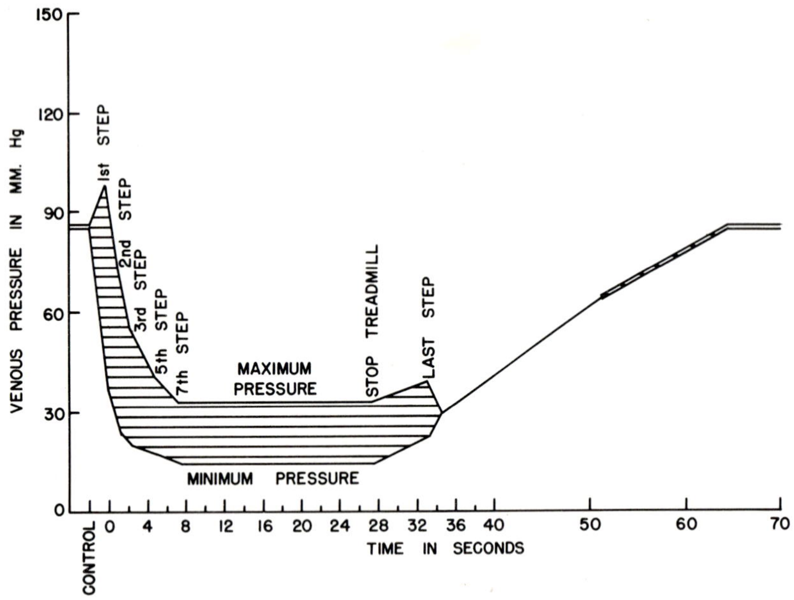

FIG. 3–20. Changes in venous pressure at the ankle of a normal man produced by walking, illustrating how compression of the deep veins causes a decrease in pressure in the superficial veins. (From Pollack and Wood: *J. Appl. Physiol.,* 1:649, 1949.)

Role of the Veins in Circulatory Control

As the blood leaves the capillaries it passes from the venules via successively larger veins to the right atrium, and in the supine subject the venous pressure decreases approximately from 15 to 4 mm Hg (Fig. 1–3). This is a small but adequate driving force which provides for the venous return.

Because under steady-state conditions the venous return is equal to the cardiac output, the resistance offered by the veins to the flow of blood is only about 15% of that on the arterial side of the circulation. As a consequence, the pre- to postcapillary resistance ratio is dominated by the degree of opening of the precapillary vessels. However, if the arterioles dilate and the venules and veins remain constricted, the resulting increase in postcapillary resistance augments the capillary pressure and may contribute to the increased extravasation of fluid (p. 263). The extreme example of a dissociation between arteriolar and venous resistances is provided by erectile tissues, where the combination of arteriolar dilation and venous constriction combines to fully distend the venous sinuses of the corpora cavernosa, which provides the turgor necessary for sexual performance.

The systemic veins are not simply a series of passive tubes for the transport of blood back to the heart. They are a reservoir of variable capacity whose compliance is about 30 times greater than that of the arterial tree; they act in

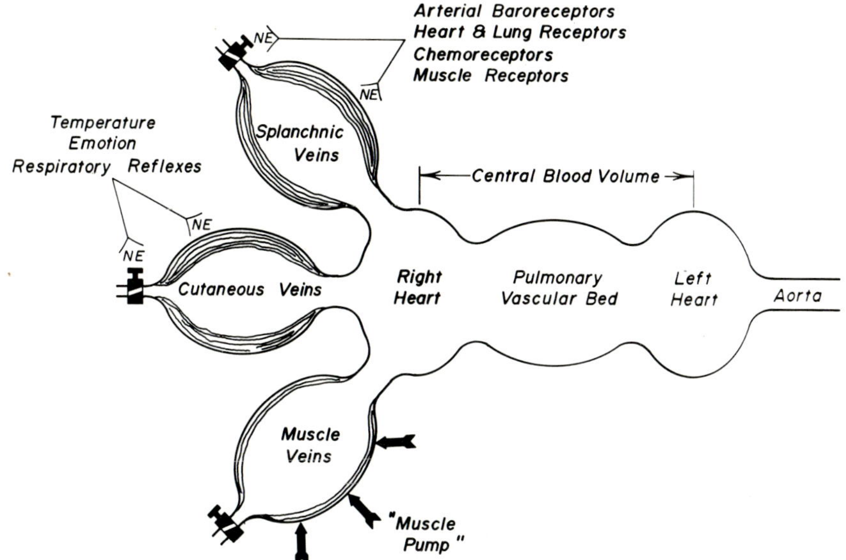

FIG. 3–21. Control of central blood volume and cardiac filling pressure by the systemic veins. Active changes in filling of the heart are brought about by contraction of the smooth muscle cells of the venous wall, in particular the splanchnic veins. The cutaneous veins play a role mainly in thermoregulation. Passive changes in capacity result from any change in distending pressure whether due to gravity or to changes in arteriolar resistance.

conjunction with the other parts of the low-pressure system, the right heart, the pulmonary circulation, and the left atrium. Together they contain about 85% of the total blood volume. The capacity of the peripheral veins can be actively decreased or increased when the smooth muscle cells in their walls contract or relax, respectively.

The three main components of the peripheral venous system are the cutaneous, the muscle, and the splanchnic veins. By active and passive changes in capacity they continuously regulate the amount of blood contained in the right heart, pulmonary vessels, and left atrium (central blood volume), and thus the filling pressure of the atria and ventricles. Cutaneous veins also play an important role in thermoregulation (Fig. 3–21).

SELECTED REFERENCES

Bishop, V. S., Peterson, D. F., and Horwitz, L. D. (1976): Factors influencing cardiac performance. In: *International Review of Physiology, Cardiovascular Physiology II,* Vol. 9, edited by A. C. Guyton and A. W. Cowley Jr., p. 239. University Park Press, Baltimore.

Blinks, J. R., and Jewell, B. R. (1972): The meaning and measurement of myocardial contractility. In: *Cardiovascular Fluid Dynamics,* Vol. 1, edited by D. H. Bergel, p. 225. Academic Press, New York.

Brooks, C. M., Hoffman, B. F., Suckling, E. E., and Orias, O. (1955): *Excitability of the Heart.* Grune & Stratton, New York.

Brutsaert, D. L., de Clerck, N. M., Goethals, M. A., and Housmans, P. R. (1978): Relaxation of ventricular cardiac muscle. *J. Physiol. (Lond),* 283:469.

Elzinga G., and Westerhof, N. (1979): How to quantify pump function of the heart. *Circ. Res.,* 44:303.

Folkow, B., and Mellander, S. (1970): Measurements of capillary filtration coefficient and its use in studies of the control of capillary exchange. In: *Alfred Benzon Symposium on capillary permeability,* Vol. II, p. 614. Munksgaard, Copenhagen.

Gibbs, C. L. (1978): Cardiac energetics. *Physiol. Rev.,* 58:174.

Glantz, S. A., and Parmley, W. W. (1978): Factors which affect the diastolic pressure-volume curve. *Circ. Res.,* 42:171.

Guyton, A. C., Granger, H. J., and Taylor, A. E. (1971): Interstitial fluid pressure. *Physiol. Rev.,* 51:527.

Haddy, F. J., Scott, J. B., and Grega, G. J. (1976): Peripheral circulation: fluid transfer across the microvascular membrane. In: *International Review of Physiology, Cardiovascular Physiology II,* Vol. 9, edited by A. C. Guyton and A. W. Cowley Jr., p. 63. University Park Press, Baltimore.

Jewell, B. R. (1977): A reexamination of the influence of muscle length on myocardial performance. *Circ. Res.,* 40:221.

Landis, E. M., and Pappenheimer, J. R. (1963): Exchange of substances through the capillary walls. In: *Handbook of Physiology, Sect. 2: Circulation,* Vol. II, p. 961. American Physiological Society, Washington, D.C.

Mayerson, H. S. (1963): The physiologic importance of lymph. In: *Handbook of Physiology, Sect. 2: Circulation,* Vol. II, p. 1035. American Physiological Society, Washington, D.C.

McDonald, D. A. (1974): *Blood Flow in Arteries,* 2nd ed., Edward Arnold, London.

Milnor, W. R. (1975): Arterial impedance as ventricular afterload. *Circ. Res.,* 36:565.

Noble, M. I. M. (1978): The Frank-Starling curve. *Clin. Sci. Mol. Med.,* 54:1.

Patel, D. J., Vaishnav, R. N., Gow, B. S., and Kot, P. A. (1974): Hemodynamics. *Annu. Rev. Physiol.,* 36:125.

Sagawa, K. (1978): The ventricular pressure—volume diagram revisited. *Circ. Res.,* 43:677.

Shepherd, J. T., and Vanhoutte, P. M. (1975): *Veins and Their Control.* Saunders, London.

Wiederhielm, C. A. (1968): Dynamics of transcapillary fluid exchange. *J. Gen. Physiol.,* 52:29S.

4

Local Control of Cardiovascular Function

The response of myocardial and vascular muscles can be modulated at the local level by the composition of the extracellular fluid, the local physical conditions to which they are exposed, and, particularly in the blood vessel wall, by locally produced active substances (autocoids).

LINK BETWEEN TISSUE FUNCTION AND BLOOD SUPPLY

The primary goal of the circulation is to ensure a proper *milieu intérieur* for the tissue cells; if the cardiovascular system fails to do so, the lack of oxygen and the resulting local accumulation of metabolites causes cellular intoxication and dysfunction. The myocardium and the central nervous system are the best illustrations of this principle. The metabolism of the myocardial and cerebral cells is the major factor controlling their blood supply, and the latter is adjusted so finely that in normal life the extracellular environment of these cells remains remarkably constant. Even when it is necessary to make overall adjustments in the cardiovascular system to counteract stress, and in particular when the blood supply cannot be maintained to all tissues, the driving pressure in the coronary arteries and the cerebral blood vessels is maintained by decreasing the blood supply to the other organs. Thus metabolic depression of myocardial contractility and cerebral function occurs only in cardiovascular failure, in conditions of severe metabolic alterations in the composition of the blood, or during mechanical impairment of coronary and cerebral blood flow (p. 227).

Perfusion of the tissues depends on their degree of activity. The smooth muscle cells of the precapillary vessels (resistance vessels) normally are partly contracted when the tissue they subserve is at rest. This inherent tone depends on the automaticity of these cells. From this resting condition (myogenic tone) they are capable of further constriction and of relaxation. The degree of relaxation is proportional to the metabolic activity of the tissue cells and permits the flow to increase in proportion to the fourth power of the radius (Fig. 1–6). For example, during graded muscular exercise the blood flow through the working muscle increases progressively by as much as 25-fold.

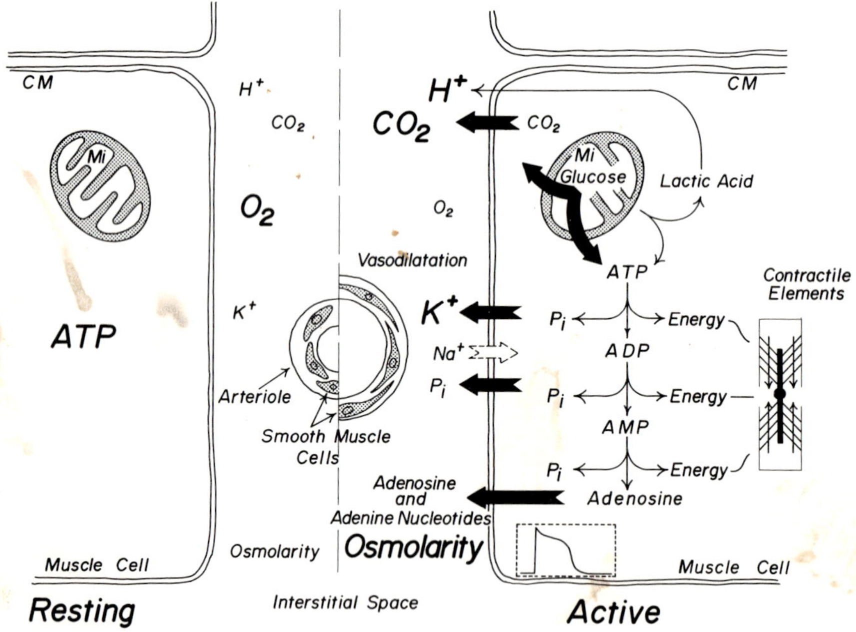

FIG. 4–1. Major changes in the composition of the interstitial fluid during contraction of muscle cells. When the muscle is inactive **(left)** the arterioles are constricted, the concentration of metabolites and carbon dioxide in the interstitial fluid is low, and little oxygen is used. When the muscles become active **(right):** (1) the depolarization of the cell membrane (CM) increases the K^+ concentration in the extracellular space; (2) the regeneration of adenosine triphosphate (ATP) by the mitochondria (Mi) augments the production of carbon dioxide, which diffuses to the extracellular space; (3) the anaerobic production of ATP in the cytoplasm results in the formation of lactic acid, which slowly diffuses out of the cell; (4) the increased amounts of lactic acid and carbon dioxide causes an increase in H^+ concentration of the extracellular fluid and thus a decrease in pH; (5) the breakdown of ATP to diphosphate (ADP) and monophosphate (AMP) and to adenosine, with liberation of inorganic phosphate (Pi), augments the concentration of adenosine and adenine nucleotides in the extracellular space; and (6) the osmolarity of the extracellular fluid increases. Each of these changes can cause relaxation of contracted smooth muscle cells, and it is likely that their combination is responsible for the adjustment of the blood flow to the metabolic needs of the tissues.

The precise link between metabolism and blood flow is unknown. Presumably substances formed by the metabolically active cells act on the resistance vessels in their vicinity to depress the myogenic tone. For a single substance or a combination of such substances to be responsible: (1) they should be capable of causing dilation of the resistance blood vessels as great as that which occurs during the increased activity of the tissues; (2) they should not enter the general circulation in amounts sufficient to alter flow to any other area; and (3) when they are injected into a systemic artery, the increase in blood flow should not be accompanied by any sensation (e.g., pain, itching). Many substances produced by metabolically active tissues, and in particular by contracting muscle, can be detected in the venous effluent from such tissues and have been examined as potential mediators of metabolic vasodilatation (hyperemia). These include: carbon dioxide, lactic acid, hydrogen ions, potassium ions, phosphate ions, polypeptides, prostaglandins, adenosine, and adenine nucleotides (Fig. 4–1). In addition, the oxygen tension of the venous blood from contracting muscle is reduced and its osmolarity increased. Of the factors mentioned above, adenosine and the adenine nucleotides best meet the criteria outlined.

Animal experiments demonstrate that in contracting skeletal muscle the resis-

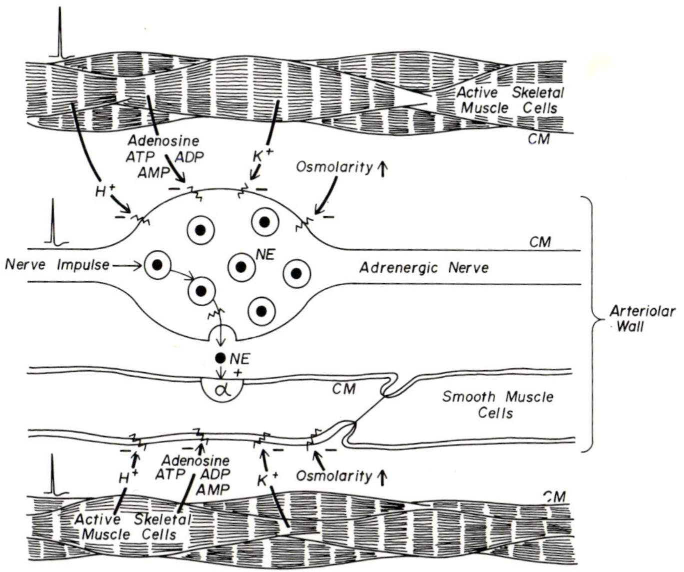

FIG. 4–2. The products of cellular activity cause dilatation of the arterioles not only because of their direct inhibitory effect on the smooth muscle cells but also because they interrupt the vasoconstrictor impulses of the sympathetic nerves. The arteriolar wall is shown as one layer of smooth muscle cells, with an adrenergic nerve ending and one of its varicosities, containing the adrenergic neurotransmitter norepinephrine (NE). AMP = adenosine monophosphate. ADP = adenosine diphosphate. ATP = adenosine triphosphate. CM = cell membrane. + = activation. − and ∿∿ = inhibitory effect. α = alpha-adrenergic receptor.

tance vessels are less sensitive to sympathetic nerve stimulation, and that substances released by contracting skeletal muscle cells (H^+, K^+, adenosine, and adenine nucleotides) act on the adrenergic nerve endings in the blood vessel wall to inhibit the release of norepinephrine (p. 113). Thus as the activity of the tissues increases, the resistance vessels are progressively disconnected from sympathetic control to help ensure the appropriate blood supply (Fig. 4–2).

The capillaries are passive tubes whose diameters are controlled by the precapillary resistance and the postcapillary pressure. They are not very distensible because of the stiffness of their basal membrane and their small diameter. Their permeability increases when the tissues become severely hypoxic.

The veins are little affected by increases in metabolic activity which lead to dilation of the resistance vessels, presumably because substances like adenosine are broken down rapidly by the red blood cells. The reactivity of the veins is unaltered by the usual fluctuations in oxygen content of the venous blood.

PHYSICAL FACTORS

Of the local physical factors which affect cardiac and vascular muscles, the transmural pressure and the local temperature are the most important.

Transmural Pressure

Heart

The degree of distention of the heart, which depends on the transmural pressure, is one of the major determinants of the stroke volume (Starling's law of the heart; Fig. 3–6.)

Resistance Vessels

The myogenic activity of the resistance vessels, particularly in the kidneys and brain, can be modulated by changes in transmural pressure. When the transmural pressure increases, the vessel constricts, which tends to maintain a constant flow; the reverse is true when the pressure decreases. The exact mechanism underlying this "autoregulation" is uncertain. It could serve as a local regulator to provide a constant capillary perfusion pressure and to avoid increases in blood flow in "nonactive" tissues when the blood pressure or the hydrostatic pressure are increased. Conversely, it maintains adequate perfusion of organs such as the brain if the perfusion pressure suddenly decreases (Fig. 4–3). An extreme example is the giraffe lifting its head; the perfusion pressure to the brain falls from about 200 to less than 100 mm Hg, but the cerebral flow is unchanged.

Below the autoregulation range the flow decreases as the perfusion pressure is reduced. In vascular beds such as the kidney and the skin, when the perfusion

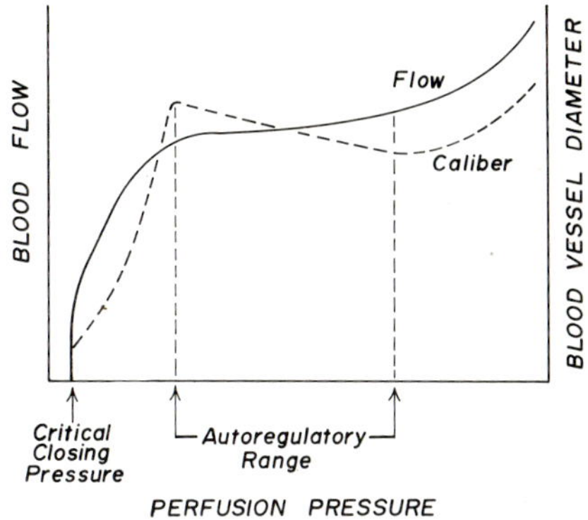

FIG. 4–3. Relationship between blood flow and perfusion pressure in systemic vascular beds. The flow remains relatively constant over a pressure range around the normal blood pressure. This is known as autoregulation and is characteristic of the brain, kidney, splanchnic, and limb circulations. For autoregulation to occur, the smooth muscle of the resistance vessels must relax as the arterial pressure decreases and vice versa. These changes in smooth muscle tone are mediated by a local mechanism whose nature remains obscure. Autoregulation permits tissue blood flow to remain constant despite changes in perfusion pressure. Above the autoregulatory range, which varies in individual beds from 60 up to 180 mm Hg, the flow increases. Below this range, as the pressure falls the flow decreases progressively. In certain vascular beds it suddenly drops to zero although the perfusion pressure approximates 20 to 40 mm Hg (critical closing pressure).

pressure falls below a critical value of about 20 to 40 mm Hg the arterioles may close and flow ceases (critical closing pressure) (Fig. 4–4). If the blood vessels are actively constricted, closure occurs at higher perfusion pressure. Critical closure may be explained by the resultant of the pressure difference across the wall (transmural pressure) and the wall tension; the relationship between these forces is defined by Laplace's law (Fig. 3–14).

The vasodilatation following temporary arrest of the circulation (reactive hyperemia) involves a myogenic response and the metabolic stimulus of tissue hypoxia. During the period of circulatory arrest the pressure in the distal vessels decreases, leading to a reduction in wall tension and consequently in myogenic activity. At the same time unidentified substances produced in the ischemic cells accumulate around the blood vessels, leading to further relaxation (Fig. 4–1). On restoring the circulation, there is an immediate increase in flow as the blood pours into the relaxed arterioles. The flow rapidly returns to the control levels as the metabolites are washed away and the normal transmural pressure is regained (Fig. 4–4).

In the contracting myocardium the compression of the vessels within the muscle causes varying degrees of impairment to flow depending on the strength of the systole. The metabolic needs must be met by the onrush of blood during diastole (Fig. 4–5). In the normal heart during ventricular systole, the intramyocardial pressure is least at the outer surface and increases throughout the ventricular wall to reach a maximum in the subendocardial muscle layers. During systole, blood flow still occurs in the outer layers but falls abruptly in the subendocardial myocardium. This is compensated for in diastole by the larger size of the small subendocardial intramuscular arteries, which permits a greater blood flow through them than through those in the outer layers (Fig. 4–6). If mechanical obstruction develops in any of the main coronary arteries, the result-

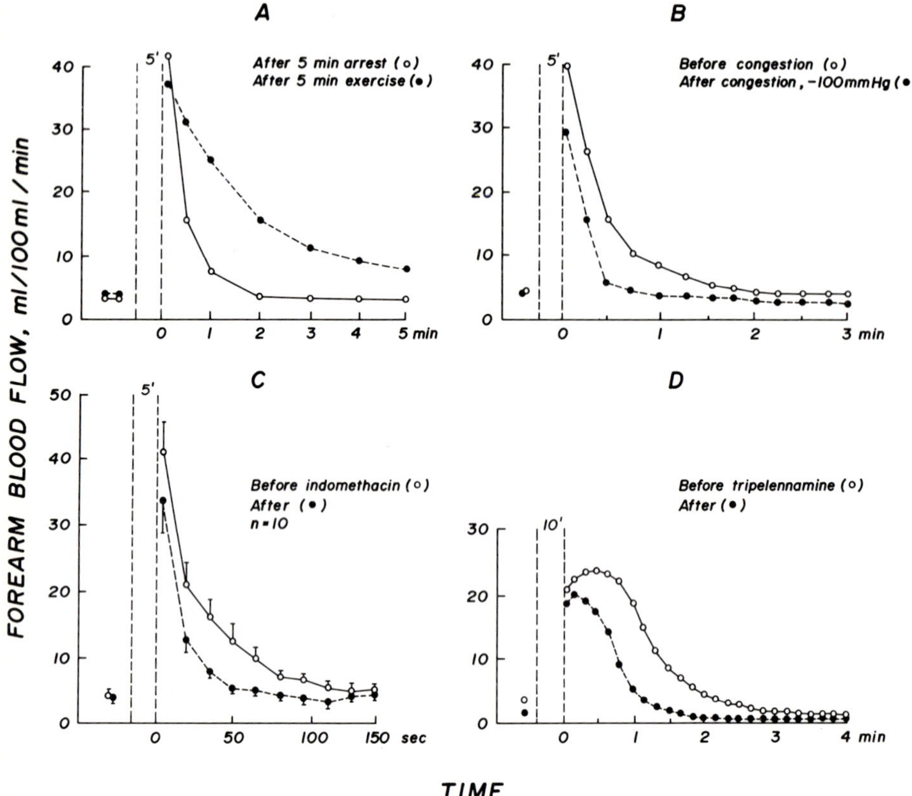

FIG. 4–4. Changes in blood flow following temporary arrest of the circulation to the human forearm (reactive hyperemia). The vertical dotted lines indicate the period of arrest by a pneumatic cuff around the arm inflated to suprasystolic pressure. **A:** Following release of the vascular occlusion, there is an immediate increase in blood flow, which returns rapidly to the preocclusion level. By comparison, after exercise of the forearm muscles the flow returns more slowly to the resting value. **B:** When the transmural pressure in the forearm vessels is maintained at a higher level by congesting them with blood prior to circulatory arrest, the subsequent hyperemia is less. This is due to a local action of the intravascular pressure on the smooth muscle of the arterioles, resulting in a greater wall tension (myogenic response). **C:** Inhibition of prostaglandin synthesis (p. 103) by the drug indomethacin reduces the hyperemia, demonstrating that prostaglandins are partly responsible for the hyperemia following circulatory arrest. **D:** The antihistaminic drug tripelennamine diminishes the reactive hyperemia following prolonged circulatory arrest, indicating that in these circumstances histamine is partly responsible (p. 102). (From Shepherd: In: *Mechanisms of Vasodilation,* edited by Vanhoutte and Leusen, p. 1. Karger, Basel, 1978.)

ing pressure drop in the distal vessels makes the subendocardial tissues particularly vulnerable to ischemia (p. 228).

In skeletal muscle during rhythmic exercise the flow also is phasic (Fig. 4–7). Very strong sustained contractions can be maintained only for a limited time because of the impairment of the blood supply to the active muscle cells.

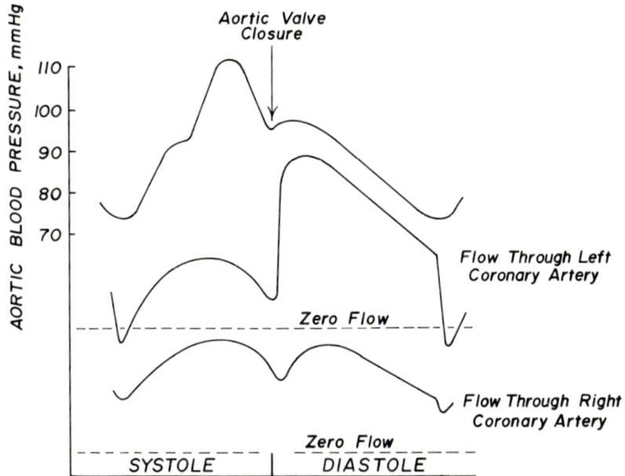

FIG. 4–5. Relationship between phasic changes in aortic blood pressure and blood flow in the left and right coronary arteries. During systole the increased intramyocardial pressure resulting from the contraction of the thick-walled left ventricle hinders blood flow into the heart muscle but facilitates venous drainage by compressing the coronary sinus and other veins. Brief retrograde flow may occur at the time mechanical compression is greatest and aortic pressure least. With the onset of isometric relaxation immediately after closure of the aortic valve, the rate of flow rapidly increases to attain a maximal level in early diastole, from which it gradually declines. In the right coronary artery the phasic changes in flow resembles the pressure pulse in the aorta. Retrograde flow does not occur since the intramural tension of the right ventricle is only moderate.

Capacitance Vessels

In the venous system changes in transmural pressure cause either passive mobilization or pooling of blood (p. 89). In the myogenically active splanchnic veins increased distention results in progressive augmentation of the amplitude and frequency of the spontaneous contractions (Fig. 4–8). This is due to the depolarizing effect of stretch, which brings the membrane potential closer to the threshold for spontaneous firing, leads to bursts of action potentials, and/or decreases the interval between them. Although not proved, a similar mechanism would explain the autoregulatory behavior of the resistance vessels. In the portal mesenteric veins the rhythmic activity is proportional to the degree of distention. Hence when more blood returns from the intestine the function of these veins in assisting the return of blood to the portal circulation of the liver is improved (portal venous pump). In other veins myogenic activity is not a normal phenomenon and thus plays an insignificant role in the overall response of the capacitance vessels. However, the response of these veins to vasoconstrictor stimuli depends on the distending pressure in analogy with Starling's law of the heart (Fig. 2–32). If during a sustained contraction of the smooth muscle there is a change in venous distending pressure, it will modify the active tension secondary to a shift in the length–tension relationship. This means that when the veins are well filled but not overdistended a greater volume of blood is displaced toward the heart for a given degree of smooth muscle activation.

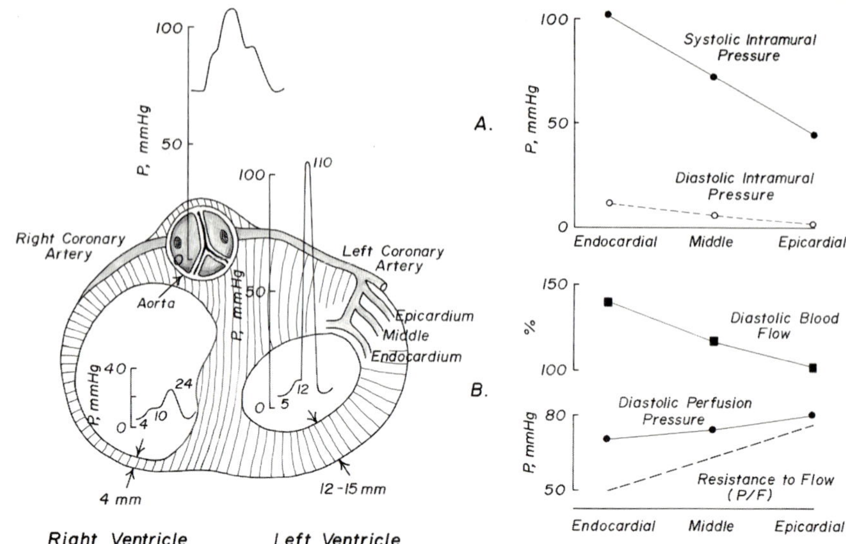

FIG. 4–6. Left: Distribution of blood flow within the myocardium. The left and right coronary arteries give rise to branches which penetrate the myocardium at right angles. In the left ventricle the intraventricular pressure generated during systole, and thus the intramural pressure in the ventricular wall, is higher than in the right ventricle. **A:** During systole and diastole the intramural pressure decreases from the subendocardial to the subepicardial parts of the ventricle. This has two consequences: (1) during systole the coronary flow is directed to the outer layers of the heart; and (2) during diastole the effective perfusion pressure (aortic pressure minus intramural pressure) is smaller in the subendocardial layers of the myocardium. **B:** Despite the lower systolic and diastolic perfusion pressure, the blood flow to the subendocardial parts of the heart is slightly more than that to the middle and subepicardial regions. This is because the subendocardial resistance to flow is lower owing to the structurally larger arterioles and the presence of more vasodilator metabolites because the innermost layers of the heart have to perform more work.

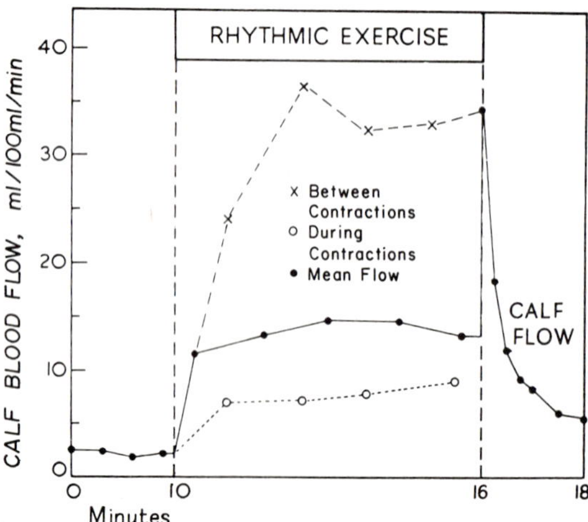

FIG. 4–7. During severe rhythmic exercise the blood flow to the active muscles is temporarily impeded during each contraction. (From Barcroft and Swan: *Sympathetic Control of Human Blood Vessels.* Edward Arnold, London, 1953.)

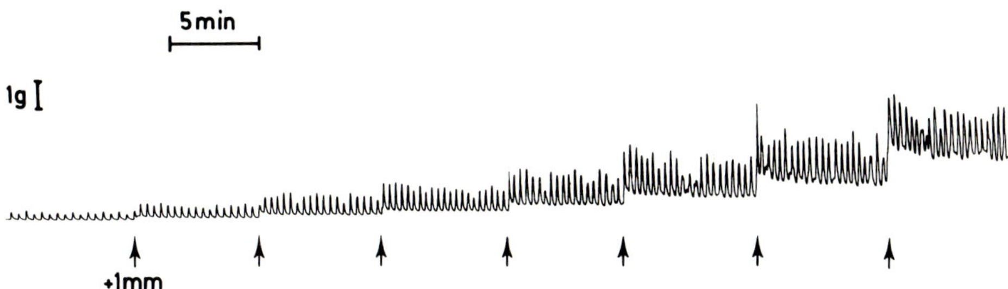

FIG. 4–8. Distention augments the myogenic activity in vascular smooth muscle as illustrated by the effect of stretch on rhythmicity and amplitude of spontaneous contractions in an isolated mesenteric vein. At each arrow the length of the preparation is increased by 1 mm; the experiment starts at zero tension. (From Shepherd and Vanhoutte: *Veins and Their Control.* Saunders, Philadelphia, 1975.)

Temperature

Heart

The increase in heart rate seen with fever is due in part to the direct effect of temperature on the sinus node, causing it to fire more frequently.

Blood Vessels

Cooling the blood below 37°C depresses myogenic activity of vascular smooth muscle cells and the responsiveness of deep blood vessels to vasoconstrictor stimuli. However, in cutaneous vessels the intracellular depressing effect of cooling is offset by a marked increase in sensitivity to norepinephrine and epinephrine (Chapter 5). When a cutaneous vessel is cooled from 37° to 25°C, its response to sympathetic nerve stimulation or circulating catecholamines is augmented (Fig. 4–9). This potentiating effect is due to an increased affinity of the cell membrane of the cutaneous vascular smooth muscle cells for the vasoconstrictor substances. If cutaneous vessels are warmed to 40°C, they become unresponsive to sympathetic nerve activation and circulating catecholamines; thus local warming disconnects these vessels from nervous control. The skin vessels are exposed to wide variations in temperature in normal life; for example, the temperature of the blood in cutaneous veins can be as low as 20° to 25°C. The constriction which results from such a decrease in temperature represents an immediate response of the organism to limit the loss of heat from the body when exposed to a cold environment and plays an important role in thermoregulation (p. 147). In animals chronically exposed to high environmental temperatures the cutaneous vessels constrict less vigorously when exposed to cold, suggesting that the ability to do so is an environmental adaptation. Conversely, certain subjects are abnormally sensitive to the local effect of cold on cutaneous vessels (Raynaud's disease; p. 218).

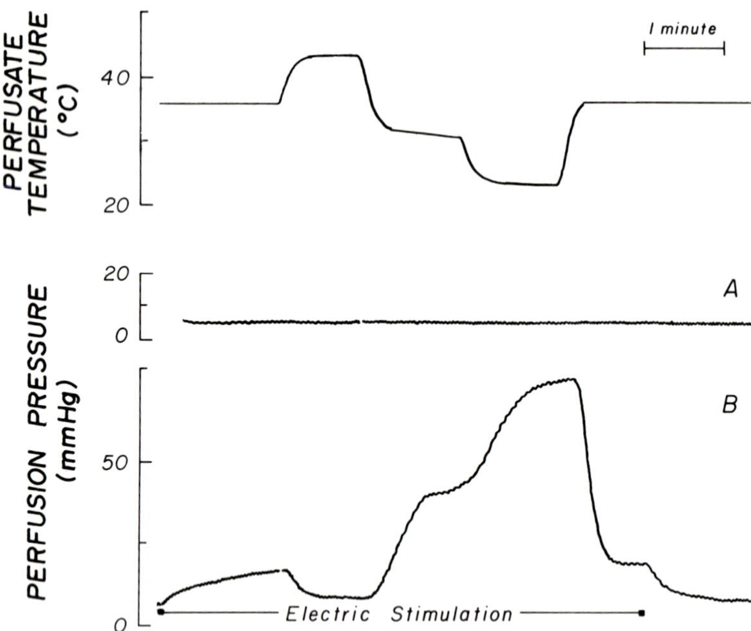

FIG. 4–9. In skin blood vessels local warming decreases and moderate cooling augments the response to sympathetic nerve stimulation, as illustrated for an isolated cutaneous vein. The vessel is perfused at constant flow, and an increase in perfusion pressure indicates a venoconstriction. When the temperature of the perfusate is altered between 20° and 42°C in the absence of stimulation, no changes in perfusion pressure are noted **(A).** When the sympathetic nerves to the vein are stimulated (electrical stimulation) **(B),** the preparation constricts slightly. Warming the perfusate abolishes the constriction, whereas decreasing the temperature greatly augments it. (From Vanhoutte and Shepherd: *Am. J. Physiol.,* 218:187, 1970.)

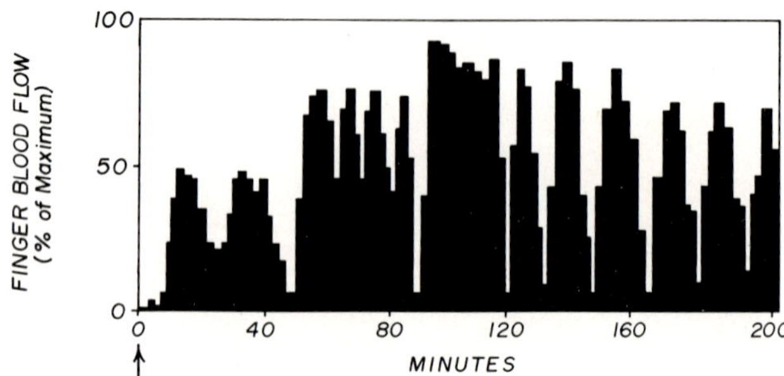

FIG. 4–10. Cold vasodilatation in the index finger during its immersion in water at 2°C. At the time of insertion into the cold water *(arrow),* the finger vessels constrict and the blood flow ceases. After 5 to 10 min the vessels dilate and the blood flow is restored (cold vasodilatation). This is followed by alternating periods of vasoconstriction and vasodilatation (hunting reaction). (From Greenfield et al.: *Irish J. Med. Sci.,* 309:415, 1951.)

If the temperature falls to about 5°C, all blood vessels, including cutaneous, dilate (cold vasodilatation). This is most pronounced when the body core is warm and only the peripheral parts are exposed to the cold. In these conditions the vasodilatation in the extremities helps maintain their function. For unknown reasons, the cold vasodilatation is interrupted periodically by abrupt and transient constrictions. This alternation of dilatation and constriction is referred to as the "hunting reaction" (Fig. 4–10). Cold vasodilatation is particularly pronounced in people accustomed to working in cold surroundings.

AUTOCOIDS

"Autocoids" refer to the vasoactive molecules which are present in certain cells or which can be formed in the tissues from cell constituents. Among the most important are histamine, 5-hydroxytryptamine, the kinins, and the prostaglandin-like substances.

Histamine

Most blood vessels contain histamine in mast cells and in nonmast cell stores. Its function is unknown. When tissues are injured, histamine is liberated. It relaxes arteriolar vascular muscle, increases capillary permeability by contracting the endothelial cells, and constricts the veins. These actions combine to cause abnormal exudation of fluid from the capillaries (p. 233) (Fig. 4–11).

In certain tissues, particularly skeletal muscle, the histamine-containing cells are quiescent, as long as the sympathetic nerves are active and liberate norepinephrine. When the sympathetic tone is withdrawn, they release histamine, resulting in vasodilatation, which complements that due to the decrease in vasoconstrictor nerve activity.

5-Hydroxytryptamine

5-Hydroxytryptamine (serotonin) is liberated from aggregating platelets during clotting; it plays an important role in the vasoconstriction following disruption of blood vessels and thus in the reduction of the blood loss (p. 23). Tissues such as brain and lung contain 5-hydroxytryptamine. In the former its release may be involved in certain vascular spasms (migraine; p. 220), and in the latter it contributes to the vascular changes seen during allergic reactions.

In the gastrointestinal wall 5-hydroxytryptamine can be released from enterochromaffin cells by mechanical compression, by acetylcholine released by the vagus nerve, or by gastrointestinal hormones such as gastrin. 5-Hydroxytryptamine dilates the arterioles, interrupts adrenergic neurotransmission, increases capillary permeability, and constricts the venules and veins (Fig. 4–12). These actions combine to make more fluid available to the exocrine glands of the gastrointestinal tract.

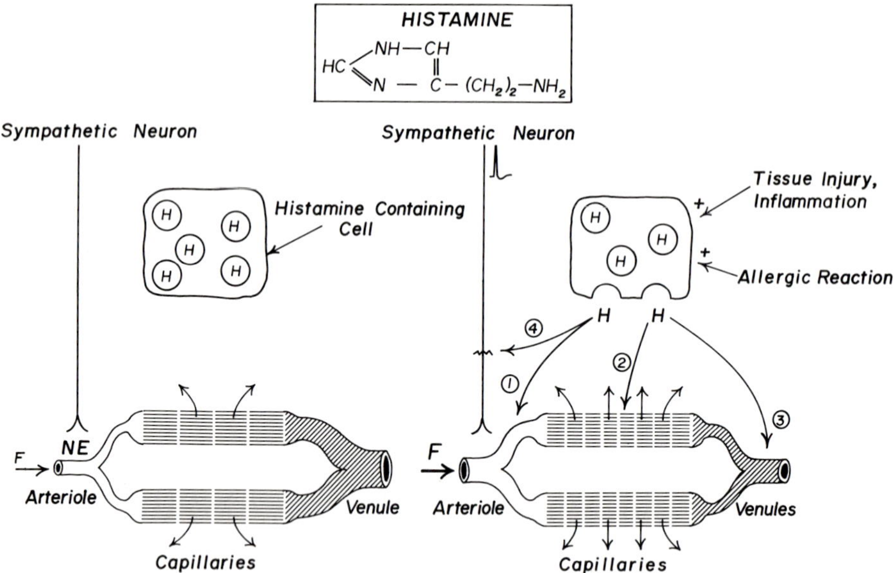

FIG. 4–11. Mechanisms of release and the vascular effects of histamine. There are cells in the blood vessel wall that contain histamine (H), which is released by injury, inflammation, and allergic reactions. This causes (1) dilatation of the arterioles; (2) increased capillary permeability; (3) constriction of the venules; and (4) inhibition of adrenergic neurotransmission (p. 113). The arteriolar dilatation results in an increase in blood flow (F). If this occurs in the skin, the affected area becomes red owing to the larger amounts of oxyhemoglobin passing through the subcutaneous microvessels. The increased capillary permeability and the increased capillary pressure, caused by arteriolar dilatation and the increased resistance offered by constricted venules, augment the exudation of fluid to the tissues, thereby causing local edema (p. 233). Because histamine inhibits adrenergic neurotransmission, the vasodilatation it causes is prolonged since it is unopposed by norepinephrine (NE) released from the sympathetic nerve endings.

Kinins

The body fluids contain a globulin, kininogen, which when acted on by the enzyme kallikrein is transformed into the decapeptide kallidin (lysin bradykinin). Kallikrein is formed in certain cells or in the plasma (Fig. 2–10). Kallidin is transformed into bradykinin by proteolytic enzymes (aminopeptidases) contained in plasma and tissues. Bradykinin in turn is metabolized into inactive peptides by carboxypeptidase (kininase I) or by the enzyme that converts angiotensin I into angiotensin II (converting enzyme or kininase II) (Fig. 4–13).

The kinins (kallidin and bradykinin) cause relaxation of arteriolar smooth muscle, increase capillary permeability, and constrict the veins. The local production of kallikrein (p. 146) by exocrine glands, and the resulting formation of kallidin and bradykinin contributes to the vasodilatation which permits the increased glandular secretion (Fig. 4–14).

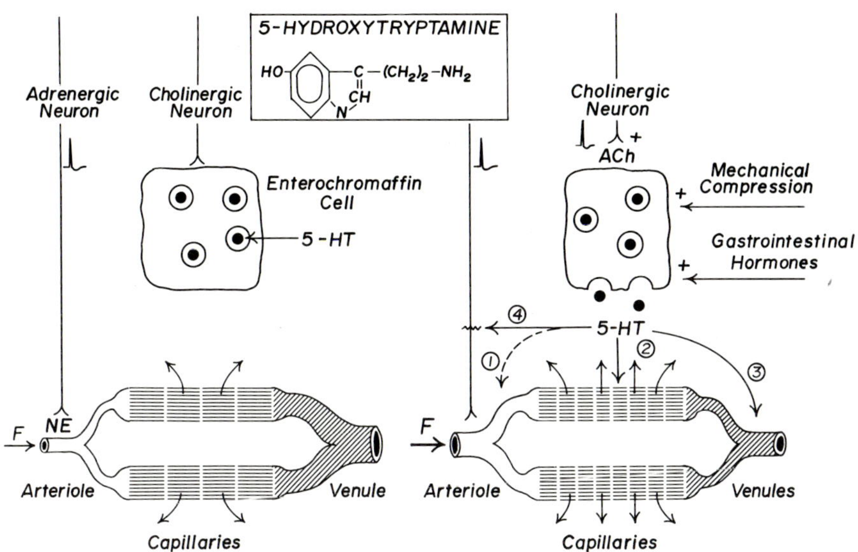

FIG. 4–12. Mechanisms of release and vascular effect of 5-hydroxytryptamine (5-HT) in the gastrointestinal wall. Mechanical compression by the contraction of the gastrointestinal muscle, or release evoked by vagal nerve activity or gastrointestinal hormones (e.g., gastrin), cause the enterochromaffin cells to discharge 5-hydroxytryptamine. The released 5-hydroxytryptamine: (1) dilates arterioles; (2) increases capillary permeability; (3) constricts venules; and (4) inhibits adrenergic neurotransmission. These effects combine to increase the blood flow (F) and the exudation of fluid to meet the metabolic requirements of the gastrointestinal wall and sustain the secretion of the gastrointestinal juices. ACh = acetylcholine. NE = norepinephrine.

Prostaglandins

The membranes of all cells contain the long-chain fatty acid arachidonic acid in their phospholipid fraction. This is synthesized from lineolic acid, an essential fatty acid present in food. Arachidonic acid can be enzymatically liberated from the phospholipids and transformed to labile endoperoxides, which in turn give raise to prostacyclin, prostaglandins (E_2, F_2, D_2), or thromboxane A_2 (Fig. 4–15): (1) *Prostacyclin:* Prostacyclin is a powerful inhibitor of platelet aggregation and causes vasodilatation in various vascular beds (Fig. 2–9). (2) *Prostaglandins:* The prostaglandins have been subgrouped depending on their solubility. In general, prostaglandins of the E-series are vasodilators and those of the F-series vasoconstrictors. Tissue injury releases arachidonic acid. This initiates the synthesis of prostaglandins, which contribute to the local vascular changes. The release of arachidonic acid can be blocked by glucocorticoids. In certain patients the excessive production of prostaglandins in the blood vessel wall inhibits the constriction caused by sympathetic nerve activity, circulating catecholamines, and angiotensin II (Bartter's syndrome). (3) *Thromboxane:* The

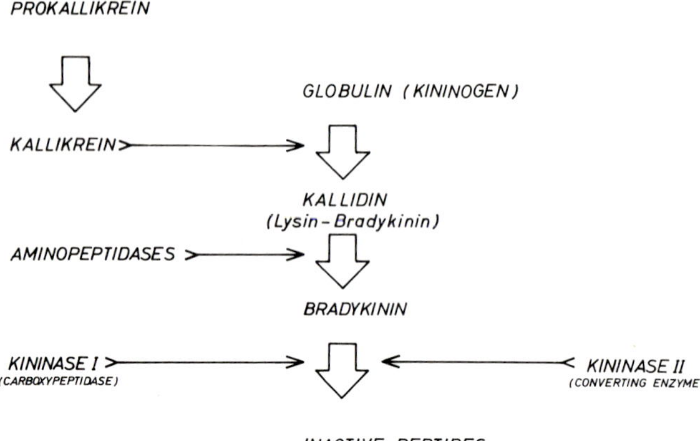

FIG. 4–13. Metabolic pathways leading to the formation and inactivation of kinins.

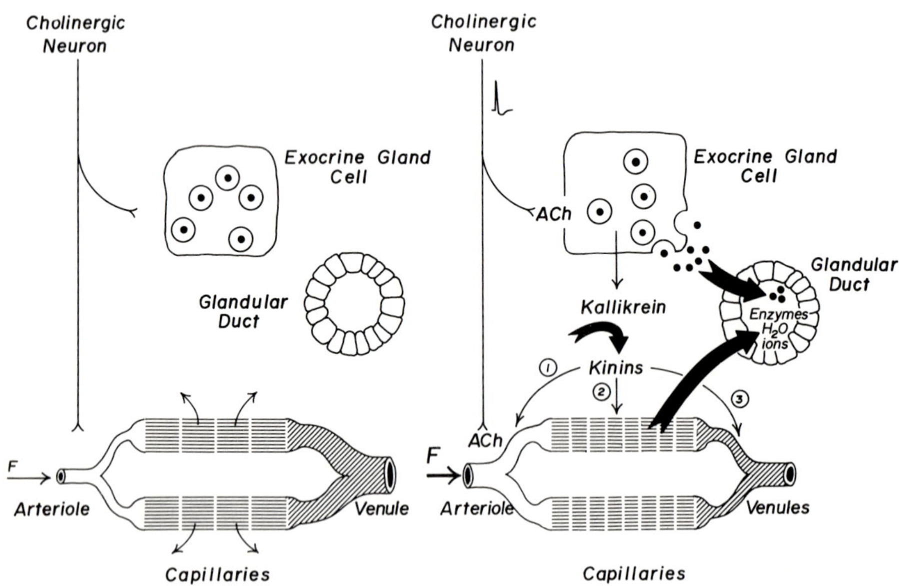

FIG. 4–14. Mechanisms of release and vascular effects of kinins in exocrine glands. When the cholinergic neurons which innervate exocrine glands (e.g., salivary glands, sweat glands) are activated, they release acetylcholine (ACh), which causes dilatation of the arterioles and stimulates the gland cells to secrete their enzymes. The gland cells also release kallikrein, initiating the formation of kinins, which: (1) dilate arterioles; (2) increase capillary permeability; and (3) constrict venules. These effects combine to augment blood flow (F) and to provide the exudation of fluid necessary to sustain the exocrine secretion.

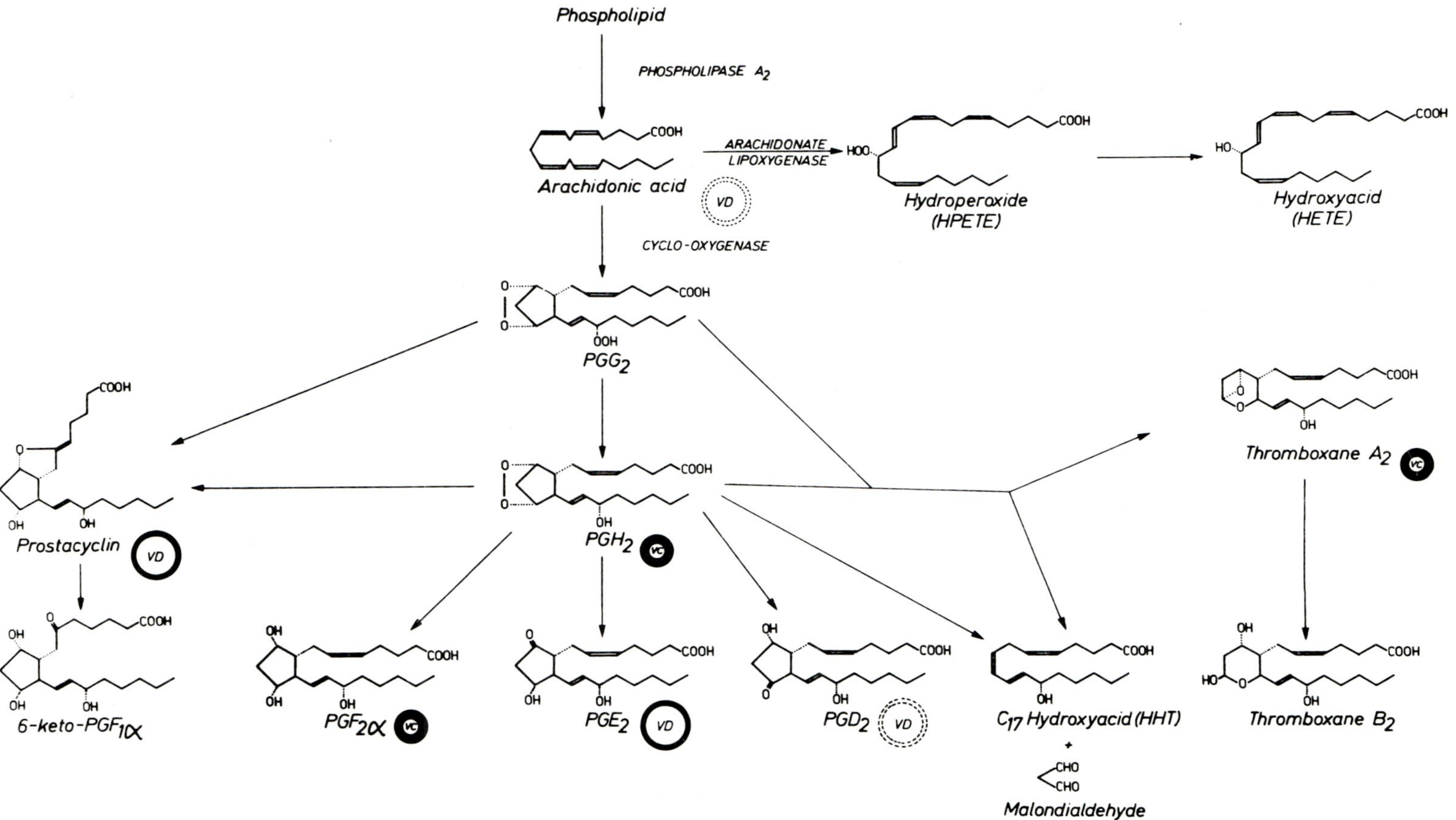

FIG. 4–15. Major metabolic pathways leading to the synthesis of prostaglandin-like substances. PG = prostaglandin. Circled symbols: causes vasodilatation (VD) and vasoconstriction (VC); dashed symbols: presumed to cause vasodilatation. (Courtesy of A. Herman.)

main effect of thromboxane is to induce platelet aggregation; in addition it causes vasoconstriction (Fig. 2–9).

SELECTED REFERENCES

Alexander, R. S. (1977): Critical closure re-examined. *Circ. Res.,* 40:531.

Belloni, F. L. (1979): The local control of coronary blood flow. *Cardiovasc. Res.,* 13:63.

Berne, R. M., and Rubio, R. (1978): Role of adenosine, adenosine triphosphate and inorganic phosphate in resistance vessel vasodilatation. In: *Mechanisms of Vasodilatation,* edited by P. Vanhoutte and I. Leusen, p. 214. Karger, Basel.

Brody, M. J. (1978): Histaminergic and cholinergic vasodilator systems. In: *Mechanisms of Vasodilatation,* edited by P. Vanhoutte and I. Leusen, p. 266. Karger, Basel.

Burton, A. C. (1962): Physical principles of circulatory phenomena: The physical equilibria of the heart and blood vessels. In: *Handbook of Physiology, Sect. 2: Circulation,* Vol. I, p. 85. American Physiological Society, Washington, D.C.

Duling, B. R. (1978): Oxygen, carbon dioxide, and hydrogen ion as local factors causing vasodilatation. In: *Mechanisms of Vasodilatation,* edited by P. Vanhoutte and I. Leusen, p. 193. Karger, Basel.

Gregg, D. E., and Fisher, L. C. (1963): Blood supply to the heart. In: *Handbook of Physiology,* Sect. II, Vol. 2, p. 1517. American Physiological Society, Washington, D.C.

Haddy, F. J., and Scott, J. B. (1968): Metabolically linked vasoactive chemicals in local regulation of blood flow. *Physiol. Rev.,* 48:688.

Johnson, P. C. (1977): The myogenic response and the microcirculation. *Microvasc. Res.,* 13:1.

McGiff, J. C., and Nasjletti, A. (1976): Kinins, renal function and blood pressure regulation. *Fed. Proc.,* 35:172.

McGrath, M. A., and Shepherd, J. T. (1978): Histamine and 5-hydroxytryptamine—inhibition of transmitter release mediated by H_2 and 5-hydroxytryptamine receptors. *Fed. Proc.,* 37:195.

Mellander, S., and Lundvall, J. (1978): Vasodilatation mediated by hyperosmolarity. In: *Mechanisms of Vasodilatation,* edited by P. Vanhoutte and I. Leusen, p. 206. Karger, Basel.

Moncada, S., and Vane, J. R. (1978): Prostacyclin (PGI_2), the vascular wall and vasodilatation. In: *Mechanisms of Vasodilatation,* edited by P. Vanhoutte and I. Leusen, p. 107. Karger, Basel.

Olsson, R. A. (1975): Myocardial reactive hyperemia. *Circ. Res.,* 37:263.

Richards, C. J., Mark, A. L., Van Orden, D. E., and Kaloyanides, G. J. (1978): Effects of indomethacin on the vascular abnormalities of Bartter's syndrome. *Circulation,* 58:544.

Verhaeghe, R. H., Lorenz, R. R., McGrath, M. A., Shepherd, J. T., and Vanhoutte, P. M. (1978): Metabolic modulation of neurotransmitter release—adenosine, adenine nucleotides, potassium, hyperosmolarity, and hydrogen ion. *Fed. Proc.,* 37:208.

5

Neurohumoral Regulation

To provide the necessary blood supply to active tissues, the local vasodilatation caused by metabolic demand must be combined with maintenance of an adequate perfusion pressure. This is accomplished by the central nervous system, which integrates information from various sensors within the cardiovascular system and modulates its components via the peripheral autonomic nerves and certain endocrine cells. The arterial pressure is determined by the product of cardiac output and total systemic vascular resistance. The central nervous system can maintain pressure in the face of an alteration in resistance in a given vascular bed by changing the resistance of other vascular regions in a compensatory direction and/or by changing cardiac output (Fig. 1–8). The adaptation of the cardiac output requires a concomitant adjustment of the capacity of the systemic veins.

FROM THE CENTERS TO THE PERIPHERY

Alterations in heart rate and contractility, and in the degree of contraction of the smooth muscle cells of the resistance and capacitance vessels, are governed by the activity of nerves connecting the central nervous system with the cardiovascular periphery. Two main types of nerve are involved: (1) the nerves which release norepinephrine at their endings and activate the cardiovascular system (adrenergic nerves); and (2) the nerves which release acetylcholine at their endings and inhibit the function of the heart and certain blood vessels (cholinergic nerves). Certain vasomotor nerves may liberate transmitters other than acetylcholine or norepinephrine. For example, purinergic nerves cause vasodilatation by liberating adenosine triphosphate or adenosine, but their role is unknown.

Adrenergic Nerves

Origin of Sympathetic Nerve Activity

The sympathetic outflow to the heart and the peripheral vessels originates in neurons located in the lateral parts of the reticular formation in the bulbar area of the brainstem (vasomotor center). The axons of these neurons form the bulbospinal tract and descend in the intermediolateral column to the preganglionic neurons of the spinal cord, located in the anterolateral columns. They consist of two types. Neurons which presumably release norepinephrine activate the preganglionic cells (adrenergic neurons). Neurons which presumably release 5-hydroxytryptamine inhibit them (serotoninergic neurons). Thus activation of the "adrenergic" neurons of the vasomotor center causes an increase in heart rate and cardiac contractility. This, combined with the constriction of the resistance vessels and the systemic veins, results in an increase in blood pressure (pressor response). Stimulation of the "serotoninergic" neurons causes changes in the opposite direction, with a resulting fall in blood pressure (depressor response). The interplay between the pressor and depressor neurons provides the major control of vasomotor tone by increasing or decreasing the number of impulses leaving the spinal cord through the final common pathway, the preganglionic adrenergic neuron. The central sympathetic outflow is ultimately conveyed to the heart and vessel wall by means of the cell bodies of the paravertebral ganglia and their postganglionic axons; the synaptic transmission between the preganglionic and the ganglionic neurons is cholinergic (Fig. 5–1).

Distribution of Sympathetic Nerves

Postganglionic sympathetic nerves run to the heart where they impinge on the sinus and atrioventricular nodes, and innervate the atria and ventricular myocardium. Heart rate and myocardial contractility are controlled by the sympathetic nervous system and increase when it is activated. Blood vessels, except umbilical and placental, are innervated by sympathetic nerves (Fig. 5–2). The density of innervation varies widely and is a reflection of the degree of participation of the individual vessels in centrally controlled responses. The resistance vessels, splanchnic veins, and cutaneous veins are densely innervated, and when

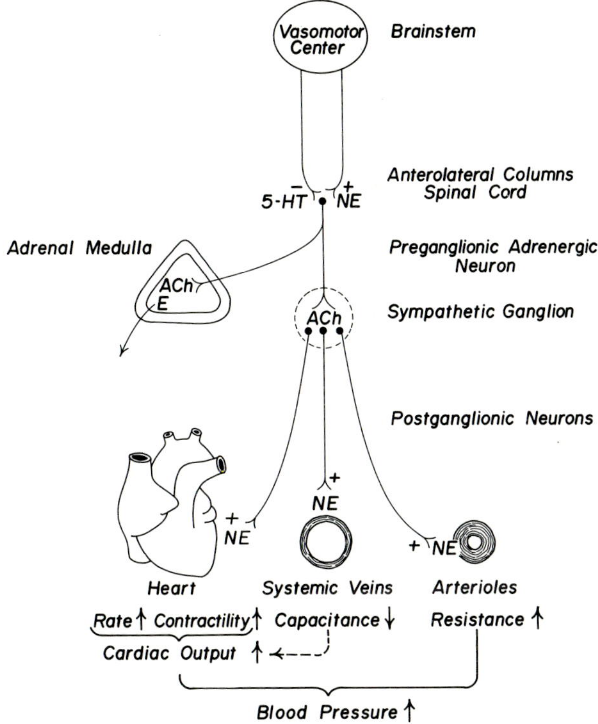

FIG. 5–1. Interaction of the pressor neurons [which presumably release 5–hydroxytryptamine (5–HT)] and depressor neurons which presumably release norepinephrine (NE) in the vasomotor center of the brainstem regulating the sympathetic outflow to the cardiovascular system. The preganglionic neurons liberate acetylcholine (ACh) at their endings in the sympathetic ganglia and the adrenal medulla. This leads to activation of the postganglionic neurons which control the response of the heart, resistance blood vessels (arterioles), and capacitance vessels (veins) by the amount of norepinephrine they liberate. In the adrenal medulla, acetylcholine causes release of catecholamines, mainly epinephrine (E), into the blood.

the sympathetic nerves to these vessels are stimulated strong constrictions occur. By contrast there is little response to sympathetic stimulation of the coronary arteries, the vessels of the brain, the large conduit vessels, the veins draining skeletal muscle, and the lung vessels. This is appropriate because: (1) The muscle of the heart is continuously active; it cannot sustain an oxygen debt; and its supply of blood in normal conditions is governed by local metabolic factors. (2) The function of the brain depends on a continuous supply of oxygen, and therefore the brain vessels are controlled by the metabolic needs of the surrounding cells. The choroid plexuses of the cerebral ventricles are highly vascularized and constitute the major site for the production of cerebrospinal fluid. Their blood vessels are richly endowed with sympathetic nerves, the stimulation of which reduces the rate of formation of cerebrospinal fluid. (3) Reducing the caliber of the distributing vessels would impair flow throughout the body. (4)

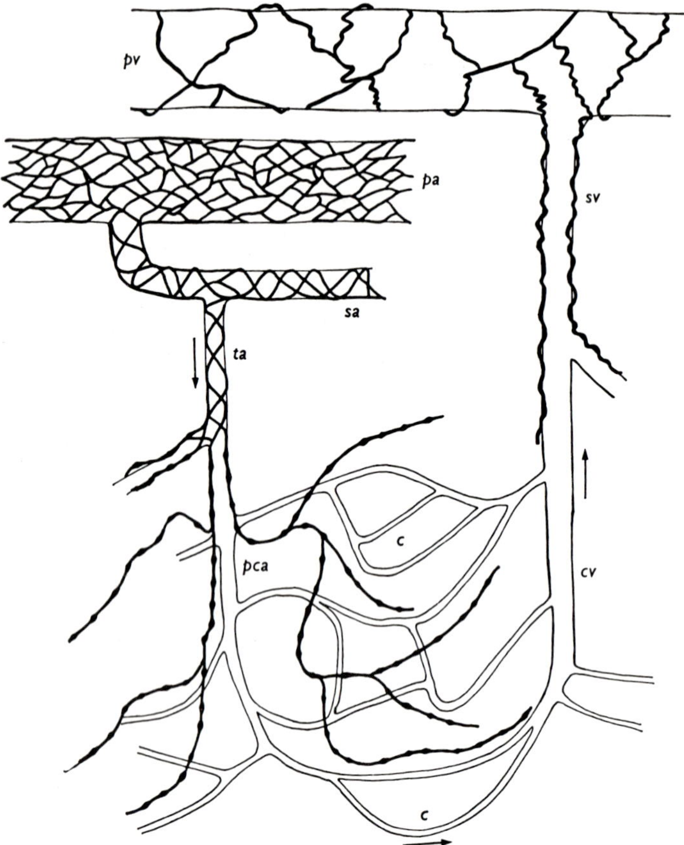

FIG. 5–2. Relationship between adrenergic nerves and the mesenteric blood vessels. pa = principal artery. pv = principal vein. sa = small artery of the microvasculature. ta = terminal arteriole. pca = precapillary arteriole. c = capillary. cv = collecting venule. sv = small vein. The adrenergic nerves are represented by the heavy lines. Arrows indicate the direction of blood flow. Note that the precapillary arterioles and the collecting venules are not innervated. [From Furness and Marshall: *J. Physiol. (Lond)*, 239:75, 1974.]

Constriction of the veins draining skeletal muscle, which form 40% of the body mass, would cause excessive transudation of fluid at the capillary level (p. 235). (5) The lung vessels are low-resistance channels designed to distribute blood evenly to the alveolar air, and it would be detrimental to decrease pulmonary capillary perfusion by constricting the pulmonary arterioles or to cause pulmonary congestion by constricting the postcapillary vessels.

The postganglionic sympathetic nerve endings form a network of unmyelinated slender processes (about 0.1 micron in diameter) which widen at regular intervals into varicosities (about 1 micron in diameter). The varicosities, which are denuded of Schwann cells, contain small granular vesicles (40 to 60 nm in diameter) in which the transmitter is stored. The varicosities are in close apposition to the myocardial and smooth muscle cells they innervate. In the heart they terminate in a depression of the sarcolemma; in the blood vessels there is a minimal distance of 80 to 100 nm (junctional cleft) between the varicosities and the smooth muscle. In most arteries the nerves do not penetrate beyond the adventitial–medial border; in veins the nerve endings usually penetrate into the media (Figs. 2–21 and 5–3).

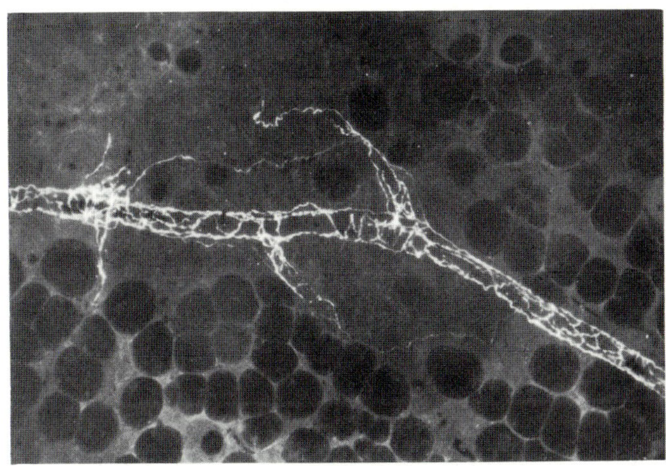

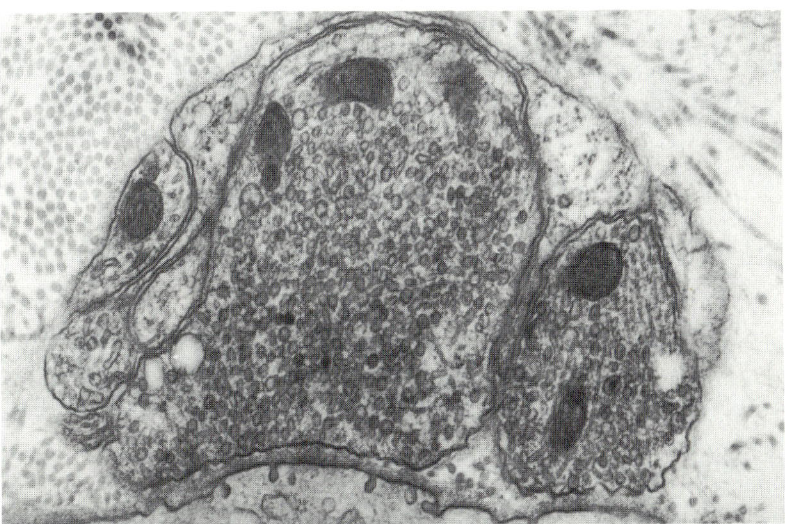

FIG. 5–3. Top: Dense network of fluorescent nerves around an arteriole, as demonstrated by a catecholamine-specific fluorescence technique (glyoxylic acid-induced fluorescence). The arrows indicate the presence of collateral nerves. ×90. (From Waris and Partanen: *Histochemistry,* 41:369, 1975.) **Bottom:** Relationship of adrenergic nerve endings (A) and smooth muscle cells (M) in the arterial wall. The nerve cells are devoid of Schwann cytoplasm (S) on the side facing the muscle and approach the muscle surface as closely as 80 nm. There are many synaptic vesicles and mitochondria in terminal varicosities. [From Burnstock et al.: *Circ. Res. (Suppl 2),* 27:5, 1970, by permission of The American Heart Association.]

Adrenergic Neuroeffector Interaction

The neuroeffector junction is the last relay station for the controlling impulses that originate in the central nervous system and thus is a vital link in the genesis of cardiovascular responses.

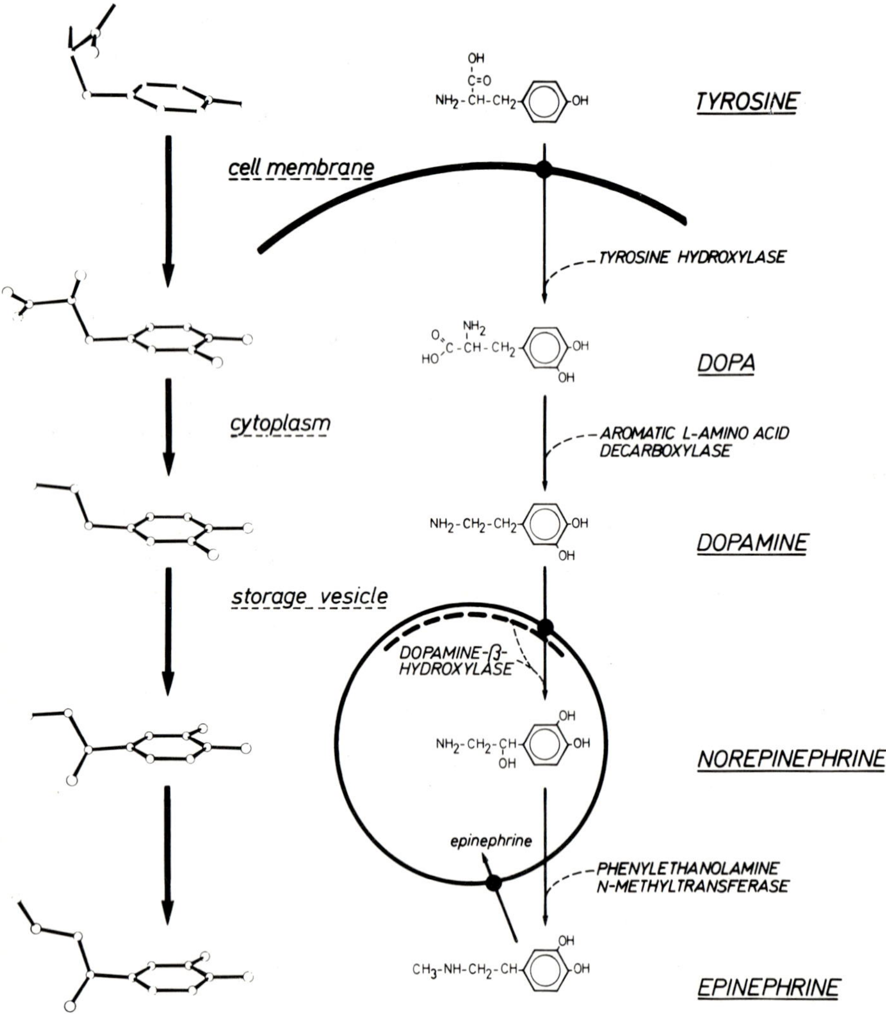

FIG. 5–4. Biosynthesis of norepinephrine and epinephrine from tyrosine in adrenergic nerve endings and the medulla of the adrenal gland. **Left:** Perspective drawings of the structure of tyrosine, DOPA, dopamine, norepinephrine, and epinephrine derived from X-ray crystallographic data; for the sake of clarity hydrogen atoms are omitted. (Modified from Tollenaere et al.: *Atlas of the Three-Dimensional Structure of Drugs.* Elsevier North-Holland, Amsterdam, 1979). **Right:** Enzymatic processes involved.

The adrenergic nerve endings take up tyrosine from the extracellular fluid and transform it in the neuroplasm to dopamine by successive enzymatic reactions. The dopamine is then taken up by the storage vesicles that are formed in the cell body and descend to the periphery with the axonal flow. In the storage vesicles dopamine is converted to norepinephrine by the enzyme dopamine-β-hydroxylase (Fig. 5–4).

The release of norepinephrine is initiated by the action potentials generated in the ganglionic cell body. The action potentials are caused by the penetration of Na^+ together with Ca^{2+} into the neuroplasm. As a consequence of the increased intraneuronal Ca^{2+} concentration, the vesicles migrate toward and fuse with the neuronal cell membrane, and empty their content of norepinephrine and dopamine-β-hydroxylase into the junctional cleft (exocytotic release) (Fig. 5–5).

The neuronal membrane senses the concentration of norepinephrine in the junctional cleft because a fraction of the neurotransmitter activates receptors on the nerve endings (presynaptic or prejunctional alpha-adrenergic receptors; p. 203), which exert a negative feedback on the exocytotic process. The alpha-adrenergic prejunctional feedback inhibition of norepinephrine release can also be initiated by exogenous or circulating catecholamines; it prevents excessive liberation of the adrenergic transmitter (Fig. 5–6).

Given a constant activity of the sympathetic neuron, the amount of norepinephrine released can be either augmented or decreased by substances which bind on the neuronal membrane (Fig. 5–6). The most important facilitatory modulator of adrenergic neurotransmission is angiotensin II. Among the inhibitory modulators are acetylcholine (p. 128), the products of cellular metabolism (Fig. 4–2), and autocoids such as histamine (Fig. 4–11), 5-hydroxytryptamine (Fig. 4–12), and prostaglandins of the E series.

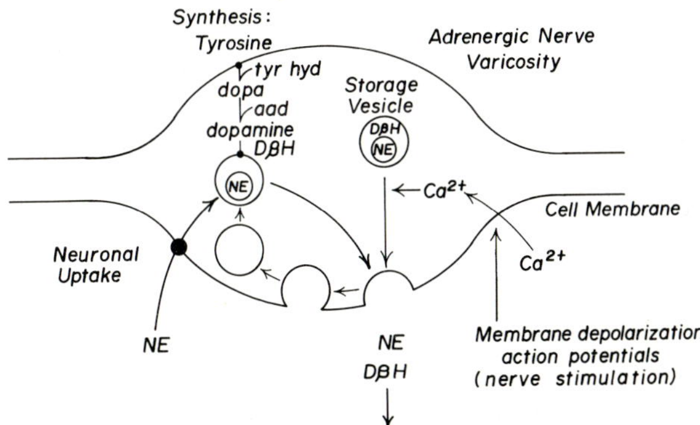

FIG. 5–5. Synthesis and exocytotic release of norepinephrine and recycling of the storage vesicles at the sympathetic (adrenergic) nerve varicosities. NE = norepinephrine. tyr hyd = tyrosine hydroxylase. aad = aromatic L-amino decarboxylase. DβH = dopamine-β-hydroxylase. ● = active carrier. (Modified from Vanhoutte: *Fed. Proc.,* 32:181, 1978.)

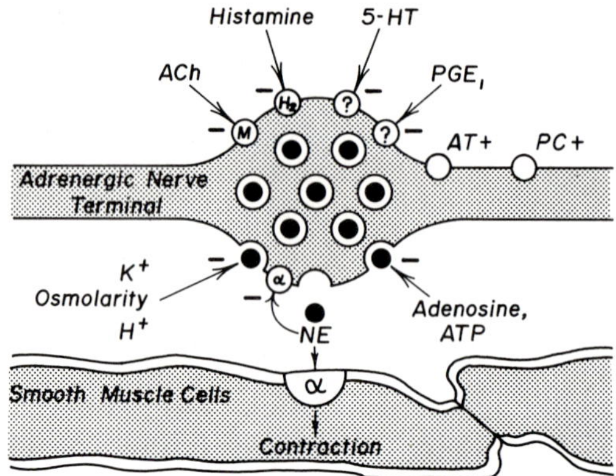

FIG. 5–6. Various excitatory (+) and inhibitory (−) influences on adrenergic neurotransmission. NE = norepinephrine. M = muscarinic. ACh = acetylcholine. AT = angiotensin II. PC = prostacyclin. PGE_1 = prostaglandin E_1. 5-HT = 5-hydroxytryptamine. H_2 = histamine$_2$ receptor. ? = unknown mechanism. α = alpha-adrenergic receptor. (Modified from McGrath and Vanhoutte: In: *Mechanisms of Vasodilatation,* edited by Vanhoutte and Leusen, p. 248. Karger, Basel, 1978.

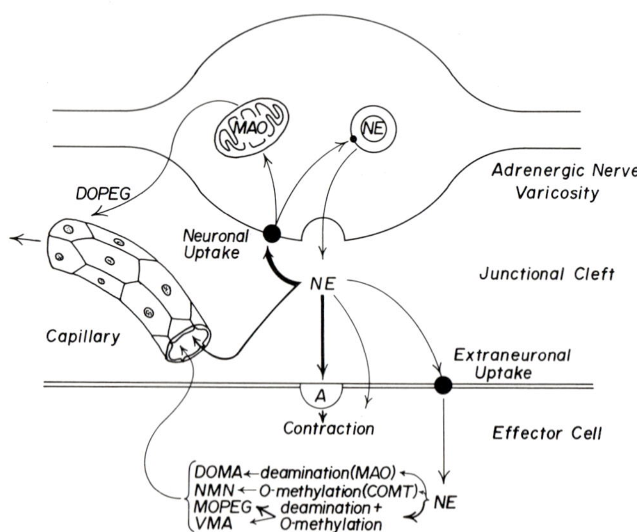

FIG. 5–7. Norepinephrine (NE) released from the adrenergic nerve varicosity enters the junctional cleft and activates the adrenergic receptors (A) on the effector cells. It is removed by (1) uptake in the nerve endings where part of it is enzymatically degraded by the intraneuronal monoamine oxidase (MAO) to 3,4-dihydroxyphenylglycol (DOPEG), but most is recycled to the storage vesicles; (2) diffusion to the capillaries; and (3) uptake by the effector cells and enzymatic degradation by the enzymes monoamine oxidase and catechol-O-methyltransferase (COMT) to 3,4-dihydroxymandelic acid (DOMA), normetanephrine (NMN), 3-methoxy-4-dihydroxyphenylglycol (MOPEG), and 3-methoxy,4-hydroxymandelic acid (VMA). The metabolites of norepinephrine are inactive and diffuse to the extracellular fluid and the capillaries. ● = active carrier.

The exocytotic emptying of the vesicles creates a concentration difference of norepinephrine between the nerve terminal and the muscle cells. This is the driving force for neurotransmitter diffusion and thus for activation of the innervated cells. With an increase in the frequency of the action potentials, more nerve varicosities are recruited and more norepinephrine is released. The distance over which norepinephrine diffuses and thus its potential to activate successive muscle cells depends mainly on the width of the junctional cleft. Not all vascular smooth muscle cells need to be directly activated by the released norepinephrine; the neurogenic signal can be propagated from "innervated" pacemaker cells to "noninnervated" cells through cell-to-cell conduction (Fig. 5–7).

When norepinephrine reaches the muscle cells it binds to lipoprotein sites on the cell membrane, which initiate their response (p. 181). The norepinephrine is removed from the junctional cleft by: (1) uptake by the neuronal cell membrane via an active carrier process linked to Na^+,K^+-ATPase; (2) seepage into the

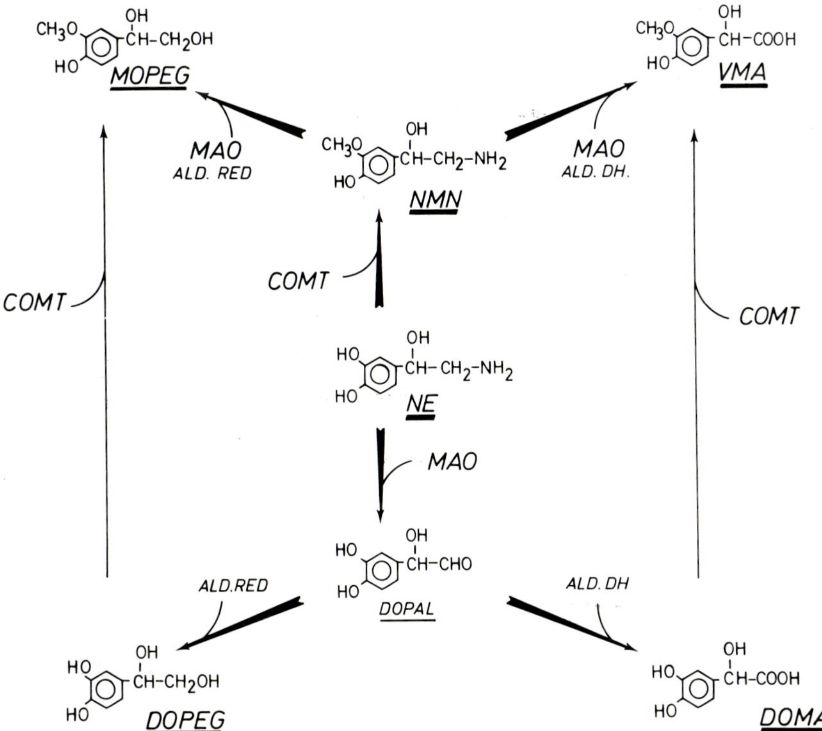

FIG. 5–8. Pathways of norepinephrine metabolism. NE = norepinephrine. MOPEG — 3 methoxy-4-hydroxyphenylglycol. DOPEG = 3,4-dihydroxyphenylglycol. VMA= 3-methoxy-4-hydroxymandelic acid. DOMA = 3,4-dihydroxymandelic acid. NMN = normetanephrine. MAO = monoamine oxidase. COMT = catechol-O-methyltransferase. DOPAL = 3,4-dihydroxyphenylglycolic aldehyde. ALD. DH = aldehyde dehydrogenase. ALD. RED = aldehyde reductase.

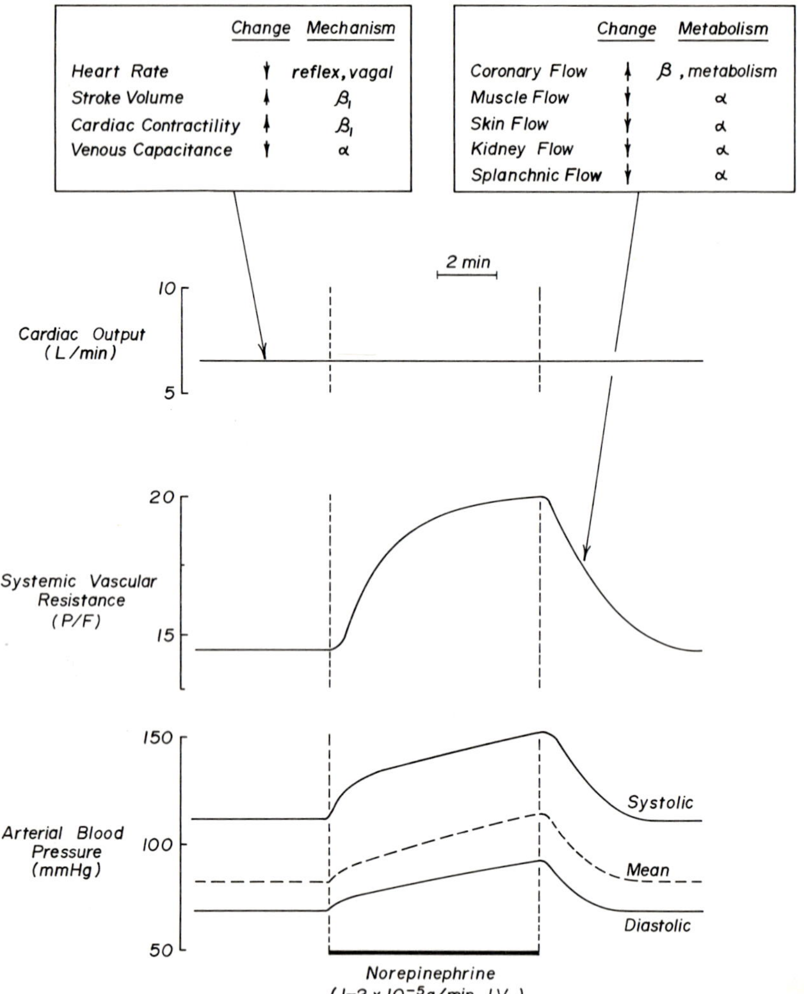

FIG. 5–9. Effects of intravenous infusion of norepinephrine on the human cardiovascular system. With the exception of the heart and brain, the blood flow to all systemic vascular beds is reduced because of activation of alpha-adrenergic receptors (α) on the resistance vessels. As a result of the increase in total systemic vascular resistance the systemic arterial systolic and diastolic pressures are elevated. The heart is reflexly slowed by increased vagal activity caused by the action of the increased pressure on the arterial baroreceptors (p. 131). Thus the cardiac output is unchanged in spite of the activation of beta$_1$-adrenergic receptors (β_1) and the resultant increased contractility of the myocardium. The increased coronary flow results from the products of increased myocardial (possibly beta) metabolism and the additional activation of the beta receptors (possibly beta$_1$) in the coronary vessels (p. 187). The constriction of the systemic veins via alpha-adrenergic receptors augments the filling pressure of the heart, and this contributes to the increase in stroke volume. F = flow, P = pressure.

capillaries; and (3) enzymatic destruction by the enzymes monoamine oxidase and catechol-O-methyltransferase after the transmitter has been taken up by either the nerve endings (neuronal uptake) or the effector cells (extraneuronal uptake) (Figs. 5–7 and 5–8).

Depending on the tissue, the binding of norepinephrine with the lipoprotein complex of the cell membrane (receptor) has different pharmacological characteristics. The adrenergic receptors have been divided into alpha- and beta-receptors (p. 184). In the heart the released norepinephrine binds mainly to beta-adrenergic receptors, causing an increase in heart rate, speed of conduction, and contractility; as a consequence, the cardiac output increases. In the blood vessels the norepinephrine released from the adrenergic terminals binds to alpha-adrenergic receptors, causing an increase in the permeability of Ca^{2+} in the cell membrane and the sarcoplasmic reticulum. This change in Ca^{2+} permeability initiates contraction of the smooth muscle cells, increasing arteriolar resistance and causing active mobilization of blood from the veins (Fig. 5–9).

Endocrine Cells Associated With the Adrenergic Nerves

Adrenal Glands

Certain preganglionic sympathetic fibers do not form synapses in the paravertebral ganglia but continue to the central part (medulla) of the adrenals, the endocrine glands situated on the upper pole of the kidneys (Fig. 5–1). They are essentially large sympathetic ganglia whose cells have lost their axons and have become specialized for the secretion of products directly into the bloodstream.

The major biochemical difference between the adrenal medullary cells and the sympathetic neurons is that in the former most of the norepinephrine synthesized is transformed to epinephrine by the addition of a methyl group; this reaction occurs in the neuroplasm and is catalyzed by the enzyme phenylethanolamine-N-methyltransferase (Fig. 5–4). This addition in the synthesis pathway occurs after birth, since the fetal adrenal medulla contains only norepinephrine. The mechanisms of storage and release of the adrenergic hormones obey the same rules as those outlined for the adrenergic nerve terminals. The secretion process is initiated by the release of acetylcholine from preganglionic sympathetic nerve fibers. The acetylcholine causes depolarization of the adrenal medullary cell, with an increased influx of Ca^{2+}. The increased cytoplasmic Ca^{2+} concentration then triggers the secretory process. The adrenal medulla contains about four times more epinephrine than norepinephrine.

The epinephrine released into the bloodstream has the following actions (Fig. 5–10): (1) An increase in the rate and the force of contraction of the heart by stimulating the beta-receptors, which are also activated by norepinephrine ($beta_1$-adrenergic receptor; p. 185). (2) A constriction of most systemic resistance vessels by stimulating the alpha-adrenergic receptors, which are also activated by norepi-

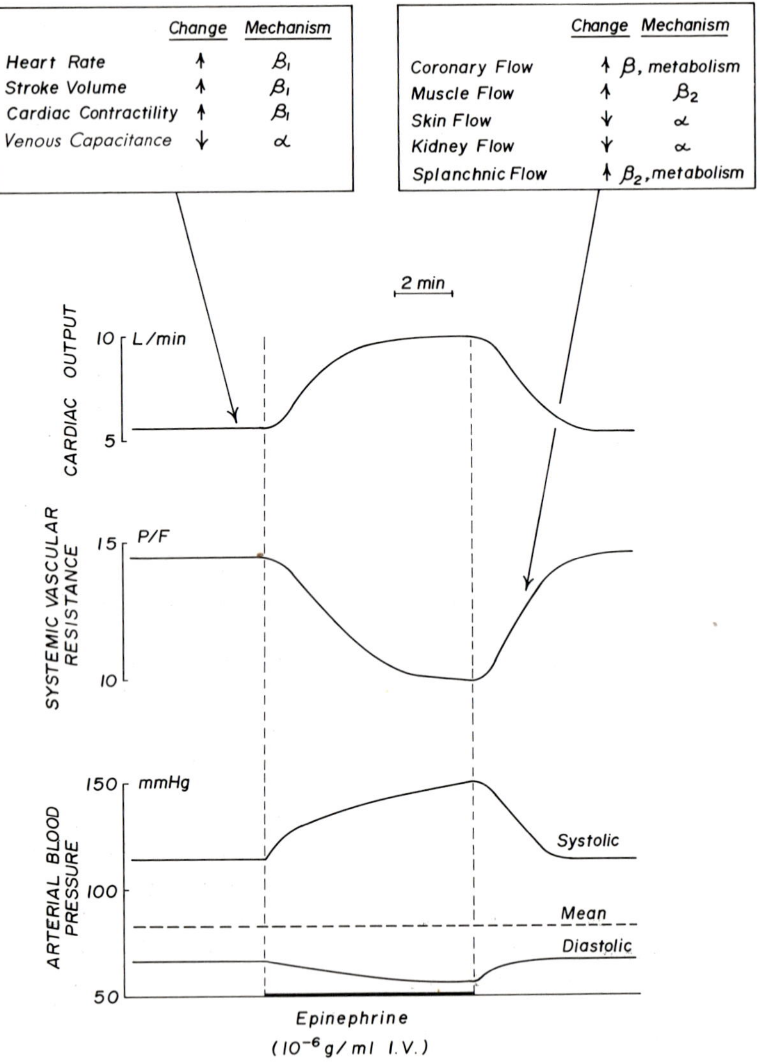

FIG. 5–10. Effects of intravenous infusion of epinephrine on the human cardiovascular system. The blood flow to the heart, brain, skeletal muscles, and splanchnic bed is increased, whereas that to skin and kidney is decreased. The total systemic vascular resistance is decreased, which is reflected in the decrease in arterial diastolic blood pressure. Cardiac output is increased owing to an increase in rate and stroke volume. This is reflected in the increase in systolic blood pressure. The constriction of the veins increases the cardiac filling pressure and, together with the increased contractility, causes the increased stroke volume. The difference between the cardiovascular effects of intravenous epinephrine and norepinephrine (Fig. 5–9) is that epinephrine, in addition to activating alpha- and beta$_1$-adrenergic receptors, also activates the beta$_2$-adrenergic receptors in the splanchnic and muscle resistance vessels, causing them to dilate.

nephrine. (3) Coronary vasodilatation mediated by beta-adrenergic receptors (p. 187). (4) Dilatation of the resistance vessels of skeletal muscle and liver due to activation of beta$_2$-receptors, which are not sensitive to norepinephrine (p. 187); in these vessels, the beta$_2$-adrenergic receptors dominate over the alpha-adrenergic receptors. (5) Constriction of the capacitance by stimulating alpha-adrenergic receptors. (6) An increase in the metabolism of the body cells brought about by an activation of glycogenolysis in liver and skeletal muscle and of lipolysis in fat cells, with a resultant increase in blood glucose and free fatty acids; the metabolic effects involve adenyl cyclase and the production of cAMP (p. 48).

The difference between circulating norepinephrine and epinephrine can be illustrated best by comparing in the normal adult the consequences of the infusion of the two catecholamines. With intravenous infusion of norepinephrine the total systemic vascular resistance is increased since all vessels, except cerebral and coronary, constrict. By contrast, infusion of epinephrine causes dilatation of blood vessels in skeletal muscle, the splanchnic area, the brain, and the heart; the resulting decrease in total systemic vascular resistance is not compensated for by constriction of the skin and kidney vessels. With both catecholamines constriction of the capacitance vessels increases the filling pressure of the heart and hence augments the stroke volume.

In normal circumstances the output of the adrenal medulla is relatively small and fluctuates during daily activities. As a rule release of adrenal catecholamines accompanies any increase in sympathetic activity and occurs particularly during mental stress, exercise, and hypoglycemia. This secretion sustains the action of the sympathetic nerves.

The epinephrine present in the blood originates from the adrenal medulla. By contrast, most of the plasma norepinephrine is due to overflow from the sympathetic nerve endings. The epinephrine is enzymatically destroyed by the liver; an important part of the norepinephrine is removed by uptake in the nerve endings of the large veins or by the pulmonary endothelium (p. 22). The catecholamines, when present in normal concentrations, do not permeate the cerebral endothelium (blood–brain barrier). The end-products of catecholamine metabolism leave the body through the kidney.

Juxtaglomerular Apparatus

The endothelium of the terminal part of the arterioles bringing blood to the glomeruli of the kidney (afferent arterioles) consists of cuboidal cells. These juxtaglomerular cells are characterized by secretory granules containing the proteolytic enzyme renin. Upon stimulation they release renin into the bloodstream (Fig. 5–11). Such stimulation can be effected by: (1) decreases in distending pressure in the afferent arterioles; (2) decreases in the amount of sodium reaching the cells of the distal tubules of the nephrons adjacent to the juxtaglomerular cells (macula densa); and/or (3) increased activity in the renal sympathetic nerves (Fig. 5–12). The cellular mechanism whereby the changes in trans-

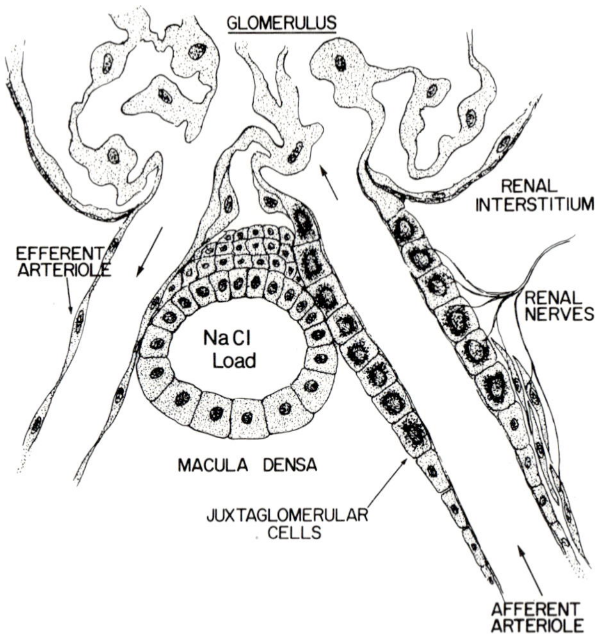

FIG. 5–11. Morphology of the juxtaglomular apparatus of the kidney. The juxtaglomerular cells of the afferent renal arteriole contain renin granules. When activated, these cells secrete renin into the circulation. (Courtesy of Dr. J. O. Davis.)

mural pressure, sodium delivery, or sympathetic activity cause changes in renin release is not known. It may involve the formation of prostaglandin-like substances. In the case of the sympathetic nerves the terminal step in the release process involves a beta-adrenergic receptor (p. 188).

The renin in the bloodstream initiates the formation of angiotensin I and II (Fig. 5–12). This occurs mainly in the lungs and peripheral blood vessels (p. 21); the components required to form angiotensin II are present in the brain, but their role is not certain. Angiotensin II has the following cardiovascular effects: (1) augmentation of the myogenic activity of the resistance vessels causing their contraction; (2) enhancement of the response of these resistance vessels to circulating and liberated norepinephrine; (3) facilitation throughout the cardiovascular system of the adrenergic neuroeffector interaction by accelerating the synthesis of norepinephrine, increasing its release by nerve impulses, and delaying its disappearance from the junctional cleft by inhibiting its uptake by nerve endings; (4) potentiation of ganglionic transmission and hence of the release of catecholamines from sympathetic nerves and the adrenal medulla; and (5) stimulation of the blood–brain barrier to stimulate neurons in discrete regions of the brain (paraventricular nuclei). The latter neurons in turn activate the cardiovascular centers to increase the sympathetic traffic to the heart and blood vessels (Fig. 5–13). The last three effects combine to increase the amount

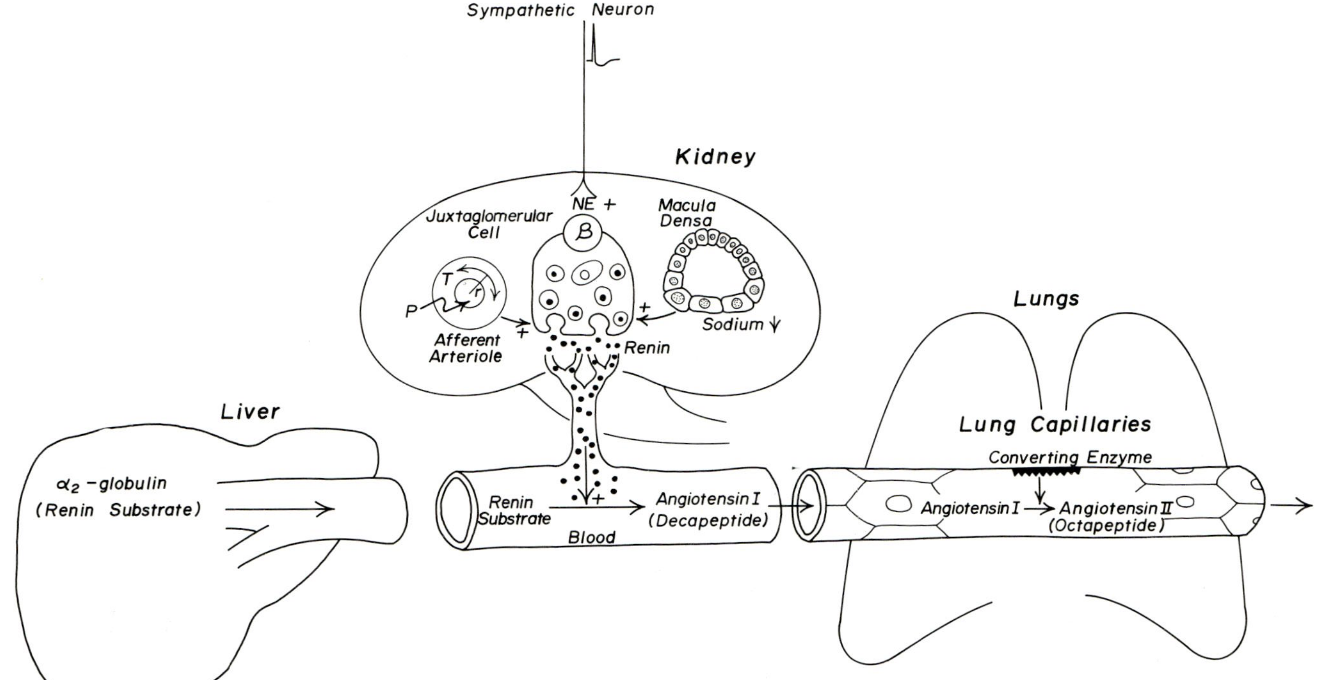

FIG. 5–12. Mechanisms of renin release from the kidney and formation of angiotensin I and II. The juxtaglomerular cells release renin from their secretory granules when stimulated by a decrease in wall tension in the afferent arteriole, an activation of their beta-adrenergic receptors, or a decrease in the amount of sodium reaching the macula densa. The proteolytic enzyme renin converts an α-globulin formed in the liver to the decapeptide angiotensin I. Converting enzyme, present mainly in the lung capillaries, converts angiotensin I to the vasoactive octapeptide angiotensin II. T = wall tension. P = transmural pressure. r = radius. β = beta-adrenergic receptor.

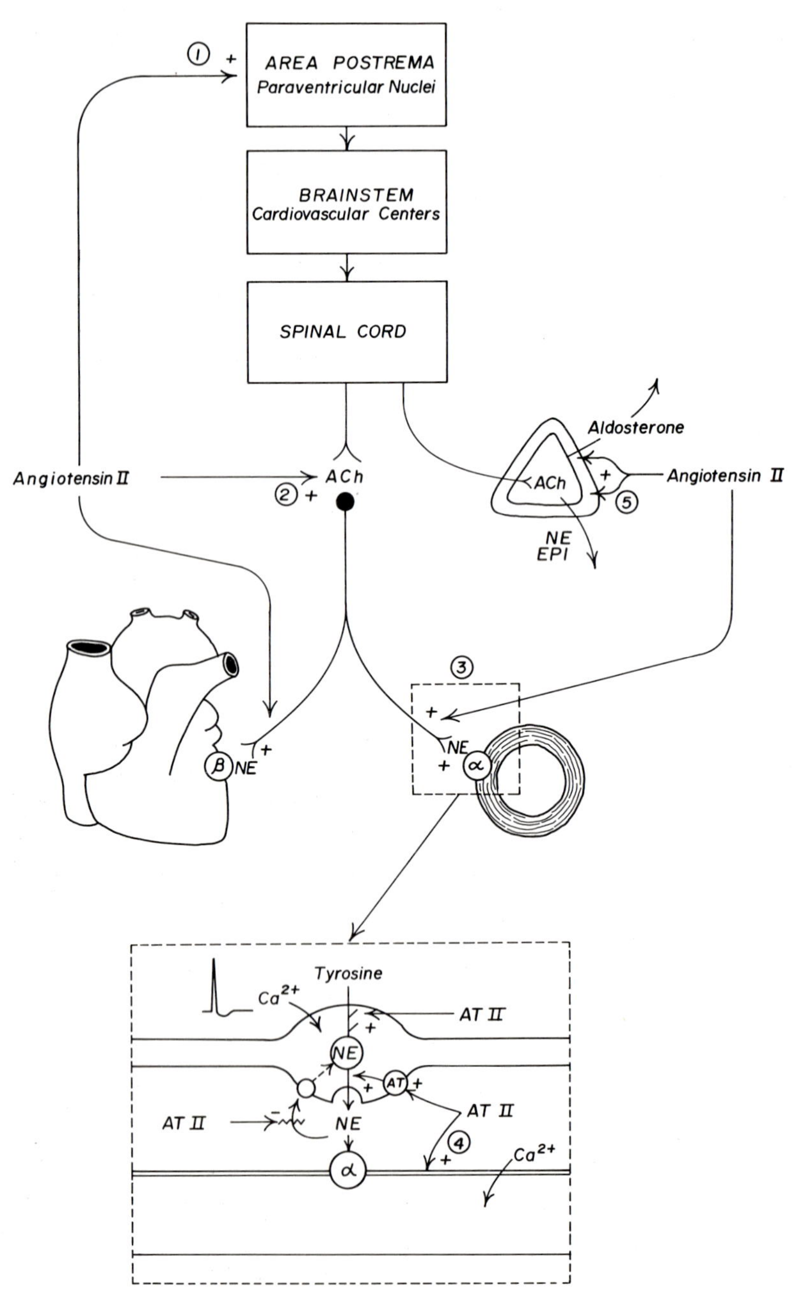

AREA POSTREMA
Paraventricular Nuclei
BRAINSTEM
Cardiovascular Centers
SPINAL CORD
Aldosterone
Angiotensin II
ACh
Angiotensin II
ACh
NE
EPI
NE
NE
Tyrosine
Ca2+
AT II
NE
AT
AT II
AT II
NE
Ca2+

of norepinephrine available for the effector cells; these actions occur with relatively low concentrations of angiotensin II and may be more important physiologically than the direct effects it exerts on the vascular smooth muscle cells. The net effect of injection, or of endogenous production, of angiotensin II is to cause a marked increase in arterial blood pressure. In addition to its cardiovascular effects, it accelerates the formation of the mineralocorticoid hormone aldosterone by the outer part of the adrenal gland (adrenal cortex). This hormone increases the reabsorption of sodium by the renal tubules in exchange for potassium.

Thus angiotensin II, which in many instances is formed as a consequence of increased sympathetic activity, exerts a positive feedback on sympathetic control. The renin–angiotensin–aldosterone system plays an important role in blood pressure regulation, not only through its direct effects on the cardiovascular system but also indirectly by helping to determine the extracellular volume via regulation of the sodium–potassium balance (p. 212).

Cholinergic Nerves

There are two sites of origin (cranial and sacral) for parasympathetic nerves supplying the cardiovascular system. Other nerve fibers release acetylcholine at their terminals and can travel with the sympathetic nerves (Fig. 5–14).

Origin and Distribution

The cholinergic outflow to the heart arises from the vagal nucleus in the medulla oblongata. The neurons of this area (cardioinhibitory center) have no inherent tone, and their activity is determined by the input from the peripheral sensors. The axons (preganglionic fibers) of the cardioinhibitory neurons pass to the heart in the cardiac branches of the vagal nerves. In the wall of the heart they synapse (ganglionic synapse) with the ganglionic neurons. The sinus node is supplied mainly from the right vagus nerve, and the atrioventricular node and bundle mainly from the left vagus nerve. Postganglionic neurons are also distributed to other parts of the atria. The ventricular myocardium is con-

---

FIG. 5–13. Mechanisms by which angiotensin II increases systemic arterial blood pressure. (1) Stimulation of neurons in the brain leading to increased activity in the sympathetic nerves to the heart, blood vessels, and adrenal medulla. (2) Potentiation of ganglionic transmission. (3) Increased synthesis and release of norepinephrine at the sympathetic nerve endings and inhibition of its reuptake into the nerves *(inset)*. Together these actions cause a marked increase of the amount of norepinephrine available to activate the alpha- and beta-receptors. (4) Direct constrictor action on the smooth muscles of the resistance blood vessels. (5) Increased formation and release of aldosterone from the adrenal cortex, with a resultant increase in reabsorption of sodium by the renal tubules. This, if excessive, can serve to "stiffen" the resistance vessels (p. 210). ACh = acetylcholine. NE = norepinephrine. EPI = epinephrine. α = alpha-adrenergic receptor. β = beta-adrenergic receptor. AT = angiotensin II receptor. AT II = angiotensin II. ⌊ = action potential in sympathetic nerve.

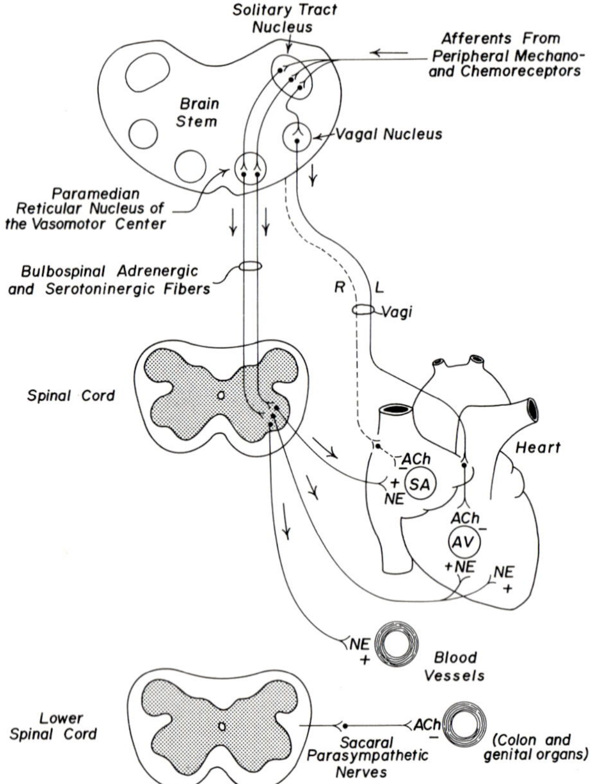

FIG. 5–14. Origin and distribution of the adrenergic and cholinergic nerves to the cardiovascular system. The vagal fibers to the heart arise from the vagal nucleus in the brainstem. This nucleus is governed by the solitary tract nucleus, which is the main receiving station for afferent information from the peripheral mechano- and chemoreceptors. (For further details see page 129 and Fig. 5–19.) The cholinergic fibers to the blood vessels of the colon and genital organs arise from centers in the lower part of the spinal cord. Not shown are vagal fibers that innervate blood vessels (p. 126) and nerve fibers that in certain species originate in the higher centers of the brain, relay in the hypothalamus, and pass directly to the spinal cord. The latter fibers innervate the resistance vessels of the skeletal muscles and, when the higher brain centers are subjected to strong emotions, liberate acetylcholine at their terminals to cause vasodilatation (p. 156). The solitary tract nucleus also has interneurons connecting it to the vasomotor center. From this center bulbar spinal fibers descend to the spinal cord and synapse with the preganglionic noradrenergic fibers to the heart and blood vessels (p. 109). ACh = acetylcholine. NE = norepinephrine. SA = sinus node. AV = atrioventricular node.

trolled by the vagal nerves to a much lesser extent, but the ventricular conducting tissues receive a rich cholinergic innervation.

Cholinergic fibers running in the wall of *resistance vessels* have the following origin: (1) the cranial parasympathetic fibers descending from the vagal nucleus, which subserve vessels of the head and viscera including the heart, lungs, gastrointestinal tract; (2) the sacral parasympathetic fibers, which subserve the blood vessels of the colon and the genital organs; and (3) cholinergic fibers, which travel with the sympathetic nerves. The latter fibers originate in the cortical areas, relay in the hypothalamus, and descend to the spinal cord without passing through the medullary cardiovascular centers. After synapsing in the sympathetic ganglia, they innervate the precapillary vessels of the skeletal muscle. These "sympathetic cholinergic vasodilator" fibers have been described in several but not all species.

There is no cholinergic innervation of the systemic veins, except those of erectile tissues.

Cholinergic Neuroeffector Interaction

The cholinergic nerve endings actively take up choline from the extracellular fluid; in their mitochondria they form another precursor, acetyl coenzyme A. The formation of acetylcholine from choline and acetyl coenzyme A occurs in

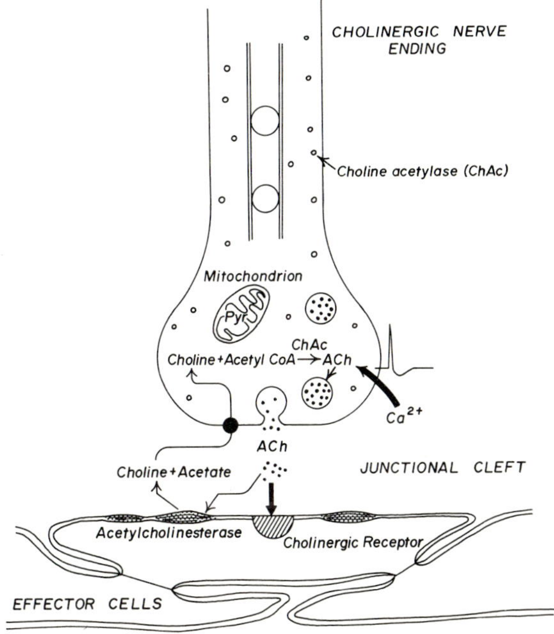

FIG. 5–15. Formation and release of acetylcholine at the parasympathetic nerve endings, and its action and breakdown at the effector cells. Acetyl coenzyme A (Acetyl CoA) is formed in the mitochondria; it diffuses to the cytoplasm where it combines with choline, which has been taken up from the extracellular fluid, to form acetylcholine. This reaction is catalyzed by the enzyme choline acetylase (ChAc). The acetylcholine is stored in vesicles. Activation of the nerve cell increases the concentration of Ca^{2+} in the neuroplasm, and this triggers the release of acetylcholine. The acetylcholine diffuses to the effector cell and binds to a cholinergic (muscarinic) receptor. The released acetylcholine is rapidly converted to choline and acetate by the enzyme acetylcholinesterase.

the neuroplasm and is catalyzed by the enzyme choline acetylase. Acetylcholine is present in a freely diffusible form in the cytoplasm and is kept in storage vesicles. When the nerve ending is activated, the neuroplasmic Ca^{2+} concentration increases and the stored acetylcholine is released into the junctional cleft. The released acetylcholine diffuses to the effector cells where it binds to receptors on the cell membrane (muscarinic receptor; p. 190). The acetylcholine is broken down by the enzyme acetylcholinesterase to choline and acetate. All tissues innervated by cholinergic nerves possess a high acetylcholinesterase activity, so the liberated acetylcholine is rapidly destroyed. The cholinergic nerve endings cannot take up acetylcholine themselves but can recycle the choline moiety (Fig. 5–15).

Role in Cardiovascular Control

The release of acetylcholine alters cardiovascular function as follows:

1. In the heart the released acetylcholine causes hyperpolarization of the pacemaker cells (Fig. 5–16) and the cells of the atrioventricular conducting tissue by increasing the permeability for potassium. As a consequence the heart rate decreases and atrioventricular conduction slows; vagal activation also decreases atrial and, to a lesser extent, ventricular contractility. The coronary vessels dilate.

2. In the gastrointestinal tract, where blood vessels dilate upon stimulation of the cholinergic nerves, it is difficult to distinguish between the direct vasodilator effect caused by the liberation of acetylcholine and the vasodilatation secondary to the increased tissue activity caused by the cholinergic transmitter.

3. In the animal species which possess sympathetic cholinergic vasodilator

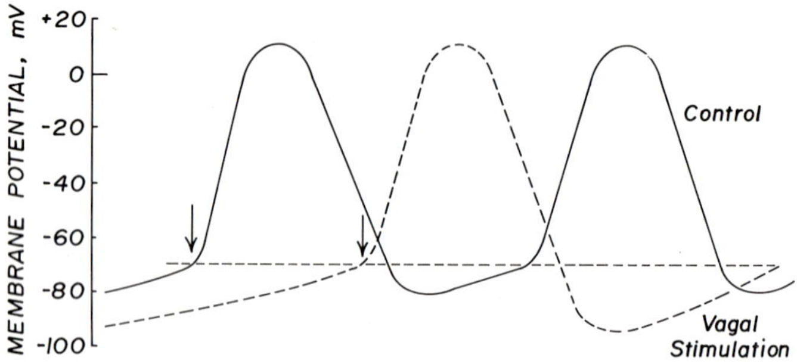

FIG. 5–16. Effect of vagal nerve stimulation on the membrane potential changes of the sinus node. By causing hyperpolarization acetylcholine released from the vagal nerve endings delays the time at which the threshold potential for the regenerative action potential *(arrow)* is reached, which causes slowing of the sinus node and thus of the heart. Changes in pacemaker activity can be caused either by lowering or increasing the membrane potential, altering the slope of the rate of diastolic depolarization, or altering the threshold for the generation of action potentials.

fibers, activation of the corticohypothalamic pathway (defense reaction, fight-or-flight reaction) causes dilatation of the resistance vessels in skeletal muscle. In the skeletal muscles of the human, dilatation of the resistance vessels occurs during emotional stress, which is due not only to circulating epinephrine but also to activation of vasodilator fibers traveling with the sympathetic nerves. The available pharmacological evidence suggests that these fibers are cholinergic (Fig. 5–17).

4. In tissues such as the salivary and sweat glands, the release of acetylcholine causes vasodilatation and activates the glandular cells. The latter in turn generate

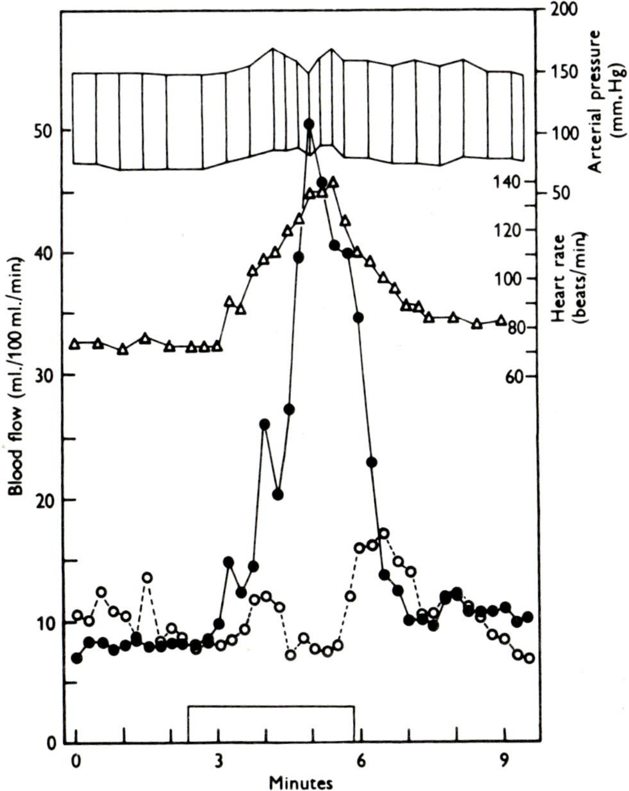

FIG. 5–17. Effect of severe emotional stress on systemic arterial blood pressure, heart rate (△), forearm blood flow (●), and hand blood flow (○) in a normal medical student. During the time indicated by the rectangle, it was suggested to the subject that he was suffering from severe blood loss. The marked increase in heart rate is due to increased sympathetic nerve activity to the sinus node and to circulating catecholamines (mainly epinephrine) released from the adrenal medulla. The striking increase in forearm blood flow is due to the circulating epinephrine stimulating beta$_2$-adrenergic receptors in the skeletal muscle resistance vessels and to activation of cholinergic fibers that travel with the sympathetic nerves to these vessels. [From Blair et al.: *J. Physiol. (Lond),* 148:633, 1959.]

kallikrein, which acts on the proteins of the interstitial fluids to produce kinins (Fig. 4–14). The resulting increase in flow allows for filtration through the fenestrated capillaries, which is a prerequisite for the formation of sweat or saliva.

5. In the erectile tissues of the penis and the clitoris the released acetylcholine causes arteriolar vasodilatation but strong constriction of the veins draining the sinusoids. As a consequence, when the parasympathetic nerves fire, the sinusoids fill with blood and the corpora cavernosa harden.

The physiological role of the cholinergic innervation of cerebral and pulmonary vessels is unknown.

Interaction With Adrenergic Transmission

In the heart and the blood vessels, acetylcholine released in the vicinity of adrenergic nerve endings binds to muscarinic receptors of the adrenergic neuronal cell membrane. As a consequence the neuronal membrane hyperpolarizes, making it more resistant to activation. Thus if acetylcholine reaches the adrenergic endings while the latter are stimulated, it causes an abrupt reduction in the release of norepinephrine. This prejunctional effect of the cholinergic transmitter greatly reinforces its direct inhibitory effect on cardiac and vascular effector cells (Fig. 5–18).

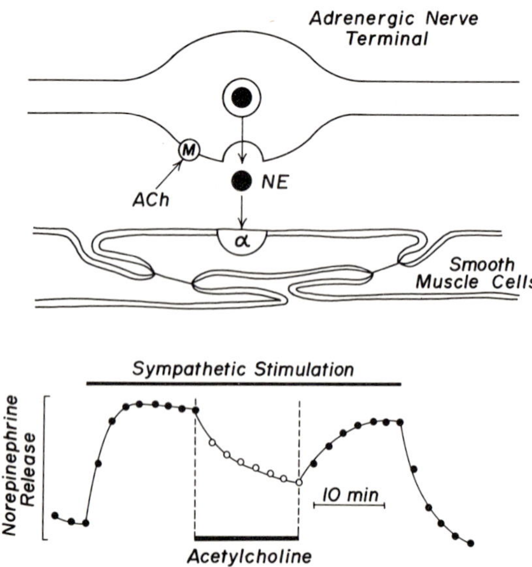

FIG. 5–18. Role of muscarinic receptors on the adrenergic nerve terminal. When the sympathetic nerves are stimulated, the output of norepinephrine is increased. Acetylcholine causes an abrupt decrease in the output by binding to a muscarinic receptor on the neuronal cell membrane. ACh = acetylcholine. NE = norepinephrine. α = alpha receptor. M = muscarinic receptor.

BRAIN CENTERS REGULATING THE CARDIOVASCULAR SYSTEM

The brain has complex networks of interneurons which, by liberating chemical transmitters to excite or inhibit each other, cause differential changes in the autonomic outflow to the components of the circulatory system. Somehow the interneurons in the brainstem relay the afferent inputs from the peripheral sensors to appropriate areas of the brain, receive information from these areas, and finally inhibit or excite discrete autonomic motor neuron pools to permit the various target organs to respond appropriately to the changing stresses imposed on the body. Although the understanding of these mechanisms is still rudimentary, certain facts are emerging (Fig. 5–19):

1. Chemical transmitters in the brain include norepinephrine, epinephrine, dopamine, and 5-hydroxytryptamine (which are classified as the monoaminergic transmitters) and acetylcholine. Many central neurons, both autonomic and somatic, probably utilize other substances which still remain to be identified. Each transmitter acts on a specific receptor of the succeeding neuron to cause its excitation or inhibition. The norepinephrine-containing neurons closely resemble the postganglionic sympathetic noradrenergic nerves morphologically and biochemically. The release of norepinephrine by the nerve impulse is calcium-dependent, and it triggers the response of the postsynaptic cell by interaction with alpha-adrenergic receptors (p. 113).

2. The majority of the afferent fibers from the arterial and cardiopulmonary mechanoreceptors terminate in the solitary tract nucleus. It is likely that input from the other receptors which modulate the circulation, such as the chemoreceptors and the trigeminal afferents (p. 165), also terminate at this site. The nucleus tractus solitarius is richly innervated by catecholamine- and 5-hydroxytryptamine-containing nerve terminals.

3. The neurons from the solitary tract nucleus relay information concerning the activity of the peripheral receptors to the vagal nucleus (see legend, Fig. 5–19) and the vasomotor center for appropriate adjustments in the autonomic outflow. The vasomotor center is part of the reticular formation, with the paramedian reticular nucleus as a major component. Unlike the solitary tract nucleus, it does not have a significant adrenergic innervation, and it selectively adjusts the sympathetic outflow to the heart and blood vessels depending on the degree of excitation or inhibition of its neurons by the chemical transmitter liberated (Figs. 5–1 and 5–14).

4. Fibers pass from the solitary tract nucleus to the hypothalamus and regulate the release of hormones such as antidiuretic hormone. They also aid in integrating the complex patterns of cardiovascular responses seen during emotion (p. 156).

5. A nucleus in the pons, the locus ceruleus, has adrenergic neurons which ascend to the posterior hypothalamus. Activation of these neurons is followed by an increase in arterial blood pressure.

6. Fibers pass from the hypothalamus to the solitary tract nucleus and the vasomotor center. The fibers from the temperature-sensitive cells of the anterior

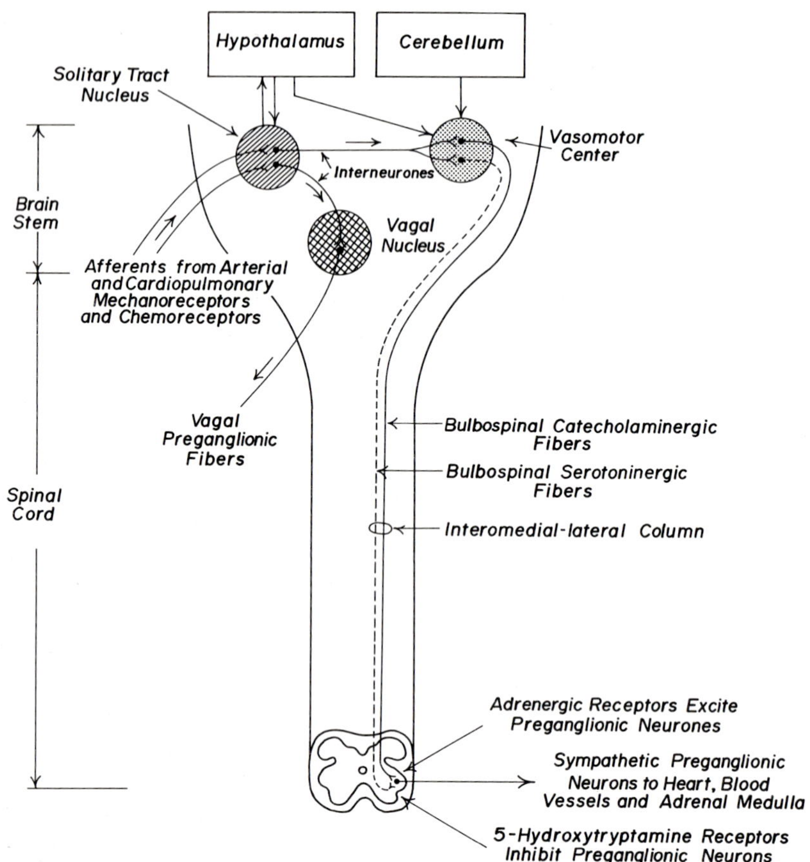

FIG. 5–19. Some central nervous structures thought to have a key role in regulation of the circulatory system. The main groups of cells in the brainstem are the solitary tract nucleus, the vagal nucleus, and the paramedian reticular nucleus that together with adjacent nuclei, constitutes the vasomotor center. Here as in Fig. 5–14, the dorsal nucleus of the vagus and the nucleus ambiguus are combined and shown as "vagal nucleus." While the nucleus ambiguus appears to play the major role in controlling the vagal outflow to the heart, in some species, the dorsal nucleus of the vagus also contributes. The solitary tract nucleus is linked by interneurons to the vagal nucleus and the vasomotor center and in turn regulate the autonomic outflow. These nuclei also are linked to suprapontine structures, in particular the hypothalamus. The fastigial nucleus of the cerebellum also relays to the vasomotor center. Although these various nuclei are bilateral (Fig. 5–14), they function as single units. For simplicity, possible connections between the hypothalamus and the higher brain centers are omitted, as are the direct connections to the spinal cord centers of the sympathetic afferents from the heart and lungs (p. 139), and the afferent receptors arising in the thoracic cage (p. 176). For details see text.

hypothalamus may pass directly to the spinal cord for the control of cutaneous blood vessels and sweat glands (p. 146).

7. A group of neurons in the cerebellum (fastigial nucleus) receive input from the vestibular apparatus in the inner ear (labyrinth), which gives rise to

reflexes orienting the body in space. On assumption of the upright posture, the fastigial nucleus sends impulses to the vasomotor center, which helps increase the sympathetic drive to the heart and blood vessels (p. 158).

8. Centers in the limbic system and the cerebral cortex presumably participate in cardiovascular control. Thus the circulation is governed by a longitudinal system of control extending from the cerebral cortex to the spinal cord and the autonomic nerve terminals in the effector organs.

PERIPHERAL SENSORS, CENTRAL INPUTS, AND CARDIOVASCULAR FUNCTION

A number of inputs modulate the activity of the vasomotor center and the vagal nucleus (Fig. 5–19). These inputs can be:

1. Generated in higher centers. This is the case in particular for the changes in circulatory behavior seen with emotion (p. 156). Other examples are the excitatory influence of the paraventricular nuclei sensitive to angiotensin II and the central adrenergic neurons, which originate in the anterior hypothalamus and cause inhibition of the medullary cardiovascular centers (p. 129).

2. Conveyed directly from a peripheral sensor to the medullary center; this involves a true "reflex arc" with a peripheral receptor, a signal to the centers, and an alteration in the activity of the cardiovascular system. The main cardiovascular reflexes are those originating from mechanoreceptors situated in the carotid sinus and the aortic arch (arterial pressoreceptors), and mechanoreceptors situated in the heart and lungs (cardiopulmonary pressoreceptors).

3. Of mixed origin, whereby information provided by a peripheral sensor is integrated with signals from other nervous centers to cause the cardiovascular response. Such mixed responses are exemplified best by chemoreception, thermoregulation, and exercise adaptation.

Carotid and Aortic Mechanoreceptors

These are receptors situated in the walls of the major blood vessels whose activity is determined by the arterial pressure. Strictly speaking they do not act as presso- or baroreceptors to measure blood pressure but are "stretch receptors." They are stimulated when they are distended. Since the pressure within the blood vessel is a determinant of wall tension, the amount of stretch to which the receptors are submitted is a function of the pressure level in the blood vessel where they are located (Laplace's law). An increased stretch of the mechanoreceptors initiates increased traffic in the afferent nerves connecting them with the solitary tract nucleus. As a consequence the vagal center and the inhibitory neurons of the vasomotor center are activated. This, on the one hand, causes an increase in vagal traffic to the heart and, on the other hand, depresses the sympathetic outflow to heart and blood vessels. The reverse occurs when the pressure falls within the blood vessels where these mechanoreceptors are situated.

Anatomy

The arterial mechanoreceptors are an arborization of nerve endings located in the adventitia at the widening of the internal carotid artery (carotid sinus) upstream from the bifurcation of the common carotid artery, and in the wall of the ascending aorta. These endings are the origin of myelinated (fast conducting) and unmyelinated (slowly conducting) afferent nerve fibers, with the latter being more numerous. The nerve fibers from the carotid sinuses form the carotid sinus nerves, which join the glossopharyngeal nerves; those from the aortic arch form the depressor nerves which join the vagus nerve (Fig. 5–20).

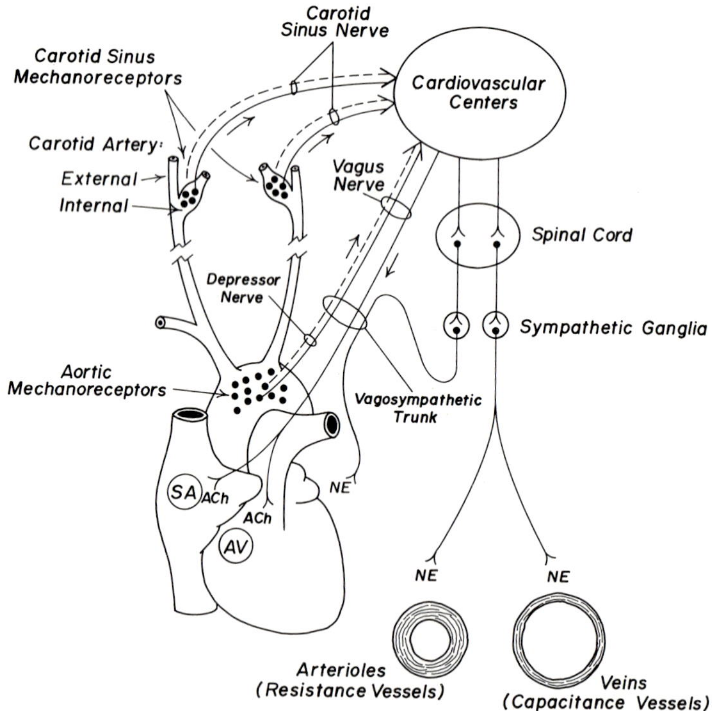

FIG. 5–20. Arterial mechanoreceptors of the carotid sinus and aortic arch. The nerve fibers from the carotid sinus form the sinus nerve, which joins the glossopharyngeal; those from the aortic arch form the depressor nerve, which joins the vagus and sympathetic to form the vagosympathetic trunk. The afferent fibers from the receptors are myelinated (———) and unmyelinated (-----). The nerves terminate in the solitary tract nucleus. Changes in the activity of those mechanoreceptors caused by alterations in the arterial blood pressure result in appropriate adjustments in the vagal and sympathetic outflow to the heart, and the sympathetic outflow to the resistance and capacitance vessels. These adjustments buffer changes in the arterial blood pressure. NE = norepinephrine. ACh = acetylcholine. SA = sinus node. AV = atrioventricular node.

Function

As the pressure is gradually increased in the carotid sinus, the first evidence of receptor activity occurs at around 65 to 70 mm Hg; below this threshold the receptors are silent. As the pressure is gradually increased, the firing augments rapidly in the myelinated afferent fibers and a sigmoidal relationship is obtained between blood pressure and receptor activity. The maximal firing is reached at around 180 mm Hg; if the pressure increases further, the activity of the receptors does not change although the vessel wall continues to expand. This means that at approximately 180 mm Hg the mechanoreceptors of the carotid sinus are maximally excited. The pressure at which one-half of the maximal firing rate is obtained corresponds to the normal blood pressure (Fig. 5–21). A similar relationship exists between distending pressure and receptor firing in the aortic arch. The main differences are that in the aortic arch the threshold pressure is higher and the pressure–response curve is displaced to the right. Thus the aortic arch does not compensate effectively for decreases in pressure below normal but reinforces the action of the carotid sinus in opposing increases in pressure above normal levels.

Greater increases in pressure cause activation of the unmyelinated afferent fibers in both regions; these fibers become involved only when the blood pressure rises abnormally (Fig. 5–22).

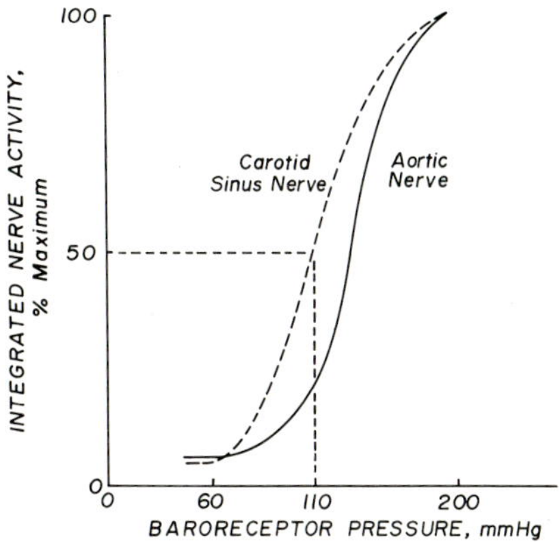

FIG. 5–21. Relation of the pressure in the carotid sinus and aortic arch to the activity in the afferent nerves from the mechanoreceptors in their walls. The aortic nerve curve is to the right of the carotid sinus nerve curve, and significant changes in nerve traffic occur at a blood pressure of 100 mm Hg for the aortic nerve compared with 70 mm Hg for the carotid sinus nerve. (Modified from Pelletier et al.: *Circ. Res.,* 31:557, 1972.)

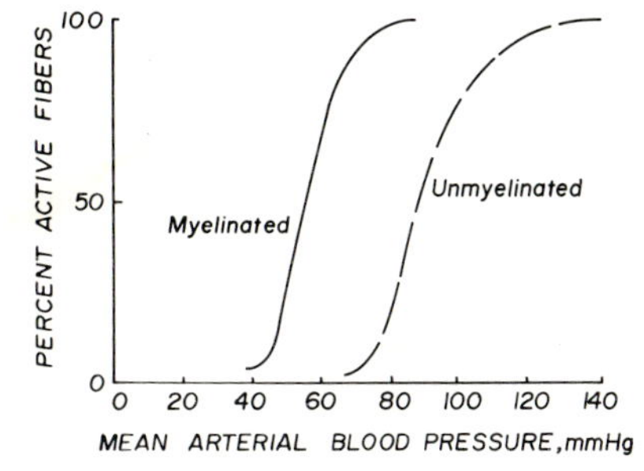

FIG. 5–22. Myelinated and unmyelinated afferent fibers from the aortic baroreceptors of the rabbit. The percentage of these fibers which have reached threshold is plotted against the mean arterial blood pressure. The myelinated afferents have a lower threshold and reach their maximal activity at a lower pressure than the unmyelinated. Thus the latter fibers are activated only when the pressure becomes abnormally elevated. (Modified from Jones and Thorén: *Acta Physiol. Scand.,* 101:286, 1977.)

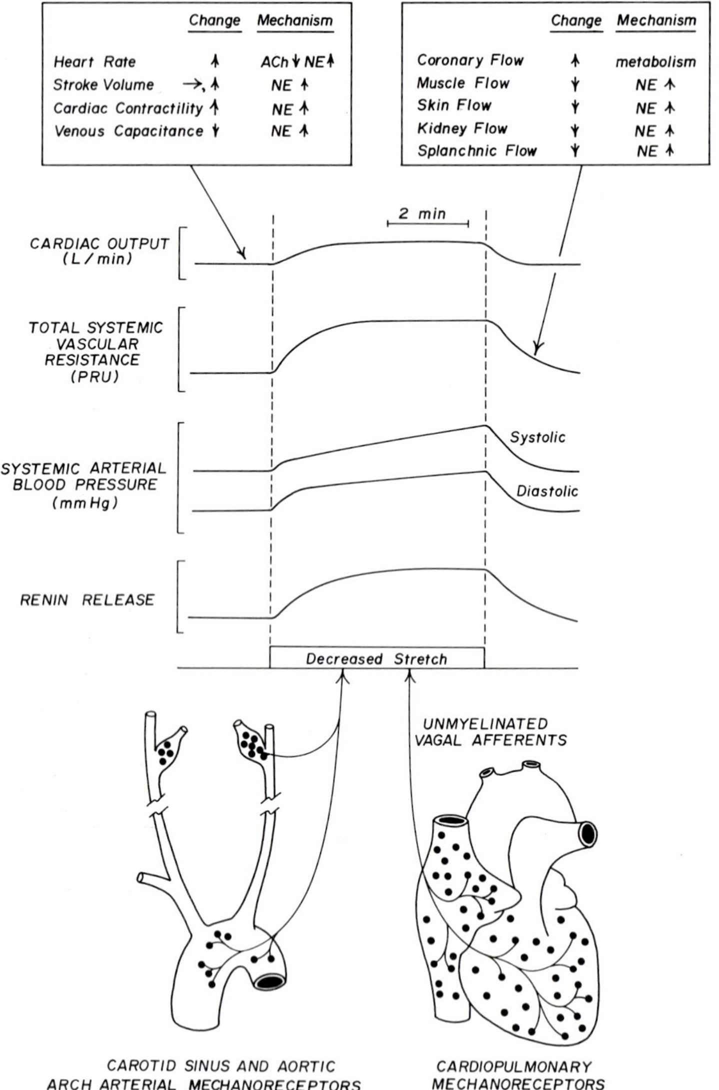

FIG. 5–23. Hemodynamic effects of a decrease in activity of the mechanoreceptors in the carotid sinus, aortic arch, and cardiopulmonary region. The continuous inhibition of the solitary tract nucleus in the medulla of the brain is lessened, and there is increased sympathetic outflow to the heart and blood vessels and decreased vagal activity to the heart. The constriction of the systemic vascular beds results in an increase in total systemic vascular resistance. The cardiac output is maintained by the increased rate and contractility, and maintenance of its filling pressure by the reflex constriction of the systemic veins. The coronary flow is increased by the increased products of metabolism of the myocardial cells and by activation of beta-receptors. The systolic and diastolic pressures are increased so an adequate perfusion pressure to the brain and coronary vessels is sustained. If the decreased pressure is due to hemorrhage, the cardiac output decreases in spite of the increase in rate and contractility because the venoconstriction is unable to provide an adequate filling pressure owing to the continuing blood loss. ACh = acetylcholine. NE = norepinephrine. PRU = peripheral resistance units.

Cardiovascular Responses

When the blood pressure falls, the firing of the mechanoreceptors becomes less, and the activity of the depressor neurons of the vasomotor center and of the vagal nucleus decreases. This results in augmented sympathetic activity to the heart and vessels and decreased vagal activity to the heart, which leads to the following (Fig. 5–23): (1) Constriction of the resistance vessels in muscle, kidney, splanchnic bed, and skin so that the total systemic vascular resistance increases. (2) Constriction of the splanchnic veins. The resulting mobilization of blood is assisted by passive expulsion following constriction of the resistance vessels. This helps maintain the appropriate filling pressure (preload) of the heart. (3) Increase in heart rate due to increased sympathetic and decreased vagal activity, and in myocardial contractility due to increased sympathetic activity. The cardiac output is maintained in the face of the greater afterload.

When the arterial blood pressure increases, the reverse occurs.

Cardiopulmonary Mechanoreceptors

Anatomy

Three sets of receptors are activated by changes in pressure in the heart chambers: (1) Discrete receptors in the endocardium at the junctions of (a) the superior and inferior vena cava with the right atrium, and (b) the pulmonary veins with the left atrium. These receptors are connected by myelinated fibers of the vagal nerves to the cardiovascular centers. (2) A diffuse receptor network of fine fibers throughout all chambers of the heart, connected to the cardiovascular centers by unmyelinated vagal fibers. (3) A diffuse receptor network of fibers (sympathetic afferents) throughout all chambers of the heart, connected to the spinal cord by myelinated and unmyelinated fibers traveling with the sympathetic nerves (Fig. 5–24).

Function

1. *Receptors at the venoatrial junctions:* These receptors are activated by atrial filling and atrial contraction. On mechanical distention of the venoatrial junctions, there is an increase in heart rate due to activation of the sympathetic outflow to the sinus node. There is no change in the activity of the efferent vagal fibers to the heart, or of the sympathetic fibers to the myocardium. The sympathetic outflow to the kidney is decreased. The caliber of the other systemic resistance vessels of the systemic veins is unchanged. The reflex increase in heart rate may help maintain cardiac volume relatively constant during an increase in venous return. In addition to the effects on the sinus node, the mechanical distention causes an increased output of water by the kidney. This diuresis is secondary to alterations in hormone liberation, most likely the inhibition of antidiuretic hormone secretion from the posterior lobe of the pituitary gland,

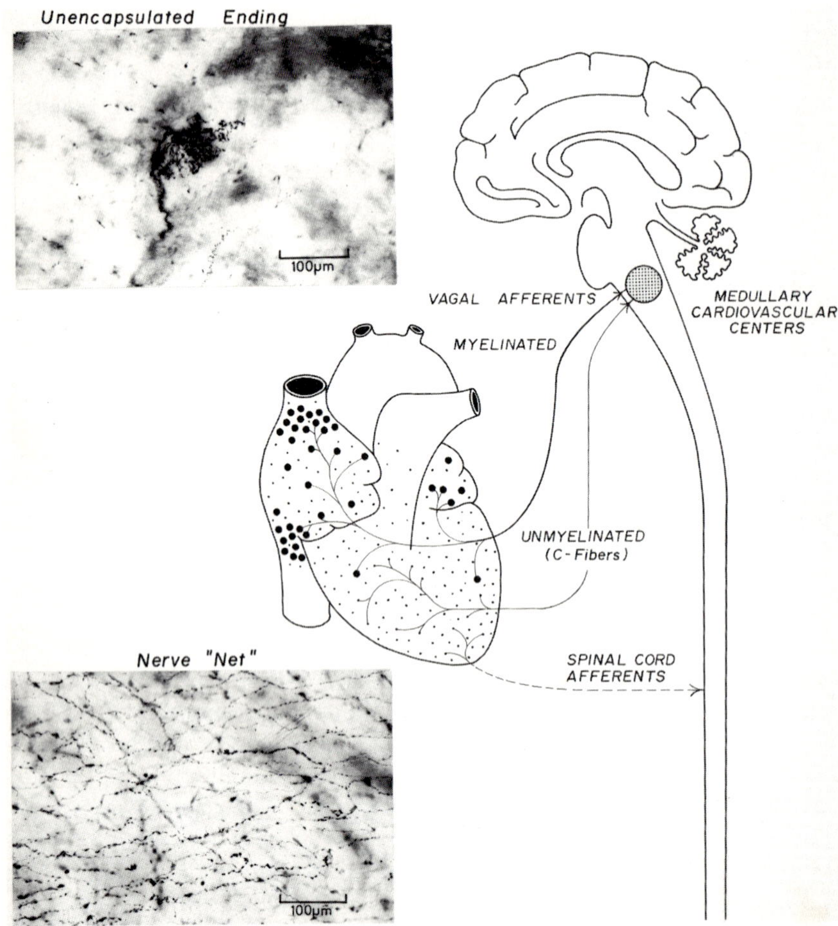

FIG. 5–24. Mechanoreceptors in the heart and their afferent fibers. Those subserved by the fast-conducting myelinated vagal afferents (8 to 30 m/sec) are localized to the junctions of (1) the caval veins with the right atrium and (2) the pulmonary veins with the left atrium. Those subserved by the slowly conducting unmyelinated afferents (less than 2.5 m/sec) arise from a widespread nerve net present in all chambers of the heart. Those subserved by the spinal cord afferents (sympathetic afferents, myelinated and unmyelinated) also arise from a diffuse network of fibers throughout the heart. **Insets:** histological appearance (methylene blue stain) of the large unencapsulated endings which are connected to the myelinated vagal afferents and the nerve "net" from which the unmyelinated vagal afferents arise. (From Linden: *Circulation,* 48:463, 1973, by permission of The American Heart Association.)

and to the increased renal blood flow. Antidiuretic hormone acts on the renal tubules to promote water reabsorption (Fig. 5–25).

2. *Receptors with unmyelinated vagal afferents:* In resting conditions these receptors have a sparse and irregular discharge, which increases as soon as the atrial or ventricular pressure rises. When activated, they behave like the

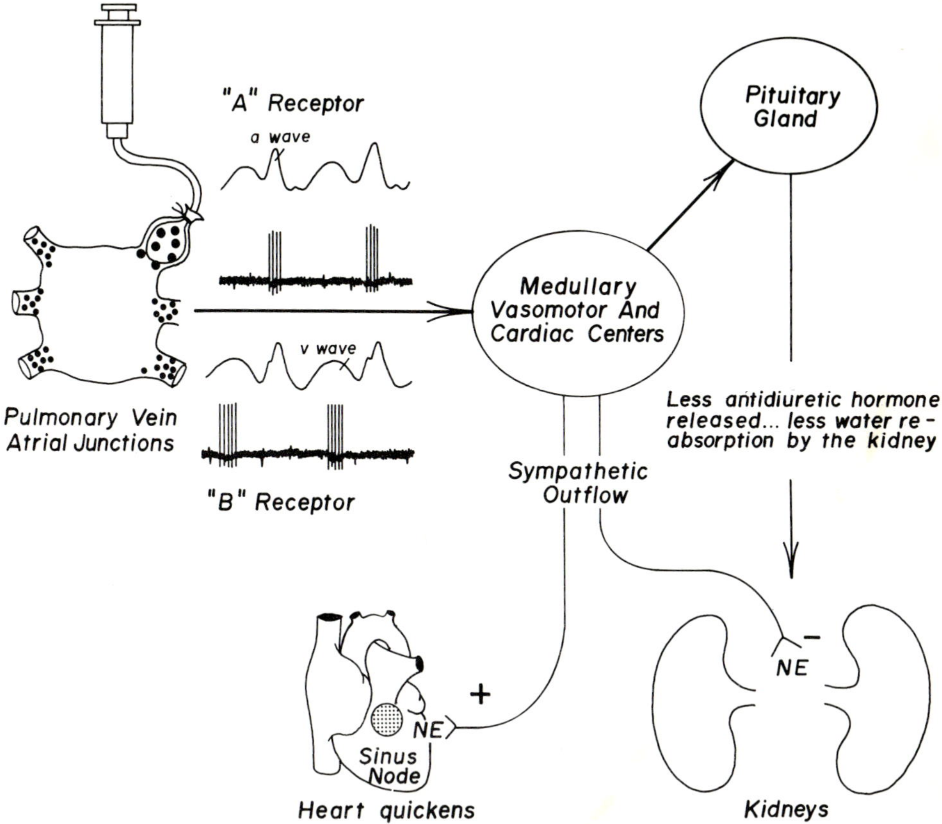

FIG. 5–25. Effect of mechanical distention (via a small balloon attached to a syringe) of the receptors subserved by myelinated vagal afferents at the pulmonary venous–atrial junction. The increased rate of firing in these fibers causes an increase in sympathetic outflow specifically directed to the sinus node so the heart quickens without a change in contractility. The output of antidiuretic hormone from the posterior lobe of the pituitary gland is reduced so less of the water filtered by the glomeruli of the kidney is reabsorbed into the blood. Normally these receptors discharge rhythmically with each cardiac cycle. The type "A" receptors discharge in unison with atrial contraction (a wave) and the "B" receptors with atrial filling (v wave) as shown by the recording of atrial pressure. Thus they signal to the brain the heart rate, the vigor of atrial systole, and the degree of atrial filling. NE = norepinephrine.

carotid and aortic mechanoreceptors by stimulating the depressor neurons of the vasomotor center and the vagal nuclei. This decreases sympathetic and increases vagal outflow, which results in a fall in blood pressure. Since about 80% of the vagal afferent fibers are unmyelinated, the aggregated activity of all these fibers from the heart, even though each has a sparse discharge, can have marked effects on the circulation. When their normal activity is interrupted, the arterial blood pressure increases owing to an increase in systemic vascular resistance, constriction of the splanchnic veins, and a maintained or increased

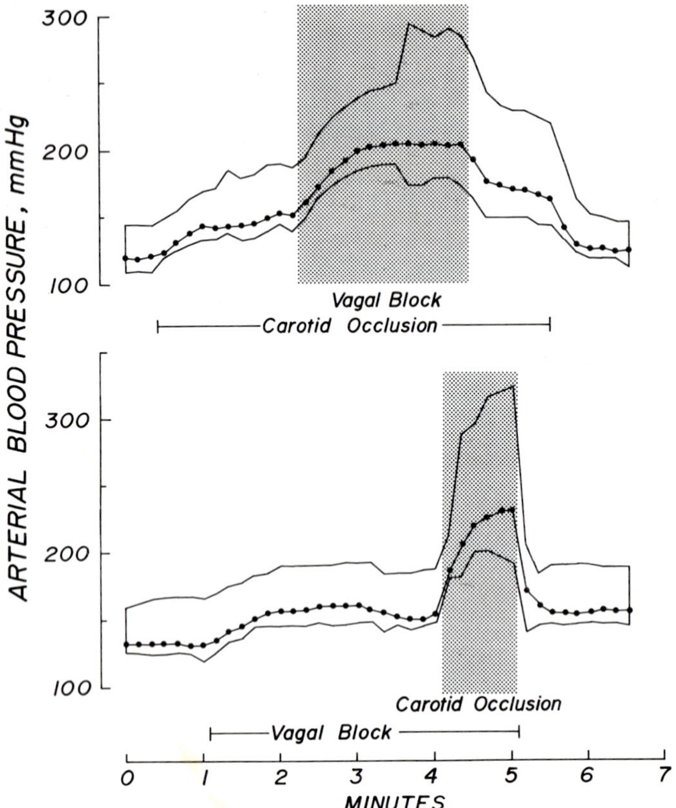

FIG. 5–26. Interaction of carotid sinus and cardiopulmonary mechanoreceptors. The arterial systolic, diastolic, and mean blood pressure increase when the carotid mechanoreceptors are unstretched by occluding the carotid arteries and when the afferent traffic from the mechanoreceptors in the heart and lungs is interrupted by cooling both cervical vagal nerves. **Top panel:** Carotid occlusion prior to vagal block. **Lower panel:** Vagal block prior to carotid occlusion. Note that the cardiopulmonary baroreflex buffers the effect of withdrawing the inhibitory influence of the carotid baroreflex and vice versa on the arterial blood pressure. (From Donald and Shepherd: *Cardiovasc. Res.,* 12:449, 1978.)

cardiac output (Fig. 5–23). Depending on the circumstances, these cardiac receptors and the carotid and aortic receptors can reinforce or oppose each other (Fig. 5–26). For example, during severe hemorrhage the pressures within the heart and the vascular system fall and the vasomotor center is freed from the inhibitory activity of both sets of receptors. This causes a marked increase in sympathetic traffic to the renal vessels, which constrict so strongly that filtration is impaired and waste products accumulate in the body. By comparison, in acute heart failure the arterial pressure decreases but the diastolic pressures in the cardiac chambers increase. The activation of the cardiac receptors opposes at the vasomotor center the reduced input from the arterial mechanoreceptors so that the renal blood flow decreases less.

3. *Sympathetic afferents:* Although these receptors are activated rhythmically during the cardiac cycle, their function is unknown. Some of them serve to convey pain sensation. When the fibers originating from these receptors are stimulated electrically, the blood pressure rises and the heart quickens.

Pulmonary Receptors

The lungs contain a variety of receptors whose precise morphology, distribution, and function have yet to be established. Some of these tonically inhibit the cardiovascular centers (Fig. 5–27).

Receptors in Airways

1. Slowly adapting stretch receptors, with myelinated vagal afferents, increase their activity as the airways widen and the lung volume augments during inspira-

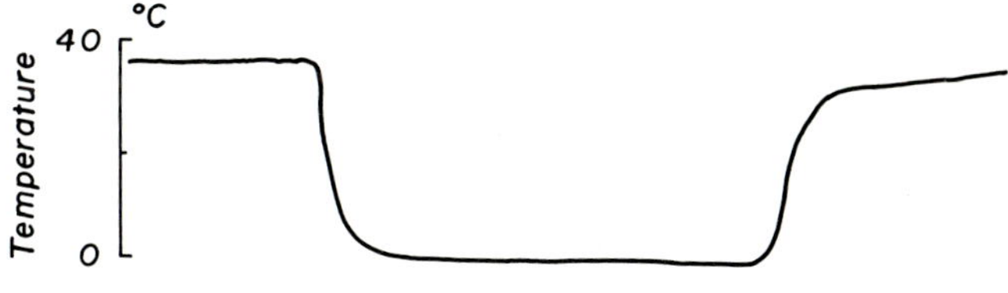

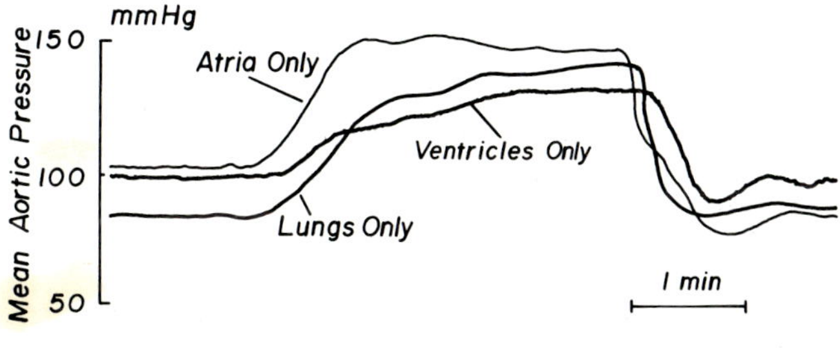

FIG. 5–27. Demonstration that the lungs, the atria, and the ventricles each exert a tonic inhibition of the cardiovascular centers. In one study the heart was removed, leaving the lungs, which were mechanically ventilated. In another the lungs and ventricles were removed, leaving the beating atria. In the third the lungs were removed and the atria denervated, leaving the innervated beating ventricles. When the traffic in the vagal afferents from the receptors in each of these structures is interrupted by vagal cooling *(top),* there is an increase in aortic blood pressure due to increased sympathetic outflow to the heart and systemic blood vessels. (Data from Mancia and Donald: *Circ. Res.,* 36:310, 1975.)

tion. The increased afferent traffic inhibits the respiratory center, causing inspiration to cease and expiration to begin. This reflex, commonly known as the Hering–Breuer inhibitory respiratory reflex, provides the optimal rate and depth of breathing for the minimal energy expenditure of the respiratory muscles. The reflex is less potent in humans than in animals. Inflation of the lungs causes acceleration of the heart and vasodilatation due to decreased vagal and sympathetic outflow, presumably by activation of the pulmonary stretch receptors (lung inflation reflex).

2. Rapidly adapting receptors in the major bronchi are connected to myelinated vagal afferents. Their function is unknown. Some of these may act as "irritant" receptors and cause the cough reflex.

3. Receptors subserved by vagal unmyelinated fibers can be activated by substances formed in the lungs (e.g., bradykinin, histamine, 5-hydroxytryptamine, and prostaglandins) during anaphylaxis (p. 101). This leads to rapid, shallow breathing (tachypnea) and bronchoconstriction.

Receptors in Lung Parenchyma

1. There are receptors connected to unmyelinated vagal afferents that respond to excessive inflation of the lungs. This causes increased vagal activity to the heart and decreased sympathetic outflow to the heart and the systemic blood vessels. Some of these receptors are located close to the pulmonary capillaries (juxtapulmonary capillary receptors; alveolar nociceptive receptors) and are activated by increases in interstitial fluid volume in the lungs. During lung edema they cause bronchoconstriction, bradycardia, hypotension, and reflex inhibition of the voluntary muscles.

2. A second type of receptor is connected to nerves which travel to the spinal cord with the sympathetic nerves (sympathetic afferents). Their function is unknown. Some are stimulated by substances released from damaged lung tissue, such as bradykinin, 5-hydroxytryptamine, and prostaglandins. They may serve to convey pain sensation. In humans whose spinal cord has been transected in the lower cervical region, lung inflation causes a reflex constriction of skin blood vessels probably by activation of these sympathetic afferents.

Chemoreceptors

An appropriate oxygen tension, carbon dioxide tension, and hydrogen ion concentration of the blood is achieved by the gas exchanges in the lungs and by the ability of the renal tubules to alter appropriately the output of fixed acids and bases from the body. Deviations of the blood gases or hydrogen ion concentration from normal are detected by groups of cells (chemoreceptors) located in the carotid and aortic bodies, which are situated adjacent to the carotid sinuses and aortic mechanoreceptors. Of these, the carotid bodies have been studied intensively because of their accessibility, and most of the information outlined below was gained from examining the structure and the function of these bodies.

Anatomy

The carotid body is a few millimeters in size and is located at the bifurcation of the carotid artery (Fig. 5–28). It contains two distinct cell types (glomal cells type I and type II), nerve fibers of varying diameter, and a rich capillary network characterized by a fenestrated endothelium. Granules with a high concentration of dopamine are found only in type I cells; the type II cells are free of granules. Each type I glomus cell is contacted by a variable number of nerve endings which unite to form the afferent nerve from the carotid body. The latter travels with the afferent nerve from the carotid mechanoreceptors and links the glomus cells to the cardiovascular and respiratory centers in the brainstem. Efferent nerve fibers from the vagus can decrease the traffic in the afferent nerves; the role of these efferent fibers is unknown. The carotid bodies

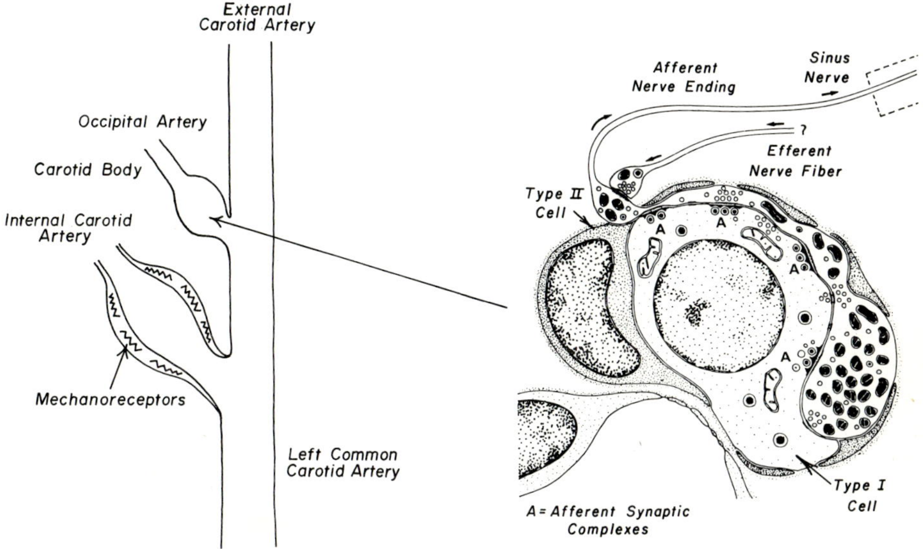

FIG. 5–28. Site, innervation, and histological structure of the carotid body. The carotid body is situated in the carotid bifurcation and gets its blood supply from the occipital artery. It contains two types of glomal cells (types I and II). Afferent nerve fibers, which run in the carotid sinus nerve, connect type I cells to the cardiovascular centers. Efferent nerves are shown to impinge upon the afferent nerve endings, but the site of their termination is unknown. Type II cells embrace type I cells with a thin cytoplasmic sheet. Arrows show the direction of the nerve impulses. (Modified from Verna: *J. Microsc. Paris,* 16:299, 1973, by permission).

receive their blood supply from the occipital artery and have a very large blood flow relative to their small size; expressed per unit of weight, the flow is about five times greater than that to the kidney and 40 times that to the brain. The blood vessels of the carotid body are richly invested with sympathetic nerves, which when stimulated cause a substantial decrease in blood flow to the carotid body. The physiological role of these nerves is unknown.

Function

The carotid chemoreceptors send signals to the medullary centers concerning decreases in the Po_2 and pH or increases in the Pco_2 of the arterial blood. In an unknown way these changes are transformed into an electrical signal. The frequency of action potentials in the afferent nerves is directly proportional to the alterations in Pco_2, Po_2, and pH, once the latter have reached a threshold level. The Po_2 must decrease from the normal value of about 95 mm Hg to about 80 mm Hg before the afferent nerve activity increases. By contrast, as soon as the Pco_2 increases above the normal value of 40 mm Hg, or the pH decreases below the normal value of 7.4, the activity of the chemoreceptors is augmented (Fig. 5–29). The slope of the increased activity and the magnitude of the increase in firing are much larger for changes in pH alone than for changes in Pco_2 alone. Usually in the intact organism changes in Pco_2, pH, and to a lesser extent Po_2 occur simultaneously and together form a powerful stimulus to the chemoreceptors.

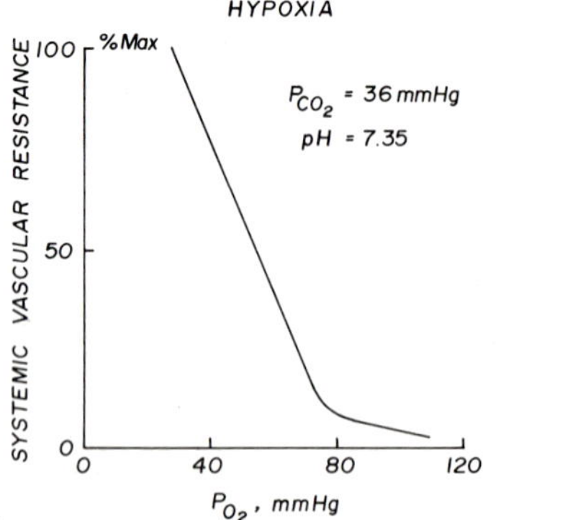

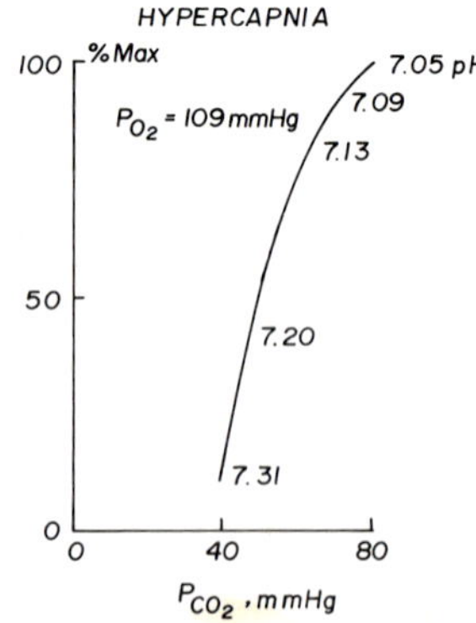

FIG. 5–29. Activation of chemoreceptors by alterations in the composition of the arterial blood, as illustrated by changes in systemic vascular resistance. With a decrease in the Po_2 of the blood perfusing the carotid bodies (hypoxia), at normal pH and Pco_2 a reflex constriction of the systemic vessels does not occur until the Po_2 decreases to 70 mm Hg. Thereafter the vessels constrict progressively as the Po_2 is decreased and thus the resistance augments. When the blood perfusing the carotid bodies is made hypercapnic, at normal Po_2, so that the pH decreases as the Pco_2 increases, the vessels constrict strongly as soon as normal values are exceeded and continue to constrict as the hypercapnia increases in severity. (Modified from Pelletier: *Circ. Res.*, 31:431, 1972.)

Response

Stimulation of the chemoreceptors causes respiration to quicken and deepen. The resulting increase in ventilation is adjusted precisely to restore the blood gases and pH to their normal values. The increased ventilation also activates

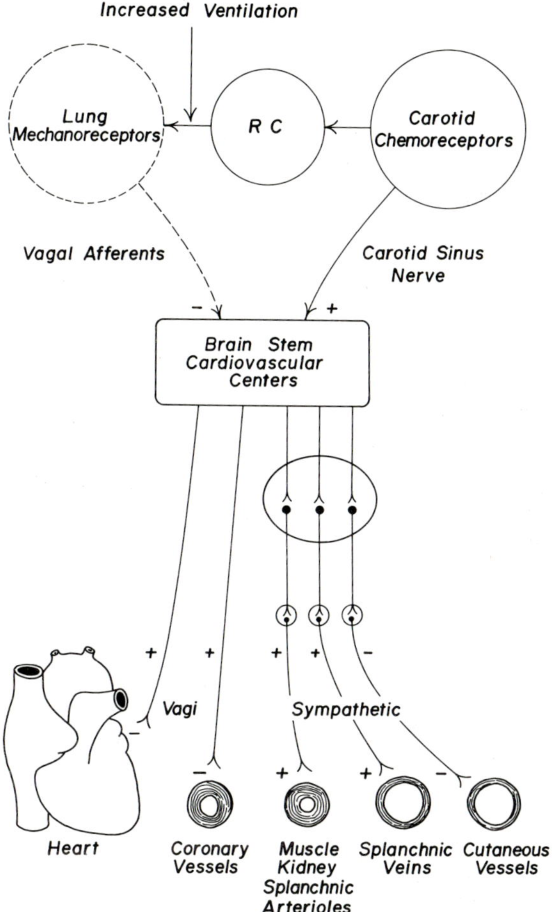

FIG. 5–30. Stimulation of the carotid chemoreceptors has effects on the respiratory (RC) and the cardiovascular centers. The resultant increase in ventilation excites mechanoreceptors in the lungs (pulmonary depressor reflex; p. 139), which has effects on the heart and systemic blood vessels opposite to the primary responses from the carotid bodies. When the latter are stimulated and ventilation maintained constant, the heart rate and cardiac contractility are decreased, and the coronary vessels are dilated owing to increased vagal activity. The increased sympathetic outflow causes constriction of the resistance vessels in skeletal muscle, splanchnic bed, and kidney as well as constriction of the splanchnic capacitance vessels. The cutaneous vessels are dilated owing to decreased sympathetic outflow. The arterial systolic and diastolic blood pressure is increased because the total systemic vascular resistance is augmented more than the cardiac output is decreased. When the ventilation is permitted to increase, these circulatory changes are attenuated. +, − = nerve traffic *(upper row)* or effector response *(lower row)* increased or decreased, respectively.

the lung mechanoreceptors, causing reflex circulatory changes which partly obscure the changes due to the stimulation of the chemoreceptors. To determine the cardiovascular response to chemoreceptor stimulation alone, lung volume and respiratory rate must be controlled. When this is done, stimulation of the chemoreceptors causes: (1) slowing of the heart and decreased cardiac output due to increased vagal activity; (2) dilation of the coronary vessels due to activation of the vagal cholinergic fibers; (3) constriction of the resistance vessels in the skeletal muscles, splanchnic bed, and kidney due to activation of their sympathetic nerves; (4) constriction of the splanchnic capacitance vessels due to activation of their sympathetic nerves; and (5) dilatation of skin vessels due to decreased activity of their sympathetic nerves (Fig. 5–30). This response increases the arterial blood pressure, so the brain and the heart are supplied with more blood and their total oxygen delivery or carbon dioxide washout is within the normal range. This is facilitated by the direct vasodilator effect that the low Po_2 (hypoxic blood) and the high Pco_2 (hypercapnic blood) have on cerebral and coronary vessels.

In the human, removal of the carotid bodies affects respiratory function in a manner similar to that seen in the animal after removal of the carotid and aortic bodies; this suggests that in the human the aortic region has little functional significance in chemoreception.

Interaction With Central Effects

Changes in Po_2, Pco_2, and pH not only alter the activity of the arterial chemoreceptors but also have direct effects on the cardiovascular and respiratory centers. As far as the cardiovascular centers are concerned, hypoxia and hypercapnia activate the vasomotor center. Hypoxia also activates the cardioinhibitory center, causing a decrease in heart rate. This occurs when there is a pathological increase in intracranial pressure.

Coronary Chemoreflexes

Injection of 5-hydroxytryptamine into the coronary arteries at their origin activates vagal afferents, which leads to transient hypertension and tachycardia. If this reflex were to be activated by 5-hydroxytryptamine derived from platelet aggregation, it could explain the transient hypertension which occasionally accompanies angina pectoris and acute myocardial infarction (p. 228). By contrast, injection of 5-hydroxytryptamine or other chemical substances into the distal coronary circulation stimulates other vagal afferents, which induce reflex bradycardia and hypotension (von Bezold–Jarisch reflex). The activation of this reflex may help explain the hypotension and bradycardia observed in most cases of coronary infarction (p. 228).

Thermoregulation

Heat is continually produced in the body, particularly in skeletal muscle, liver, and heart. During rest, sufficient heat is generated to raise the temperature of the body 1°C per hour, and during moderate work 5°C per hour, if no means were available for its dissipation. Heat is lost mainly from: (1) the skin by radiation, conduction, convection, evaporation, and sweating; and (2) the respiratory tract by warming inspired air and by evaporation. Sweating and alterations in blood flow through the skin can be rapidly and finely adjusted by the body's thermoregulatory mechanisms. In the human they are the most important modalities of heat loss for the maintenance of an optimal body temperature. The term body temperature refers to the core temperature, i.e., the temperature of the brain and the thoracic and abdominal viscera. These organs require a relatively constant temperature (37°C) to function effectively. On the other hand, the temperature of the skin, particularly in the extremities, varies widely with the changes in skin blood flow and sweat gland activity, and with the ambient temperature.

Anatomy

Temperature sensors are present in the following locations: (1) Groups of neurons in the preoptic area of the anterior part of the hypothalamus, in the bottom of the 3rd ventricle in the midbrain, are especially sensitive to small changes in temperature. They are the control center for temperature regulation of the body and function as a thermostat. (2) Receptors sensitive to heat are located in the skin. They are different from those serving thermal sensation. Their afferent fibers run to the spinal cord with the sympathetic nerves and then ascend to the hypothalamus (Fig. 5–31). (3) Other temperature-sensitive elements have been described in the deep blood vessels, the abdominal viscera, and the spinal cord.

Function and Cardiovascular Responses

The cardiovascular response to thermoregulatory stress originates in the hypothalamic center and involves mainly the skin circulation (Fig. 5–31). The changes in the latter are due to the combination of the alteration in sympathetic nerve activity and the direct effect of temperature on the blood vessel wall (p. 99). This permits effective management of increased heat production in the body and maintenance of body temperature in a wide variety of environmental conditions.

Heat Production

When the heat production of the body increases (e.g., during muscular exercise), the blood gains heat on passing through the active tissues. As the warmer

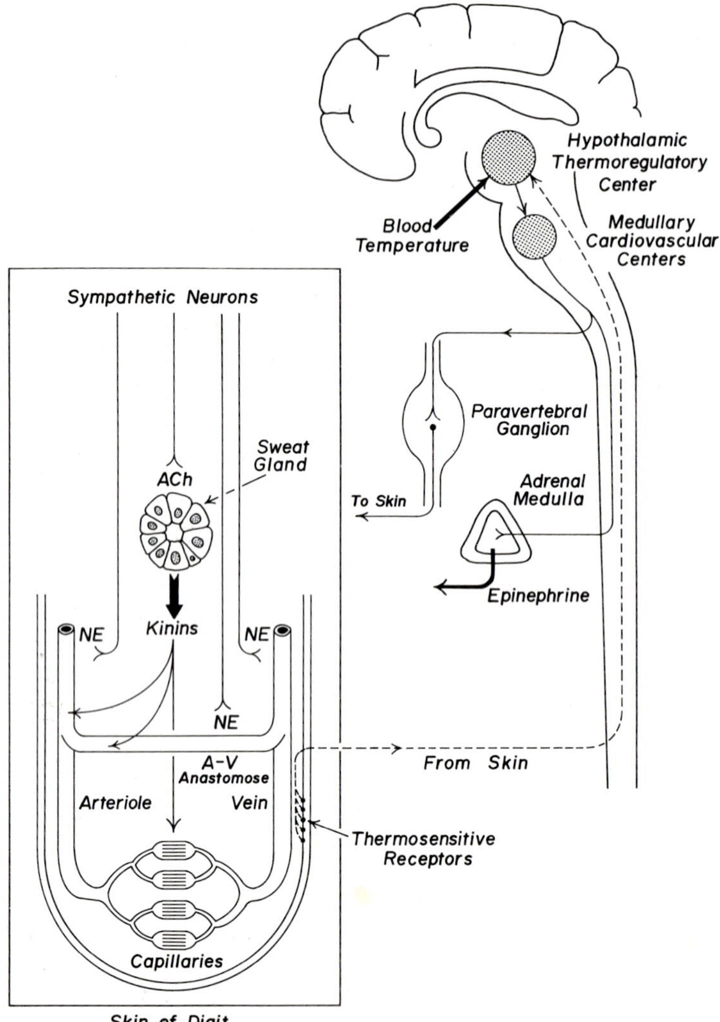

FIG. 5–31. Link between the skin and the thermoregulatory control. An increase in the temperature of blood activates temperature-sensitive cells in the hypothalamus with a resulting decrease in sympathetic activity to the cutaneous vessels and a simultaneous increase in the activity of the cholinergic fibers to the sweat glands. The decrease in sympathetic activity opens arteriovenous anastomoses and causes a large increase in skin blood flow so heat is dissipated to the surroundings. Activation of the sweat glands causes the formation and release of kinins (p. 102), which contributes to the dilation of the skin vessels. When the blood temperature decreases, opposite changes occur; the increase in sympathetic activity is sustained by the secretion of epinephrine into circulating blood. Thermosensitive receptors in the skin also provide an input into the thermoregulatory centers.

blood reaches the hypothalamus the temperature-sensitive cells increase their rate of discharge; they can respond to changes in blood temperature as small as 0.2°C. There follows by modulation of the output of the medullary centers: (1) Dilatation of the skin resistance vessels due to a decreased sympathetic activity. In the areas where sweating occurs this results in additional vasodilatation (p. 102). The direct effect of heat on the vascular smooth muscle cells of the skin vessels also causes their relaxation (p. 99). (2) In the palmar skin of hands and feet, particularly in the digits, there are direct channels (20 to 70 microns in diameter) between the small arteries and the small veins (arteriovenous anastomoses). These open because the sympathetic activity to the vascular smooth muscle in their wall decreases. The opening of these low-resistance channels directs large amounts of blood to the cutaneous veins (Fig. 5–31). During severe heat stress the blood flow through the digits of the hand can increase by 60 ml/100 ml tissue/min compared to about 20 ml/100 ml tissue/min through the body of the hand. In these circumstances the total blood flow through the skin may exceed 2 liters/m^2/min. (3) Dilatation of the cutaneous veins occurs because of the combination of decreased sympathetic activity and the direct relaxatory effect of warming on cutaneous venous smooth muscle (p. 100). The wide caliber of these vessels and their position at the surface of the skin permits large amounts of warm blood to be exposed almost directly to the environment. The cutaneous veins thus act as radiators for the dissipation of heat. (4) An increase in cardiac output due to increased sympathetic and decreased vagal activity. The increase in cardiac output is directed to the skin since the blood flow to the internal organs may even decrease as the marked reduction in skin resistance causes the blood pressure to fall slightly, resulting in an unloading of the arterial mechanoreceptors (Fig. 5–23).

Hot Environment

When the skin is exposed to a hot environment the immediate increase in skin blood flow is caused by activation of the temperature-sensitive receptors in the skin, together with the direct relaxing effect of warming on the cutaneous vessels. If the blood warms to the extent that the hypothalamic temperature increases, a response is initiated similar to that described for increased heat production (Fig. 5–32).

If the outside temperature is very high, dissipation of heat is no longer sufficient despite the maximal skin blood flow. The dilated skin vessels actually take up heat, and the body temperature continues to increase. When the brain temperature exceeds 42° to 43°C, heat stroke occurs.

Exposure to Cold

When the body is exposed to cold, the local effect of cooling (p. 99) causes constriction of the resistance vessels, the arteriovenous anastomoses, and the

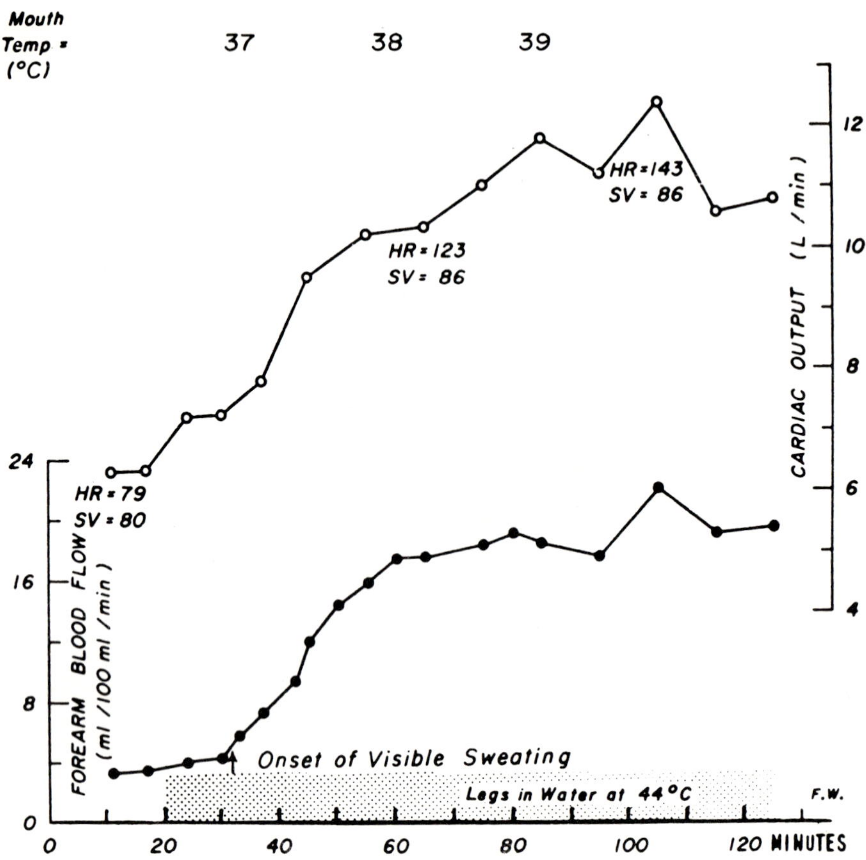

FIG. 5–32. Changes in cardiac output and forearm blood flow during body heating. The increase in forearm blood flow is due solely to an increase in blood flow in the skin of the forearm. (From Koroxenides et al.: *J. Appl. Physiol.,* 16:869, 1961.)

veins in the skin. This local effect of cooling is reinforced by a reflex increase in sympathetic activity emanating from cold receptors in the skin. The cutaneous venoconstriction decreases heat loss not only by reducing the venous surface area but it also directs venous flow through the deep veins which run alongside arteries so that transfer of heat takes place. Such a countercurrent exchange creates a thermal short-circuit that carries some of the arterial heat back to the body. If, despite these peripheral constrictions, the temperature of the blood reaching the hypothalamus is decreased, vasoconstriction occurs in the parts of the body surface which are not directly exposed to the cold. In addition, a general reaction is initiated whereby the subject usually engages in voluntary muscle activity to increase heat production; the latter may be reinforced by involuntary waves of contraction of skeletal muscles (shivering). There is also an endocrine reaction with secretion of hormones (e.g., epinephrine) which augments the metabolic rate of the tissues (Fig. 5–31). The shivering–metabolic part of the response to cold originates in the posterior hypothalamus, and the other adjustments are initiated in the anterior part.

Fever

When the setpoint of the hypothalamic thermostat is reset at a higher level, the resulting cutaneous vasoconstriction and shivering cause an increase in blood temperature (fever). This in turn initiates an increase in heart rate by a direct effect on the sinus node (p. 99) and by inhibition of the cardioinhibitory center. As the fever subsides, the opposite changes occur.

Muscle Contraction

Two neural control mechanisms are involved in the cardiovascular response to muscular contraction: (1) The higher centers in the brain that initiate the

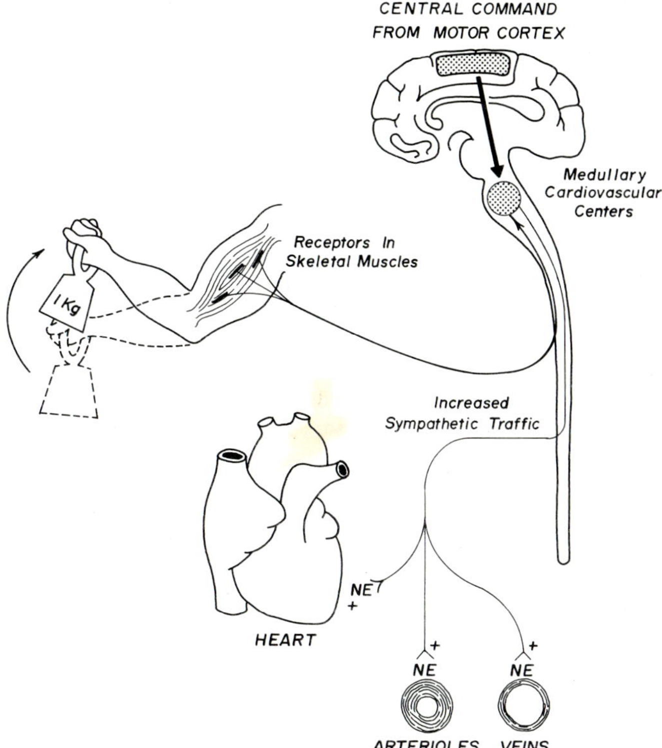

FIG. 5–33. The cardiovascular response to contraction of skeletal muscles is coordinated by the medullary centers, which receive signals from the higher centers that initiate the voluntary movement and from receptors which sense the degree of activity of the contracting muscles. The sympathetic activity to heart and blood vessels is increased. The heart rate and contractility are augmented and the splanchnic and kidney vessels constricted. These adjustments permit the increase in cardiac output to be distributed preferentially to the active muscles where vessels are dilated by the local accumulation of metabolites. NE = norepinephrine.

contraction alter the output of the medullary cardiovascular centers. The site of the former and the way they are connected to the latter is unknown. (2) Receptors, probably free nerve endings in the skeletal muscles, sense the degree of activity of the latter and signal it, through myelinated and unmyelinated afferent fibers of small diameter, to the spinal cord and the medullary centers. It is not known whether these receptors are activated by muscle tension or by the chemical events in the contracting muscle. These two mechanisms combine to maintain or increase the perfusion pressure to the active muscle. They also contribute to the adjustment of ventilation during exercise (Fig. 5–33).

Reflexes From Other Areas

Cardiovascular responses can be elicited by stimulation of a variety of other body structures. Of these, only the reflexes originating from the trigeminal area (nasal and facial receptors) appear to play a significant role (p. 165).

Selectivity of Cardiovascular Reflexes

So far in this section the separate roles of the various receptors involved in regulation of the cardiovascular system have been described. When one of these is activated, there is not a uniform change in nervous activity to all components of the cardiovascular system. Qualitative and quantitative differences occur. An example of the former is stimulation of the receptors at the venoatrial junctions causing a specific increase in the sympathetic outflow to the sinus node, whereas that to the kidney is decreased. Another example is chemoreceptor stimulation when the sympathetic outflow to most vascular beds is increased but that to the cutaneous veins is decreased. Quantitative differences are found between the cardiac receptors, which are subserved by unmyelinated vagal afferents and influence the kidney vessels more than those of skeletal muscle, and the arterial mechanoreceptors for which the opposite is true. In man the arterial mechanoreceptors predominate in the control of splanchnic as compared to skeletal muscle vessels, whereas the cardiopulmonary receptors have their major influence on the latter. These differences teach us that each of the peripheral inputs to the medullary cardiovascular centers connects with a specific combination of neurons to provide a response appropriate for combating the perturbation of the system.

INTERACTIONS BETWEEN THE CARDIOVASCULAR AND RESPIRATORY SYSTEMS

An increase in heart rate occurs during inspiration and a slowing during expiration. This is due to a variation in the depolarization frequency of the sinus node caused largely by alterations in vagal activity (Fig. 5–16) and is called respiratory sinus arrhythmia. It is most marked in children and young

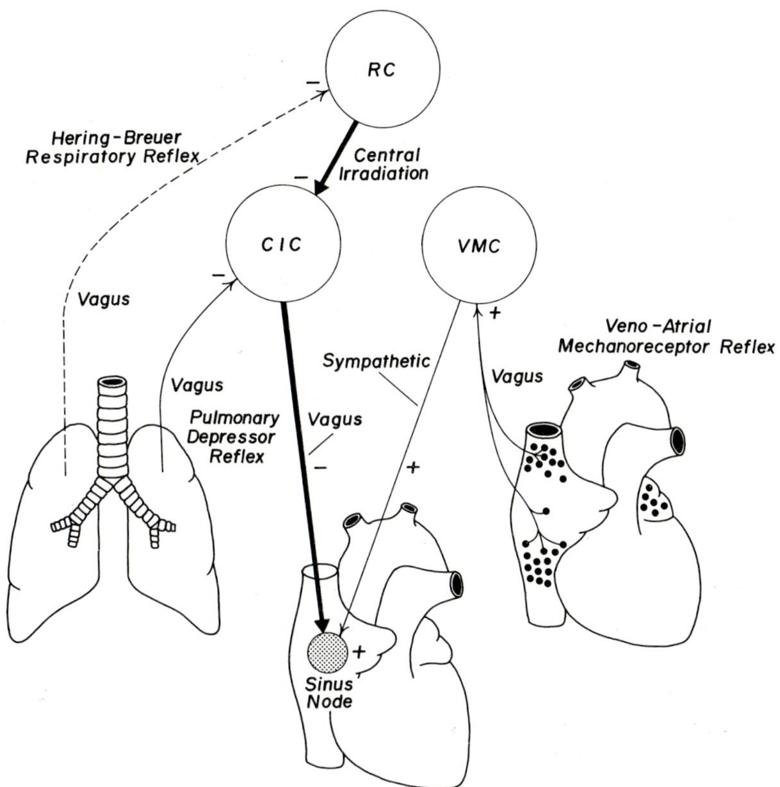

FIG. 5–34. Respiratory sinus arrhythmia. Postulated mechanisms causing quickening of the heart rate during inspiration. (For details see text). Toward the end of inspiration, the lung expansion activates the Hering–Breuer respiratory reflex, which in turn inhibits the respiratory centers. During the resultant expiration the heart slows. RC = respiratory centers. CIC = cardioinhibitory center (nucleus ambiguus and dorsal nucleus of the vagus). VMC = vasomotor center, + = activation, − = depression.

adults. Three mechanisms could explain the increase in heart rate with inspiration (Fig. 5–34): (1) reflex inhibition of the cardioinhibitory center (vagal nucleus) by the slowly adapting stretch receptors in the lungs; (2) central irradiation of inhibitory impulses from the respiratory centers to the cardioinhibitory center; (3) increased filling of the right atrium during inspiration, which activates mechanoreceptors at the junction of the great veins with the right atrium, with a resultant increase in sympathetic activity to the sinus node (p. 137).

The arterial blood pressure also fluctuates with respiration, rising during inspiration and decreasing with expiration. This is due mainly to the increased filling of the right heart caused by the lowered intrathoracic pressure during inspiration (p. 87). This increases the right ventricular and consequently the left ventricular stroke volume. A change in the set point of the arterial baroreceptors with respiration contributes to the blood pressure fluctuation.

INTERACTIONS BETWEEN CARDIOVASCULAR REFLEXES AND BLOOD VOLUME CONTROL

In health the total blood volume remains remarkably constant. The plasma volume continuously exchanges with the interstitial fluid volume through hydrostatic and osmotic forces (p. 82); together they form the extracellular fluid volume whose amount is determined by the balance of fluid intake by the gastrointestinal tract and fluid loss through the kidneys, lungs, and skin. Specialized groups of cells of the hypothalamus play a central role in regulating this fluid balance (Fig. 5–35):

1. *Osmoreceptors:* When the osmoreceptors, situated in the anterior hypothalamus, are stimulated by increased osmotic pressure of the body fluids, they initiate thirst and drinking, and trigger the release of antidiuretic hormone. The osmoreceptor cells can be activated by as little as a 2% increase in plasma osmolarity.

2. *Angiotensin II receptors:* If the plasma volume decreases without a change

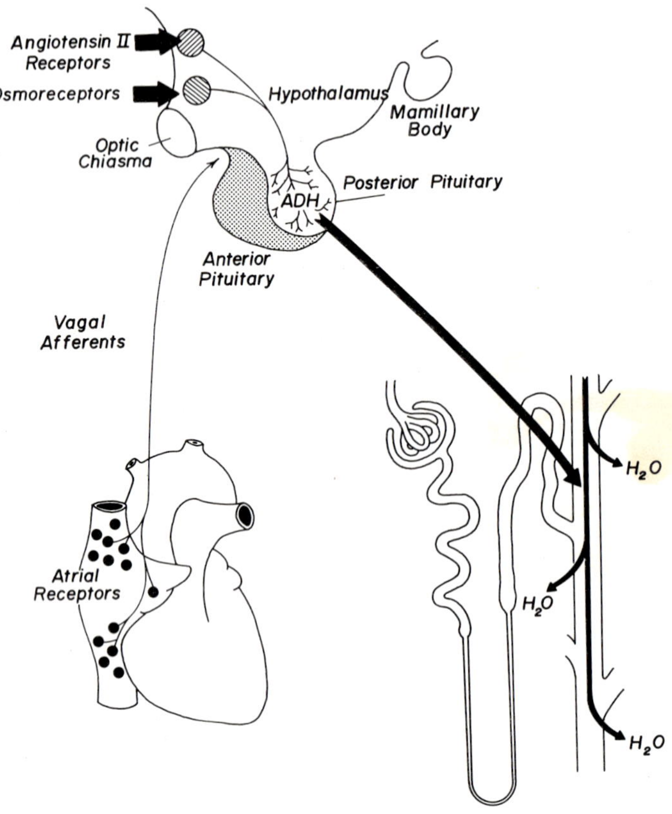

Fig. 5–35. Factors acting on the hypothalamus to modulate the secretion of antidiuretic hormone which regulates the resorption of water by the kidney and hence alters the urinary volume.

in its osmolarity, as occurs in hemorrhage, there is an increased secretion of renin from the kidneys and formation of angiotensin II. The circulating angiotensin II acts on specialized receptor cells located around the third and fourth ventricles, outside the blood–brain barrier, and stimulate the hypothalamic areas concerned with thirst and the release of antidiuretic hormone.

3. *Supraoptic and paraventricular nuclei:* The hormones of the posterior pituitary gland, oxytocin, and antidiuretic hormone (vasopressin) are synthesized in the cell bodies of neurons in the supraoptic and paraventricular nuclei. The nonapeptides are transported along the axons of these neurons to the posterior part of the pituitary gland where each is stored bound to polypeptides called neurophysins. When antidiuretic hormone is released into the bloodstream and reaches the cells of the collecting ducts of the kidney, it augments the intracellular levels of cyclic 3′,5′-adenosine monophosphate (p. 48). In an unknown way this results in an increase in the permeability of the collecting ducts so that water enters the hypertonic interstitium of the renal pyramids. As a consequence water is retained in excess of solute.

The release of antidiuretic hormone into the bloodstream is initiated not only when the hypothalamus senses an increased osmolarity of the extracellular fluid or increased plasma levels of angiotensin II, but also when the mechanoreceptors signal a decrease in blood volume. Due to their great distensibility the atria are especially suited to signal the degree of filling of the vascular system, and the large unencapsulated endings at the venous–atrial junctions are the prime sensors of small changes in blood volume (p. 135). With larger volume changes (e.g., during hemorrhage) all the mechanoreceptors participate. Release of antidiuretic hormone also occurs in other situations where the central blood volume is abruptly decreased, such as on changing from the supine to the upright position or with positive-pressure breathing. Conversely, its secretion is inhibited and more urine is formed (diuresis) when the central blood volume is increased, as seen by expansion of the blood volume, when the gravity decreases (p. 161), or when the body is immersed in water.

INTERACTIONS BETWEEN CARDIOVASCULAR AND ENDOCRINE CONTROL

Several hormones which play their major role in the regulation of other body functions also affect the cardiovascular system. Among the most important are:

1. *Insulin:* Insulin increases the oxygen uptake and the glucose consumption of cardiac and vascular muscle.

2. *Glucagon:* Glucagon has a positive inotropic effect on the heart and causes dilatation of most vascular beds, in particular the coronaries and the splanchnic area, with a resulting decrease in peripheral resistance. The cardiovascular effects of glucagon are due to activation of the enzyme adenyl cyclase, which augments the intracellular level of cyclic 3′,5′-adenosine monophosphate (p. 48).

3. *Thyroxine:* Thyroxine stimulates the oxygen consumption and the metabolism of cardiac and smooth muscle cells. It augments the heart rate in part by a direct effect on the sinus node. In the heart and the blood vessels thyroxine augments and prolongs the response to catecholamines.

4. *Gastrointestinal hormones:* The hormones which regulate gastrointestinal function (gastrin, cholecystokinin, and secretin) cause vasodilatation of the splanchnic blood vessels. In part this is secondary to the increased activity of the gastrointestinal wall and the release of 5-hydroxytryptamine (p. 101).

5. *Corticosteroids:* Aldosterone and higher concentrations of cortisol and deoxycorticosterone promote the Na^+ reabsorption and K^+ excretion by the kidney tubules. The increased reabsorption of Na^+ is accompanied by that of water. Hypersecretion of aldosterone affects the cardiovascular system by causing hypervolemia and water-logging of the vascular wall. In addition, the corticosteroids augment and prolong the action of the catecholamines because they inhibit their extraneuronal uptake (p. 117).

6. *Estrogens:* Female sex hormones, particularly estrogens, increase the distensibility of the vascular wall, inhibit the contractility of vascular smooth muscle cells, and reduce the peripheral release of norepinephrine. These effects help explain the increase in venous compliance seen during pregnancy and in women taking oral contraceptives.

SELECTED REFERENCES

Abboud, F. M., Heistad, D. D., Mark, A. L., and Schmid, P. G. (1976): Reflex control of the peripheral circulation. *Prog. Cardiovasc. Dis.*, 18:371.

Altura, B. M., and Altura, B. T. (1977): Influence of sex hormones, oral contraceptives and pregnancy on vascular muscle and its reactivity. In: *Factors Influencing Vascular Reactivity,* edited by O. Carrier Jr. and S. Shibata. Igaku-Shoin, Tokyo.

Antonaccio, M. J. (1977): Neuropharmacology of central mechanisms governing the circulation. In: *Cardiovascular Pharmacology.* Raven Press, New York.

Bevan, J. A. (1978): Norepinephrine and the presynaptic control of adrenergic transmitter release. *Fed. Proc.*, 37:187.

Brengelmann, G. (1970): Temperature regulation. In: *Physiological and Behavioral Temperature Regulation,* edited by J. D. Hardy, A. P. Gagge, and J. A. J. Stolwijk, p. 105. Charles C Thomas, Springfield, Ill.

Coleridge, H., and Coleridge, J. (1972): Cardiovascular receptors. In: *Modern Trends in Physiology,* Vol. 1, edited by C. B. B. Downman, p. 245. Appleton-Century-Crofts, New York.

Donald, D. E., and Shepherd, J. T. (1978): Reflexes from the heart and lungs: Physiological curiosities or important regulatory mechanisms. *Cardiovasc. Res.*, 12:449.

Feigl, E. O. (1969): Parasympathetic control of coronary blood flow in dogs. *Circ. Res.*, 25:509.

Ferrario, C. M., Gildenberg, P. L., and McCubbin, J. W. (1972): Cardiovascular effects of angiotensin mediated by the central nervous system. *Circ. Res.*, 30:257.

Ganong, W. F., Rudolph, C. D., and Zimmermann, H. (1979): Neuroendocrine components in the regulation of blood pressure and renin secretion. *Hypertension,* 1:207.

Gauer, O. H., and Henry, J. P. (1976): Neurohormonal control of plasma volume. In: *International Review of Physiology, Cardiovascular Physiology II.* Vol. 9, edited by A. C. Guyton and A. W. Cowley Jr., p. 145. University Park Press, Baltimore.

Hayward, J. N. (1977): Functional and morphological aspects of hypothalamic neurons. *Physiol. Rev.*, 57:574.

Heistad, D. D., and Marcus, M. L. (1978): Evidence that neural mechanisms do not have important effects on cerebral blood flow. *Circ. Res.*, 42:295.

Higgins, C. B., Vatner, S. F., and Braunwald, E. (1973): Parasympathetic control of the heart. *Pharmacol. Rev.,* 25:119.

James, T. N., Urthaler, F., Hageman, G. R., and Isobe, J. H. (1978): Further analysis of components in a cardiogenic hypertensive chemoreflex. In: *Neural Mechanisms in Cardiac Arrhythmias,* edited by P. J. Schwartz, A. M. Brown, A. Malliani, and A. Zanchetti, p. 251. Raven Press, New York.

Kirchheim, H. R. (1976): Systemic arterial baroreceptor reflexes. *Physiol. Rev.,* 56:100.

Korner, P. I. (1971): Integrative neural cardiovascular control. *Physiol. Rev.,* 51:312.

Linden, R. J. (1975): Reflexes from the heart. *Prog. Cardiovasc. Dis.,* 18:201.

Mancia, G., Lorenz, R. R., and Shepherd, J. T. (1976): Reflex control of circulation by heart and lungs. In: *International Review of Physiology, Cardiovascular Physiology II.* Vol. 9, edited by A. C. Guyton and A. W. Cowley Jr., p. 111. University Park Press, Baltimore.

Oparil, S., and Haber, E. (1974): The renin-angiotensin system. *N. Engl. J. Med.,* 291:389, 446.

Paintal, A. S. (1973). Vagal sensory receptors and their reflex effects. *Physiol. Rev.,* 53:159.

Purves, M. J., editor (1975): *The Peripheral Arterial Chemoreceptors.* Cambridge University Press, Cambridge.

Sagawa, K., Kumada, M., and Schramm, L. P. (1974): Nervous control of the circulation. In: *International Review of Physiology, Cardiovascular Physiology, I.* Vol. 1, edited by A. C. Guyton and C. E. Jones, p. 197. University Park Press, Baltimore.

Shepherd, J. T. (1963): *Physiology of the Circulation in Human Limbs in Health and Disease.* Saunders, Philadelphia.

Shepherd, J. T., Lorenz, R. R., Tyce, G. M., and Vanhoutte, P. M. (1978): Acetylcholine-inhibition of transmitter release from adrenergic nerve terminals mediated by muscarinic receptors. *Fed. Proc.,* 37:191.

Shepherd, J. T., and Vanhoutte, P. M. (1975): Skeletal muscle blood flow: neurogenic determinants. In: *The Peripheral Circulation,* edited by R. Zelis, p. 3. Grune & Stratton, New York.

Thorén, P. (1979): Role of cardiac vagal C-fibers in cardiovascular control. In: *Reviews of Physiology, Pharmacology and Biochemistry.* Springer-Verlag, Heidelberg *(in press).*

Vanhoutte, P. M. (1978): Heterogeneity in vascular smooth muscle. In: *Microcirculation,* edited by G. Kaley and B. M. Altura, Vol. II, p. 181. University Park Press, Baltimore.

Vanhoutte, P. M. (1978): Adrenergic neuroeffector interaction in the blood vessel wall. *Fed. Proc.,* 37:181.

Vatner, S. F., and Braunwald, E. (1975): Cardiovascular control mechanisms in the conscious state. *N. Engl. J. Med.,* 293:970.

Whelan, R. F. (1967): *Control of the Peripheral Circulation in Man.* Charles C Thomas, Springfield, Ill.

Zanchetti, A. S. (1977): Neural regulation of renin release: Experimental evidence and clinical implications in arterial hypertension. *Circulation,* 56:691.

6

Integrated Responses of the Cardiovascular System to Stress

In daily life humans encounter various stresses and are engaged in a variety of activities. All require rapid adjustments of cardiovascular function.

EMOTION

The cardiovascular responses to acute emotional stress are due to activation of the corticohypothalamic brain centers and vary depending on the severity of the stress and the disposition of the individual. The hypothalamus connects with the medullary cardiovascular centers, and also controls the cholinergic outflow to skeletal muscles and sweat glands. With emotion the following changes are usually seen (Fig. 6–1):

1. *Heart:* The heart rate and contractility increase, with an increase in cardiac output, in response to increased sympathetic and decreased vagal activity.

2. *Resistance vessels:* The blood flow to the skeletal muscles is increased. In the human this is due to activation of cholinergic vasodilator fibers and to the release of epinephrine by the adrenal medulla. The kidney and the splanchnic flow decrease because of increased sympathetic activity and circulating epinephrine. The skin blood flow does not change, except for those subjects who develop emotional sweating in the hands and feet where a consequent increase in flow

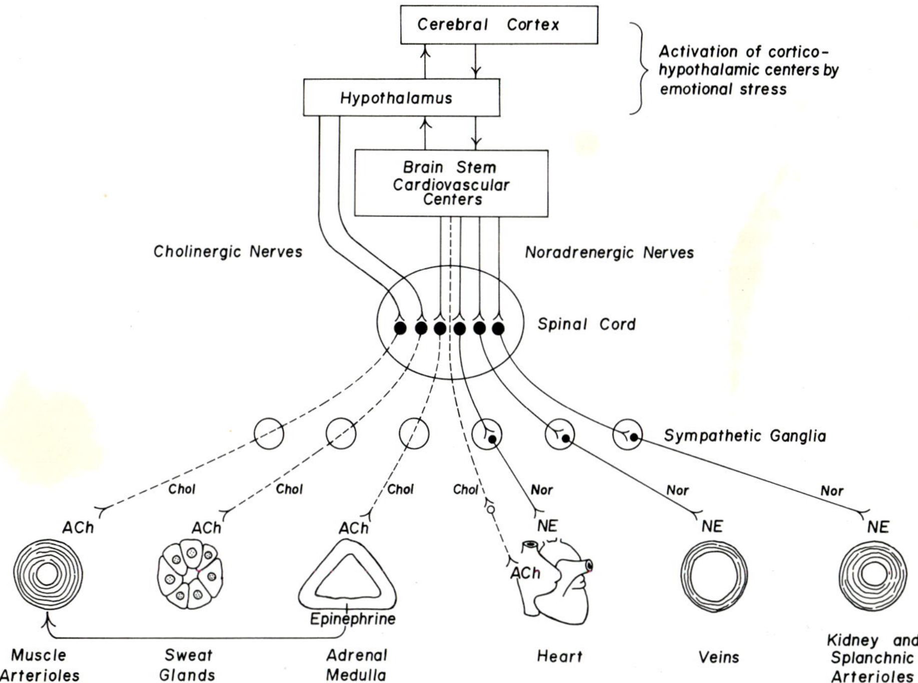

FIG. 6–1. Cardiovascular response to emotional stress involves: (1) increased activity of cholinergic fibers (Chol) to muscle arterioles causing their dilatation, (2) increased activity of cholinergic fibers to the sweat glands causing sweating and skin vasodilatation (p. 102), (3) increased activity of the preganglionic sympathetic fibers to the adrenal medulla causing secretion of epinephrine into the bloodstream which reinforces the dilatation of the muscle arterioles (Fig. 5–10), (4) reduced activity of the vagal nerve and increased activity of the sympathetic postganglionic fibers (Nor) to the heart, resulting in increased heart rate and contractility, (5) increased sympathetic outflow to the capacitance vessels causing their constriction, and (6) increased sympathetic outflow to the renal and splanchnic resistance vessels causing their constriction. ACh = acetylcholine, NE = norepinephrine.

occurs (p. 104). When the emotion involves embarrassment, abrupt dilatation occurs in the face (blushing) the mechanism of which is unknown; it may be due to the release of kinins which follows the activation of cholinergic fibers to the sweat glands (Fig. 4–14). The total systemic vascular resistance increases or decreases depending on the balance between these individual changes. The arterial blood pressure usually increases.

3. *Capacitance vessels:* The cutaneous veins are constricted, and the splanchnic capacitance is decreased.

These various changes, which prepare the body to take action, resemble the changes seen with exercise. The emotional component may persist during the physical activity and help determine the cardiovascular adaptation during the latter. The most typical example is the rise in blood pressure seen during intercourse, the amplitude of which depends on the emotional involvement.

Another response to emotional stress is characterized in certain susceptible subjects by a sudden slowing of the heart (increased vagal activity) at the time the skeletal muscle vessels dilate. This combination causes an abrupt fall in blood pressure and loss of consciousness (vasovagal syncope; p. 266). Similar responses (fight-or-flight reaction) have been identified in the animal; the hypothalamus plays the central role in their genesis.

The nature of the emotional trigger can vary widely in different people and even in the same person on different occasions. Subjects under hypnosis show similar hemodynamic changes when fear or anger are induced.

CHANGES IN GRAVITATIONAL FORCES

Increased Gravity

Standing

When changing from a lying to a standing position, about 20% of the blood in the heart and lungs is displaced to the legs. The venous filling of the heart is less, and as a consequence the cardiac output is decreased. The resultant unloading of the cardiopulmonary mechanoreceptors leads to tachycardia, constriction of the systemic resistance vessels, and an active and passive decrease in splanchnic capacitance. Despite the compensatory increase in heart rate, the cardiac output during quiet standing is less than during rest in the supine position. However, the arterial blood pressure is maintained because of the reflex constriction of the peripheral blood vessels (Fig. 6–2).

In the lungs the interrelationships between pressures in the pulmonary artery, the alveoli, and the pulmonary veins determine the force available for perfusing the pulmonary capillaries. When lying, the pressure in the pulmonary artery and veins exceeds the alveolar pressure in all parts of the lung, so the pressure available for lung perfusion is the difference in pressure between the pulmonary artery and the veins. When standing, because of gravitational forces acting on the blood vessels within the lungs, the pressure in the pulmonary artery and veins is decreased at the apex of the lungs and increases progressively from the apex to the base. The alveolar pressure remains the same throughout the lungs. Toward the apex of the lung the pulmonary artery pressure, although reduced, still exceeds the alveolar pressure. However, the latter is greater than that in the pulmonary veins, and as a consequence the blood flow through the pulmonary capillaries in the apex is determined by the difference between the pressure in the pulmonary artery and that in the alveoli. Toward the base of the lung the pulmonary artery and vein pressures exceed the alveolar pressure; hence the latter is not a determinant of the perfusion pressure in this area (Fig. 6–3).

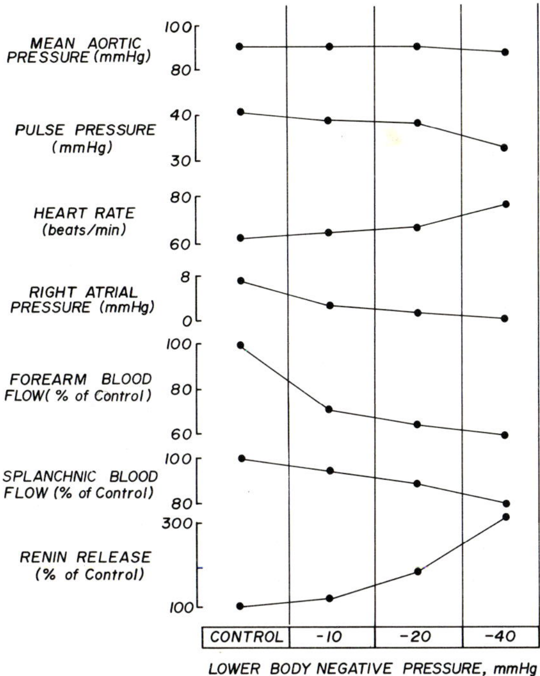

FIG. 6–2. When a normal person changes from the supine position to standing upright, about 300 to 800 ml blood moves to the lower limbs. The cardiac output is reduced by 1.0 to 2.5 liters/min. The heart rate increases, and the stroke volume decreases. A convenient method of studying the effects of displacement of blood from the heart and lungs to the legs is to apply negative pressure to the lower half of the body. As the filling pressure of the heart (right atrial pressure) and cardiac output decrease, the systemic arterial blood pressure is maintained by reflex constriction of the systemic resistance vessels, as illustrated by the decreased forearm and splanchnic blood flow. There is an increase in heart rate and in the release of renin from the kidneys. These reflex changes with negative pressures up to 20 mm Hg are due mainly to the lessened inhibition of the vasomotor center by the cardiopulmonary mechanoreceptors. The arterial baroreceptors play a minor role since the arterial mean and pulse pressure are only slightly decreased. However, when the negative pressure is increased to 40 mm Hg and more pooling of blood occurs, the aortic pulse and mean pressure decrease and the reduced input from the arterial baroreceptor to the medullary cardiovascular centers reinforces that from the cardiopulmonary receptors, causing a greater increase in heart rate, cardiac contractility, and renin release, and further constriction of the systemic resistance vessels and veins. (Data from Fasola and Martz: *Aerospace Med.,* 43:713, 1972; Johnson et al.: *Circ. Res.,* 34:515, 1974; and Zoller et al.: *J. Clin. Invest.,* 51:2967, 1972.)

Acceleration

With an increase in gravity as seen during acceleration, the cardiovascular effects are due to the resulting changes in the weight of blood. The body may be exposed to three types of acceleration: (1) Radial acceleration, when a constant speed is maintained despite a change in direction. This occurs during centrifuga-

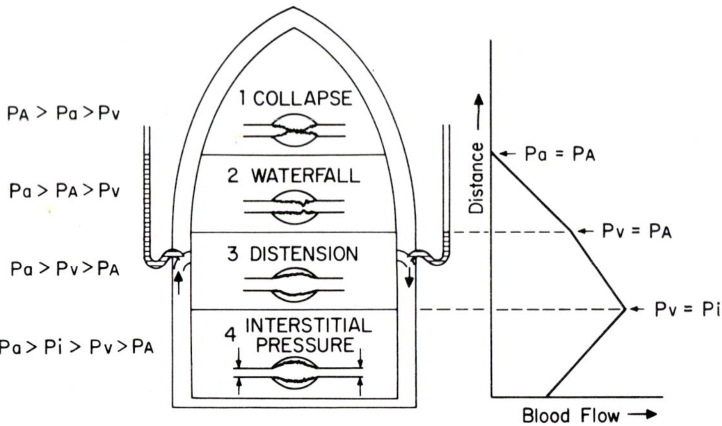

FIG. 6–3. In the upright position there is an uneven distribution of pulmonary blood flow. This is due to the increase in hydrostatic pressure from the apex to the base of the lung (approximately 1 cm H_2O/cm distance) and to the fact that the pulmonary vessels are not rigid tubes. If they were, they would behave like siphons and blood flow would be uniform throughout the lung. Blood flow distribution depends therefore on the relation between pulmonary arterial pressure (P_a), pulmonary venous pressure (P_v), alveolar pressure (P_A), and interstitial pressure (P_i). In the main pulmonary artery the mean pressure is about 15 mm Hg, at the apex of the lung about 4 mm Hg, and at the base about 26 mm Hg. Four zones can be recognized: (1) The pressure in the pulmonary alveoli is greater than that in the pulmonary vessels, the capillaries are collapsed, and there is no flow. (2) The pressure in the pulmonary artery exceeds that in the alveoli, so blood flow increases progressively through this zone. The pressure in the alveoli exceeds the pulmonary venous pressure, so the flow is independent of the latter. Hence the descriptive term "alveolar waterfall." (3) The pulmonary venous pressure exceeds the alveolar pressure, so flow is now proportional to pulmonary artery pressure minus pulmonary venous pressure, and not as in zone 2 to pulmonary artery pressure minus alveolar pressure. The pulmonary blood flow increases throughout zone 3 owing to the increasing hydrostatic pressure distending the blood vessels. (4) The interstitial pressure (P_i) increases toward the base of the lung, and if it exceeds the pulmonary venous pressure, then the pulmonary artery pressure minus the interstitial pressure determines the blood flow. (From Lenfant: In: *Physiology and Biophysics. II. Circulation, Respiration and Fluid Balance,* edited by Ruch and Patton, p. 351. Saunders, Philadelphia, 1974.)

tion or when a pilot pulls his plane out of a dive. (2) Linear acceleration, when an increase in velocity is obtained without a change in direction. (3) Angular acceleration, when an increase in speed is combined with a change in direction. In response to these three types of acceleration, a reactive force results from the inertia of the body proportional to the mass of the latter and the magnitude of the acceleration. This force acts in the direction opposite to that of the accelerating force and becomes apparent as an increase in weight.

In man the effects of acceleration are most pronounced when the direction is parallel to the long axis of the body (head-to-foot or foot-to-head) and less pronounced when perpendicular to the latter (transverse acceleration). Thus when sitting in an environment of normal gravity (1 *g*), if the systolic pressure in the left ventricle is 120 mm Hg, it would be about 96 mm Hg at the base of the brain and about 170 mm Hg in the feet. By contrast, if the gravity is augmented five times (5 *g*) in the direction of head to foot, the weight of the blood is five times as great and all hydrostatic pressure differences are increased fivefold. Thus with the same ventricular pressure of 120 mm Hg, the pressure at the base of the skull will now be 0 and at the feet about 370 mm Hg. With the rapid onset of such acceleration, the resulting decrease in arterial pressure to the brain causes a loss of vision and unconsciousness. If the gravitational stress is continued, the heart rate and arterial pressure increase, presumably because of reflexes initiated by the carotid sinus mechanoreceptors. The cardiac output remains decreased secondary to the decrease in stroke volume resulting from the pooling of blood in the veins of the extremities. In the abdomen little pooling occurs because the content of the gastrointestinal tract is submitted to the same gravitational load as the blood. The footward displacement of the abdominal contents, particularly the liver, pulls down the diaphragm and limits its normal movements during respiration, thus indirectly affecting venous return (p. 87).

With transverse acceleration, the cardiovascular consequences are slight, except in the lungs where there is redistribution of blood to the dorsal parts. For this reason spacecraft are designed with the crew exposed to transverse acceleration rather than to headward increases in gravity. During "blast-off" the reactive force is from the front to the back ("eyeballs-in" acceleration) and for 1 to 2 min the astronauts are exposed to about 10 *g*. The increased weight of the blood may temporarily occlude the alveoli in the dorsal regions of the lungs, resulting in desaturation of the arterial blood.

Space Flight and Weightlessness

During space flight the cardiovascular effects of weightlessness are similar to those of water immersion. During blast off the space traveler is subjected to gravitational stresses. When zero gravity is reached, the blood from the lower body is displaced to the upper part of the body. This is manifest to the crew by a feeling of fullness of the head, congestion of the nasal sinuses, distention of the neck veins, and puffiness of the face, especially in the periorbital region. The vascular resistance in the legs is decreased, and the limb veins are more distensible. Adaptation occurs by diuresis and reduced fluid intake, so the plasma volume is decreased; the red cell volume also decreases so the hematocrit is unchanged. As a consequence, the intrathoracic volume is restored to normal, whereas the total blood volume is decreased by about 16% (Fig. 6–4). On return to earth gravity, the blood is redistributed to the lower limbs. The central blood volume and the heart volume are reduced. The filling pressure of the heart and the stroke volume are less, and the resting heart rate faster, than before the space flight. As a result, there is a reduced tolerance for standing upright, and fainting may occur. The increased thirst and fluid intake and the increased water and sodium reabsorption by the renal tubules restore the extracel-

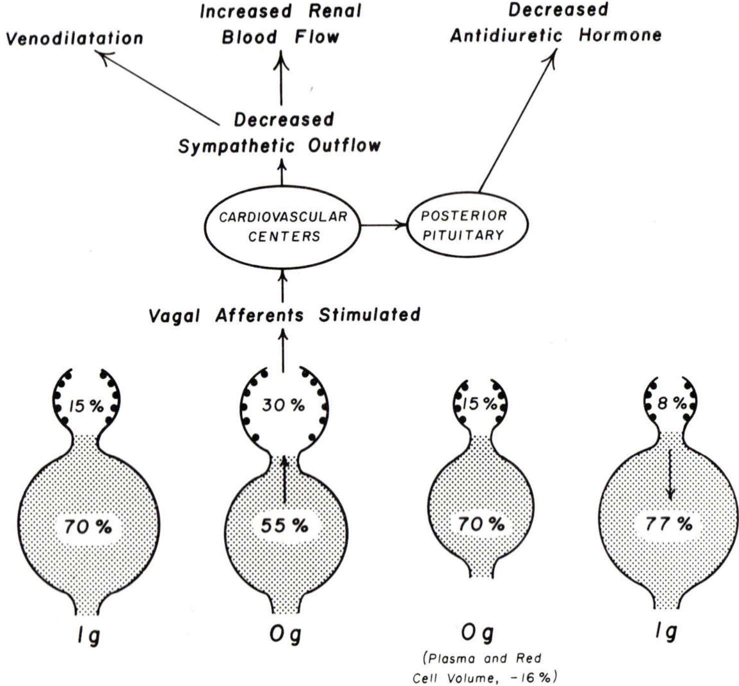

FIG. 6–4. Blood volume adjustments to weightlessness (zero gravity; 0*g*). The dotted area of each schematic represents the percent of the total blood volume in the systemic veins, and the clear area above it the percent in the heart and lungs. During space flight the shift of blood from the systemic veins to the heart and lungs at the onset of weightlessness activates the cardiopulmonary mechanoreceptors (●). As a result, less water is reabsorbed by the renal tubules and there is diuresis, which is attributed to decreased release of antidiuretic hormone from the posterior pituitary. The increased renal blood flow and the increased glomerular filtration caused by the decreased sympathetic outflow to the kidney contributes to the diuresis. There is decreased sodium reabsorption (natriuresis). Part of the natriuresis may be due to decreased renin release and hence less circulating aldosterone. As a result of these adjustments, the plasma volume is decreased by about 16%. By unknown mechanisms the red blood cell volume is decreased by a similar amount, so the hematocrit is unchanged. On return to earth's gravitational field *(right)* the total blood volume is reduced so relatively more blood is pooled in the dependent parts on standing, and the arterial blood pressure may fall (postural hypotension).

lular fluid and plasma volume within a few hours. The restoration of the red cell volume is slower but is completed within 2 weeks or less.

Similar changes occur with continuous bed rest of more than 6 to 8 weeks.

ALTITUDE

At altitudes above sea level the barometric pressure decreases and the oxygen concentration in the air is diminished. Increased ventilation, which leads to a more rapid removal of carbon dioxide and to an increased partial pressure of oxygen in the alveoli, is the most important mechanism used to compensate for the low atmospheric oxygen tension at high altitudes. At 2,000 meters above sea level the barometric pressure is decreased by 20% and the arterial Po_2 falls from 97 to 70 mm Hg, but cardiovascular function is not impaired. At 4,300 meters, with a 40% reduction in barometric pressure, the arterial Po_2 falls to 50 mm Hg, which causes temporary discomfort and reduced cardiovascular performance during mild exercise. After a few days of adaptive changes (acclimatization) the reduction in performance is seen only during more severe physical exertion. At 7,000 meters only well-acclimatized persons can tolerate the 60% reduction in arterial Po_2.

The ventilation is increased at higher altitudes in proportion to the reduction in barometric pressure because the reduced oxygen tension of the arterial blood stimulates the arterial chemoreceptors and leads to increased activity of the respiratory center in the medulla. Simultaneously there is a decrease in the carbon dioxide tension of the blood, as excessive amounts of this gas are eliminated by the increased ventilation. This, together with the resulting increase in the alkalinity of the blood, acts to oppose the increased respiratory drive by depressing the arterial chemoreceptors and the medullary respiratory center. Two mechanisms permit the increased respiratory drive to continue: (1) the pH of the cerebrospinal fluid bathing the respiratory center is restored to normal by the active transport of bicarbonate from this fluid to the blood by the cells forming the blood–brain barrier; and (2) excretion of excess bicarbonate by the kidneys returns the systemic blood pH toward normal.

During acclimatization the volume of red blood cells and plasma increases; the extra hemoglobin permits the oxygen content of the arterial blood to remain normal (about 20 ml oxygen/100 ml blood) at altitudes higher than sea level, although the percentage of saturated hemoglobin is decreased because of the reduced oxygen tension (Table 6–1).

At rest the cardiac output, systemic arterial blood pressure, and oxygen consumption in subjects acclimatized to altitude are similar to those in persons at sea level. With moderate exercise both groups show a similar increase in cardiac output and oxygen consumption for the same workload. Although the blood viscosity is increased, the systemic arterial blood pressure is not higher than during similar exercise at sea level. By contrast, when normal subjects at sea level are given air to breathe which is low in oxygen, the cardiac output for a given work load is greater since more blood must be delivered to the tissues to meet their increased oxygen requirements. This illustrates the sparing effect the additional hemoglobin has on the cardiac output in acclimatized subjects.

The main difference between subjects living at high altitudes and those at sea level is that during work which requires similar oxygen consumptions the stroke volume is less at high altitudes and the same cardiac output is achieved by a faster heart rate. The lesser stroke volume may be due to a depressant action of the chronic reduction in Po_2 on the myocardium. The maximal heart

TABLE 6–1. *Effect of altitude*[a]

Parameter	Effect according to altitude: 0 meters	2,000 meters	3,000 meters	4,300 meters
Barometric pressure (mm Hg)	760	600	523	450
Atmospheric PO_2 (mm Hg)	159	126	110	94
Alveolar PO_2 (mm Hg)	103	80	72	54
Arterial PO_2 (mm Hg)	97	70	65	50
Arterial PCO_2 (mm Hg)	41	38	36	34
Blood volume (ml/kg)	80	81	83	100
Hemoglobin (g/100 ml)	15	16	17	20
O_2 saturation (%)	97	96	91	81
O_2 content (ml/100 ml)	20	20	20.5	22
Mean pulmonary artery pressure (mm Hg)	13	16	25	28

Data are from Balke et al.: *Am. J. Cardiol.,* 14:796, 1964; Vogel et al.: *Med. Thorac.,* 19:461, 1962; and Comroe: *Physiology of Respiration,* 2nd ed., Year Book Medical Publishers, Chicago, 1974.

[a] For comparison the altitudes of various locations are as follows: Denver, Colorado, 1,600 meters; Mexico City, 2,200 meters; Leadville, Colorado, 3,000 meters; and Morococha, Peru, 4,500 meters.

rate is similar at high altitudes and sea level. Since the maximal stroke volume is diminished, the maximal cardiac output is less.

In people born and living at high altitudes, the mean pulmonary artery pressure is higher than at sea level because of the reduced oxygen tension (Table 6–1). The mean pressures in the pulmonary vein and the left atrium are normal. Since the blood flow through the lungs is normal, the increased pressure is due to increased resistance offered by the small vessels in the lungs. The contribution of the increased viscosity of the blood to the increase in resistance must be minor because people living at high altitudes, when taken to sea level, lose their excess red blood cells before the pulmonary artery pressure decreases. Natives of high altitudes retain the increased content of smooth muscle in their pulmonary arteries and arterioles which is present in all fetuses and neonates but at sea level regresses during the early months of life (p. 274).

In certain species (e.g., the cat and rabbit) the small pulmonary precapillary vessels constrict when the Po_2 in the alveolar air is low. This is a local effect of the decreased Po_2 on the smooth muscle, opposite to that seen in the systemic vessels. Many substances (e.g., 5-hydroxytryptamine, histamine, angiotensin II, and prostaglandins) have been suggested as mediators of this constriction, but the mechanism remains unknown. For the lung, it provides for efficient oxygenation of the blood by adjusting perfusion to ventilation. Thus if certain alveoli are underventilated, the blood flow to them is decreased and redistributed to the well-ventilated air sacs, avoiding a venoarterial shunt. The degree to which this mechanism operates in the human remains uncertain.

Susceptible subjects who exercise shortly after reaching higher altitudes develop pulmonary edema. The mechanism is not known.

DIVING

Mammals (including man), birds, and reptiles have the ability to redistribute their circulation during diving. This is due to the activation of two reflexes (Fig. 6–5):

1. *Trigeminal reflex*: When the face is immersed in water, the sensory endings of the trigeminal nerve are activated. This elicits a reflex cessation of respiration (apnea), vagal-induced bradycardia, and constriction of systemic vessels in the splanchnic region, skeletal muscles, and kidneys due to an increased activity in their sympathetic nerves. The splanchnic and cutaneous capacitance vessels constrict.

2. *Chemoreceptor reflex*: The apnea is followed quickly by a decrease in Po_2 and an increase in Pco_2 in the arterial blood, which stimulates the arterial chemoreceptors. The continued sensory input from the trigeminal nerve overrides

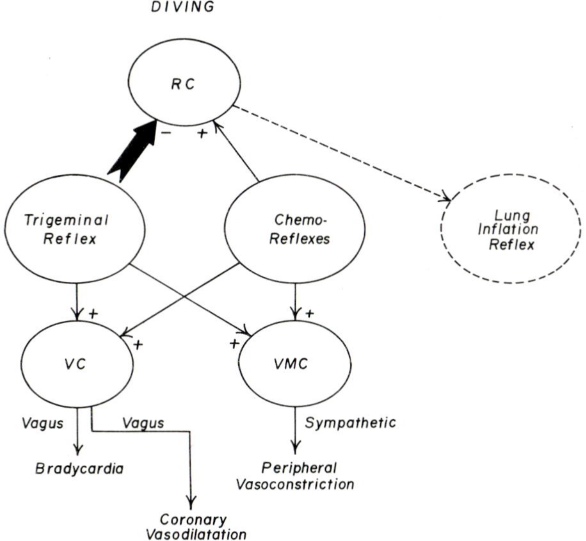

FIG. 6–5. During a dive the sensory endings of the trigeminal nerve are activated first. This initiates the trigeminal reflex, leading to cessation of respiration, and therefore eliminates the lung inflation reflex (p. 140). The trigeminal reflex also causes bradycardia by activating the vagal efferents to the sinus and atrioventricular nodes. By increasing sympathetic activity it causes constriction of the splanchnic resistance and capacitance vessels and of the resistance vessels of the kidney and the inactive muscles. The reflex bradycardia and vasoconstriction are reinforced by stimulation of the chemoreceptors from the changes in the blood gases. The coronary vessels dilate owing to activation of their cholinergic nerves. RC = respiratory center, VC = vagal center, VMC = vasomotor center, + = activation, − = depression.

the action of the chemoreceptors on the respiratory center. The circulatory effects of chemoreceptor stimulation augment those from the nose and face, leading to further cardiac slowing and constriction of systemic vessels. There is a reflex dilatation of the coronary arteries mediated by the vagal nerves. The arterial blood pressure is maintained, and the oxygen in the blood is made available to the most vulnerable systems, the heart and brain. The lactic acid formed and stored in the muscles during a prolonged dive floods into the circulation when breathing is resumed.

EXERCISE

Rhythmic Exercise

With the onset of rhythmic (isotonic) muscular exercise, a complex series of cardiovascular adjustments occur to ensure that: (1) the active muscles receive a blood supply appropriate to their increased metabolic needs; (2) the heat generated by the active muscles is eliminated; and (3) the blood supply to the brain and the heart is maintained (Fig. 6–6).

With the immediate dilatation of the resistance vessels in active muscle as a consequence of the sudden increase in metabolites surrounding them (p. 92), the systemic vascular resistance decreases in proportion to the muscle mass involved. To maintain arterial blood pressure there is an increase in sympathetic activity proportional to the work load. This causes constriction of the resistance vessels in the splanchnic bed and the kidneys (Fig. 6–7). These two beds are particularly suited for short-term adjustments of the systemic vascular resistance because their blood supply is greatly in excess of the metabolic requirements of their tissues, and their normal function can be temporarily held in abeyance. In nonworking muscles the resistance vessels constrict. In the working muscles the increasing level of metabolites progressively decreases the local release of norepinephrine and inhibits the vascular smooth muscle cells (Fig. 4–2). Thus the local modulation of the sympathetic outflow ensures that working muscles are perfused according to their needs while nonworking muscles contribute to the compensatory increase in resistance. The increased sympathetic outflow causes constriction of the splanchnic capacitance vessels, with active mobilization of blood from the liver, spleen, and intestinal veins. This, together with passive mobilization resulting from the arteriolar constriction, provides for an adequate filling pressure of the heart and maintenance or an increase of the stroke volume. The rate and contractility of the heart are augmented. The increased cardiac activity combines with the surge of venous blood from the contracting muscles (muscle pump) and the constricted capacitance vessels to augment the cardiac output in proportion to the metabolic requirements of the working muscles. As the cardiac output augments, there is a progressive increase in systemic arterial pressure. The increase in pulmonary blood flow with exercise causes a moderate increase in mean pulmonary artery pressure (Fig. 6–8). During pro-

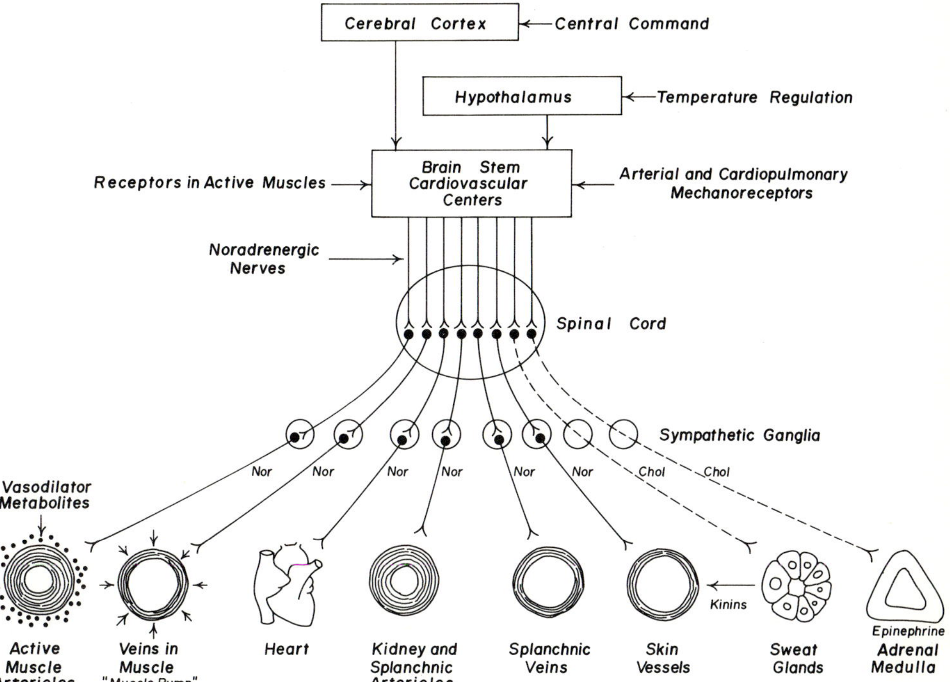

FIG. 6–6. Regulation of the circulation during exercise involves the following adaptations: (1) Local: The resistance vessels dilate in the active muscles owing to the products of muscle metabolism (Fig. 4–1). These products also disconnect the sympathetic nerves from the muscle vessels (Fig. 4–2). (2) Mechanical: During upright exercise the muscle pump returns blood from the lower limbs to the central circulation (Fig. 3–20). (3) Nervous: The sympathetic outflow to the heart and systemic blood vessels is increased. The vagal outflow to the heart decreases (not shown). This causes tachycardia, increased cardiac contractility, and constriction of the resistance vessels in the kidney and splanchnic bed, and of the splanchnic capacitance vessels. The increased sympathetic outflow is due in part to a "central command" from the cerebral cortex and to activation of receptors in the contracting skeletal muscles (Fig. 5–33). The arterial and cardiopulmonary mechanoreceptors prevent marked fluctuations in arterial pressure from normal values. As exercise continues and the body temperature begins to rise, the temperature-sensitive cells in the hypothalamus are activated; they then inhibit the sympathetic outflow to the skin vessels and stimulate the cholinergic fibers to the sweat glands. This results in dilatation of the skin vessels (Fig. 5–31). (4) Humoral: if exercise is severe, the cholinergic fibers to the adrenal medulla are activated and epinephrine is released into the bloodstream (Fig. 5–1). This enhances the heart rate and contractility as well as the constriction of the veins and the renal resistance vessels. Chol = cholinergic, Nor = adrenergic.

longed exercise the hemoglobin concentration of the blood increases consequent to a decrease in plasma volume resulting from the augmented exudation of fluid in the dilated muscle beds. This increases the oxygen-carrying capacity of the blood. The arterial and cardiopulmonary mechanoreceptors, the receptors in skeletal muscle, and the inputs from higher centers to the medullary cardiovas-

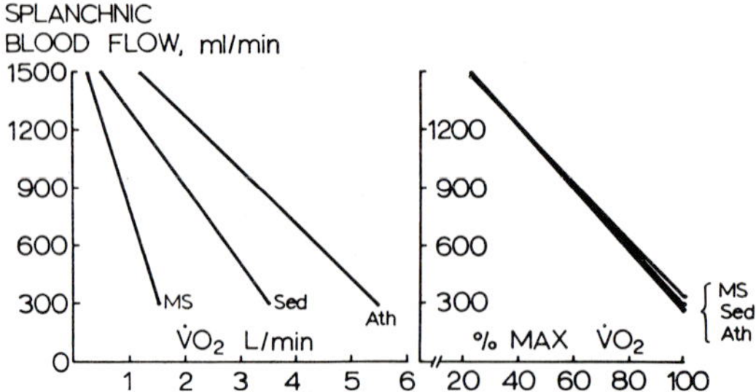

FIG. 6–7. Progressive reduction in splanchnic blood flow with increasing severity of exercise in normal sedentary young men (Sed), athletes (Ath), and patients with mitral stenosis (MS). The splanchnic viscera receive 20 to 25% of the total cardiac output at rest but extract only 10 to 25% of the available oxygen (Fig. 3–1). Thus they are well suited for reduction in blood flow without metabolic consequences and for redistribution of this flow to the working muscles during exercise. Each slope line on the left ends at the average maximal oxygen uptake of the group. On the right, slope lines become almost superimposed when oxygen uptake is expressed as the percent of maximal for each group. There is a similar relationship between renal blood flow and oxygen uptake during exercise. (From Rowell: In: *Physiology of Work Capacity and Fatigue,* edited by Simonson, p. 140. Charles C Thomas, Springfield, Ill., 1971.)

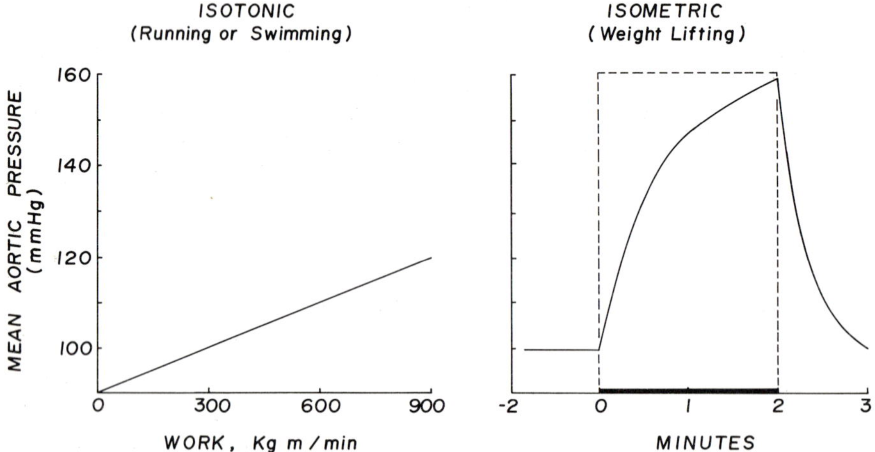

FIG. 6–8. Blood pressure response to isotonic (rhythmic) **(left)** and isometric (static) **(right)** exercise. During running or swimming there is only a moderate increase in mean aortic blood pressure since the increase in cardiac output is accompanied by a decrease in total systemic vascular resistance due to dilatation of the resistance vessels in the many active skeletal muscles. The mean pulmonary artery pressure also increases (e.g., from 12 to 18 mm Hg for an increase in oxygen consumption of about 2 liters/min). By contrast, during strong isometric exercise, as when lifting a heavy object, there is a very large increase in aortic blood pressure. Here the increase in cardiac output is not balanced by the decrease in systemic vascular resistance, since the isometrically contracting muscles mechanically impede the blood flow.

cular centers play a role in making these complex adjustments in autonomic outflow to the cardiovascular system (Fig. 6–6).

The heat generated by the active muscles causes the temperature of the blood to increase, leading to activation of the thermosensitive cells in the anterior hypothalamus which initiate dilatation of the skin vessels and sweating (p. 145). The larger blood flow to the skin necessitates a further increase in cardiac output and greater constriction of the renal resistance, splanchnic resistance, and splanchnic capacitance vessels (Fig. 6–9). This response results from an additional increase in sympathetic outflow mediated by the cardiovascular mechanoreceptors in response to the decreasing pressures in the vascular system as the skin vessels dilate.

In normal subjects the upper limit of rhythmic exercise is determined by the cardiovascular system, since neither ventilation, gas diffusion in the lungs, nor gas exchange in the capillary beds of the muscles are limiting factors. The cardiovascular performance is limited by the maximal increase in heart rate and stroke volume as well as the maximal ability to constrict resistance and capacitance vessels. It is modified by the position of the subject, the thermal environment, and the need to divert blood to tissues other than skin and muscle (e.g., during digestion, pregnancy). Differences in performance between individuals are determined by factors such as age, sex, and physical condition.

Body Position

During maximal exercise in the supine position, the stroke volume increases by 10 to 20% of the resting volume. The increase in cardiac output is due mainly to the acceleration of the heart. The maximal cardiac output usually is reached at frequencies in the range of 180 to 200 beats/min. At these heart rates the diastolic filling time is sufficient to permit the heart to maintain a

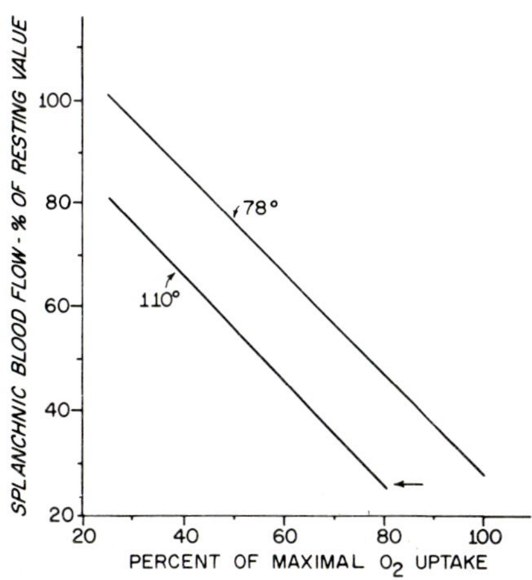

FIG. 6–9. Splanchnic blood flow in normal man during exercise as the percentage of resting splanchnic blood flow in neutral (78°F) and hot (110°F) environments *(ordinate).* The severity of the exercise is expressed as a percentage of the oxygen uptake during maximal exercise *(abscissa).* In both environments there is a progressive reduction in blood flow with increasing severity of exercise. In the heat there is a larger reduction in flow at equivalent work levels, indicating the stronger reflex constriction of the splanchnic resistance vessels to compensate for the greater dilation of the skin resistance vessels. (From Rowell: In: *Physiology and Biophysics. II. Circulation, Respiration and Fluid Balance,* edited by Ruch and Patton, p. 215. Saunders, Philadelphia, 1974.)

maximal stroke volume (p. 75). The blood volume in the heart and lungs remains relatively constant.

At the start of leg exercise in the upright position, the muscle pump returns blood from the legs to the thorax (p. 75), and the cardiac filling pressure and stroke volume increase to values approximating those at supine rest. Although the increase in cardiac output with moderate exercise is similar for a given oxygen consumption in supine and standing positions, the total cardiac output is less in the latter because the blood flow to the splanchnic bed and the kidneys is decreased. With maximal exercise the values for cardiac output become similar in upright and supine positions because maximal compensatory constrictions are reached in both situations (Fig. 6–10). When arm exercise is performed in the sitting or standing position, the blood pooled in the lower extremities is not returned to the heart and lungs, and the cardiopulmonary volume and cardiac filling pressure remain decreased. As a consequence the stroke volume and cardiac output remain lower at each level of oxygen uptake.

The capacity for leg exercise is improved in the upright position because the hydrostatic pressure load increases the local arterial pressure and the muscle pump decreases the venous outflow pressure. Hence the driving force for tissue perfusion is almost doubled in the legs.

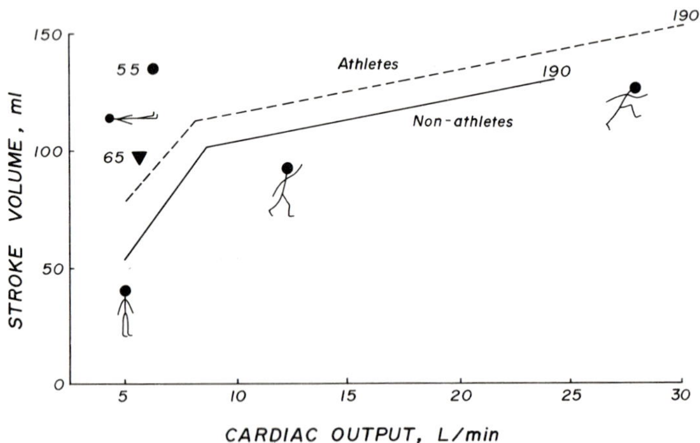

FIG. 6–10. Cardiac output and stroke volume in athletes (●) and nonathletes (▼), during resting supine, quiet standing, and graded upright exercise. Figures represent the heart rate (beats/minute). The pattern in both groups is the same, except the athletes have a larger stroke volume and a slower heart rate when resting. On standing the stroke volume decreases because of pooling of blood in the lower limbs. Even with mild exercise the muscle pump restores the pooled blood to the heart and lungs, and the stroke volume approaches the supine value. As exercise increases in severity, the stroke volume continues to increase slightly, so that as maximal exercise is approached it exceeds by about 10% the values obtained in the supine position at rest. Oxygen consumption in both groups at rest is about 300 ml/min, and at maximal effort it is about 3,000 ml/min in the nonathletes and about 5,000 ml/min in the athletes.

Thermal Environment

In a hot environment the cardiac output is greater at rest and during submaximal work than in a cool surrounding because of the increased skin blood flow. The maximal work capacity is decreased because the maximal cardiac output is reached sooner in the heat. An additional factor which reduces maximal cardiac output is the accumulation of blood in the capacious skin veins with a consequent reduction in the filling of the heart and in stroke volume. Even during prolonged moderate exercise in comfortable environmental conditions, the continuous heat production leads to dilatation of the skin veins with a consequent modest decrease in stroke volume; the heart rate increases and maintains the cardiac output (Fig. 6–11).

Digestion

Exercise performed during digestion (postprandial exercise) resembles exercise in a hot environment. At rest the heart rate and cardiac output are augmented to permit perfusion of the dilated gastrointestinal vessels. These changes are maximal 1 to 4 hr after eating large meals. Thus during moderate exercise the cardiac output is higher than in the fasting subject.

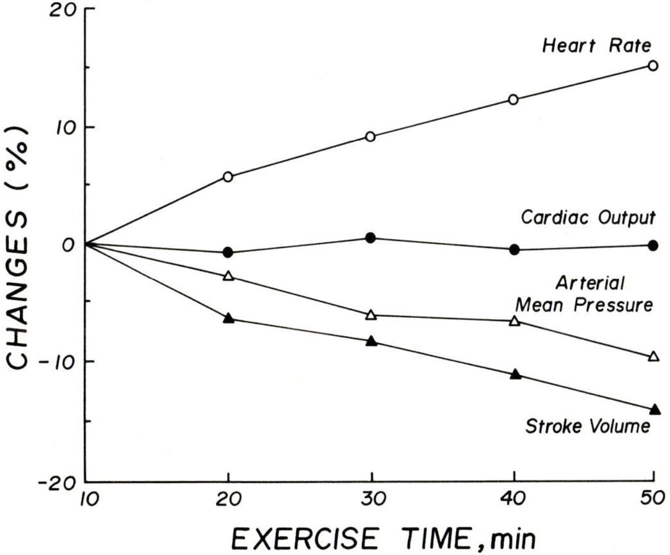

FIG. 6–11. Response to prolonged exercise. The mean arterial pressure and stroke volume decrease slightly, and the cardiac output is maintained by a further increase in heart rate. These changes are due to the increasing dilatation of the cutaneous veins to meet the need for body temperature regulation. With the consequent reduction in the volume of blood in the heart and lungs, the filling pressure decreases and stroke volume falls. (Data from Ekelund and Holmgren: *Acta Physiol. Scand.,* 62:240, 1964.)

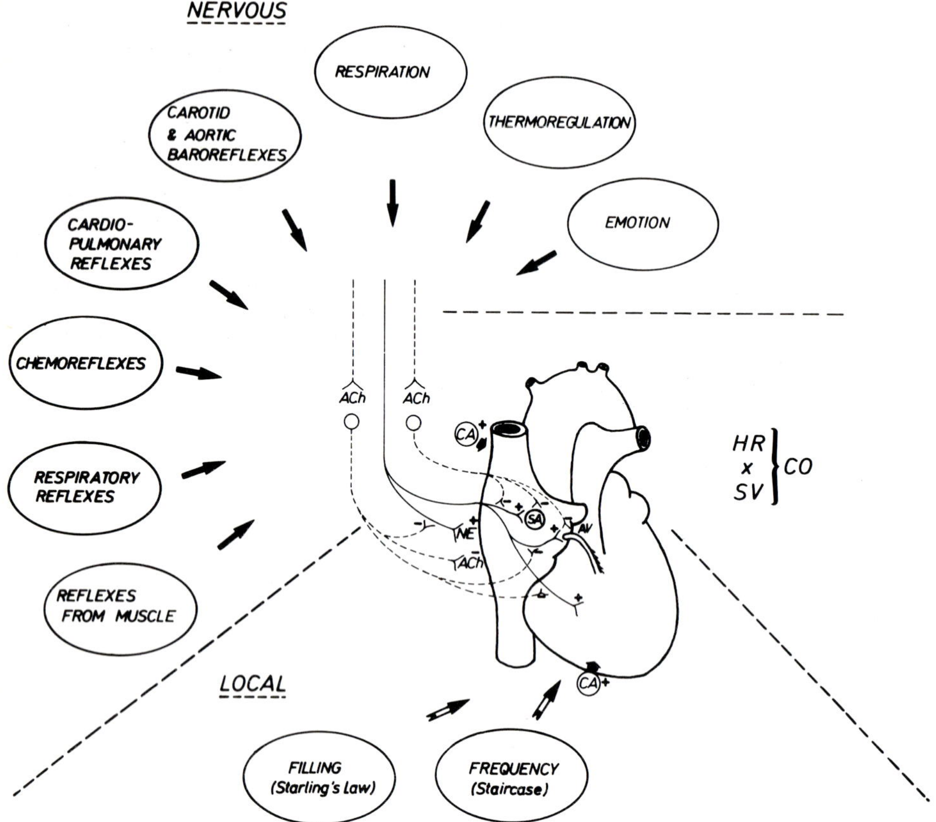

FIG. 6–12. Summary of the neurohumoral and local factors regulating cardiac function. While the cholinergic fibers *(dotted lines)* affect mainly the sinus node and the conducting tissues they also impinge on the sympathetic fibers *(solid line)* to modulate the output of norepinephrine (p. 128). ACh = acetylcholine. AV = atrioventricular node, CA = circulating catecholamines, CO = cardiac output, HR = heart rate, NE = norepinephrine, SV = stroke volume, + = activation, — = depression.

Pregnancy

The blood pressure remains within the normal range during normal pregnancy. The cardiac output gradually increases by about 25% to compensate for the increasing uterine blood flow (p. 270). The increase in heart rate is minor, usually not more than 10 beats/min. The increase in blood volume (25 to 30%) compensates for the increased distensibility of the venous wall caused by the circulating hormones (estrogen and progesterone; p. 154), so that stroke volume may actually be slightly augmented. All these changes peak around the 30th week of gestation. When the pregnant woman exercises, cardiac output is greater for a given work load because of the oxygen demands of the placental circulation.

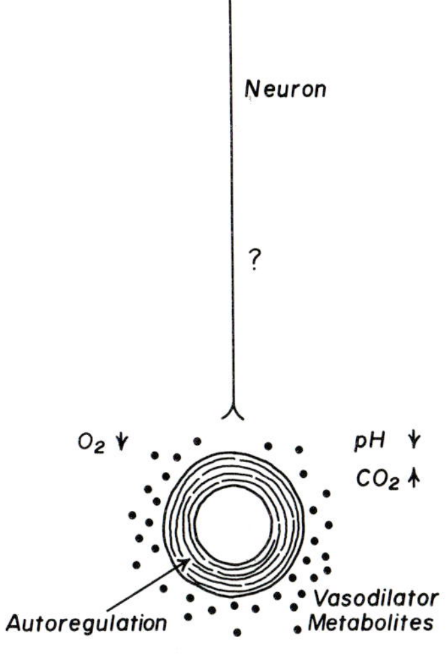

FIG. 6–13. Regulation of the cerebral circulation. Products of metabolism and changes in periarteriolar pH, P_{CO_2} and P_{O_2} act directly on the cerebral arterioles to adapt cerebral blood flow to the metabolic needs of the individual parts of the brain. When the pH of the cerebrospinal fluid decreases, the brain vessels dilate and vice-versa. In addition, to maintain a constant flow, the cerebral vessels adjust their diameter to the existing pressure (autoregulation, p. 95). The cerebral vessels are innervated by autonomic nerves, the role of which is unknown. In normal man, the average blood flow of the whole brain is remarkably constant at about 50 ml/100 g/min (white matter about 20 ml/100 g/min, grey matter about 100 ml/100 g/min) provided the P_{CO_2} does not vary.

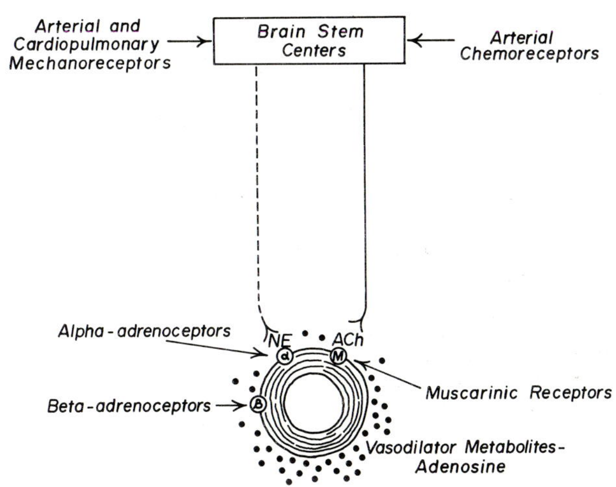

FIG. 6–14. Regulation of the coronary circulation. Products of metabolism, acting directly on the muscle arterioles, provide for the blood flow to meet the metabolic needs of the heart muscle (p. 91). Stimulation of arterial chemoreceptors, as occurs during diving, dilates the coronary arterioles by activating cholinergic fibers to these vessels (p. 165). Reflex decreases in coronary blood flow may occur, mediated by increases in sympathetic outflow to the heart and alpha-receptor (α) activation but these usually are offset by the metabolic vasodilatation resulting from the increased cardiac contractility. There are beta-receptors (β) in the coronary vessels which are not affected by norepinephrine (NE) released from the sympathetic nerve endings; their role is unknown. During systole, the flow to the left heart decreases owing to mechanical compression of the vessels within the left ventricular myocardium (p. 98), and ranges from 10 to 50% of the flow during diastole. ACh = acetylcholine, M = muscarinic receptor.

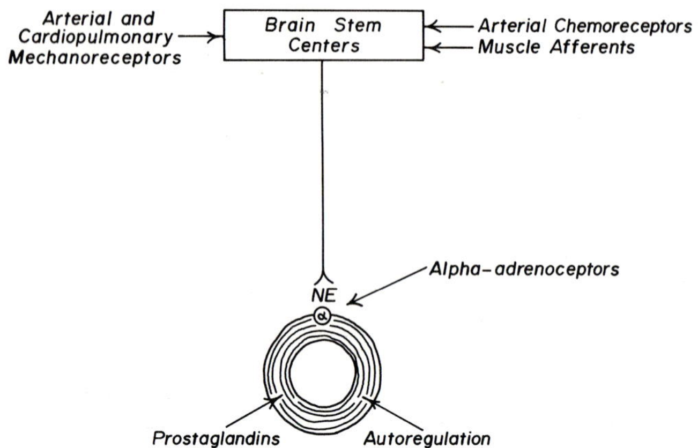

FIG. 6–15. Regulation of the renal circulation. The blood flow to the kidneys is greatly in excess of its metabolic needs (p. 63). The afferent, but probably not the efferent, arterioles to the glomeruli have a sympathetic nerve supply. Normally there is little activity in the sympathetic nerves to the kidney vessels. Changes in renal blood flow occur reflexly mainly by alterations in the activity of the arterial and cardiopulmonary mechanoreceptors (p. 131), the arterial chemoreceptors (p. 140), and afferents from the contracting skeletal muscles (p. 149). There is no evidence for a cholinergic nerve supply to the kidney vessels. The kidney vessels are especially sensitive to changes in transmural pressure (autoregulation; p. 95). Prostaglandins are formed in the kidney and depending on their nature may increase or decrease renal flow (Fig. 4–15). When the levels of circulating catecholamines and angiotensin II increase, the kidney vessels constrict.

Age

As age increases from 30 to 80 years there is little change in the relationship between cardiac output and oxygen consumption, although the maximal capacity for exercise decreases. With age the elasticity of the blood vessel wall decreases, with a resulting increase in systolic blood pressure as the viscoelasticity of the aorta and the other windkessel vessels decreases (p. 209). In addition, the blood vessels dilate less easily because of decreased ability to produce cyclic 3′,5′-adenosine monophosphate (p. 48).

Sex

The cardiovascular response to exercise is similar in men and women, but the maximal working capacity is less in the latter.

Training and Constitution

With training, the resting heart rate becomes slower owing to increased vagal activity. The mechanism by which this occurs is unknown. The relationship between cardiac output and oxygen consumption during exercise is similar before and after training, but at each level of oxygen consumption the heart rate is less and the stroke volume greater in the trained athlete. Since the maximal heart rate that can be achieved is the same in trained or untrained persons, training permits higher maximal cardiac output and oxygen consumption by increasing the maximal stroke volume (Fig. 6–10).

Although training improves cardiovascular performance in all individuals, certain people are physically predisposed to attain exceptional athletic ability. These athletes have larger stroke volumes, total amounts of hemoglobin, and blood volumes in relation to body weight, and thus larger capacity for oxygen transport.

In extremely obese persons the resting cardiac output and blood volume are increased by about 20% and 30%, respectively, because of the blood flow to

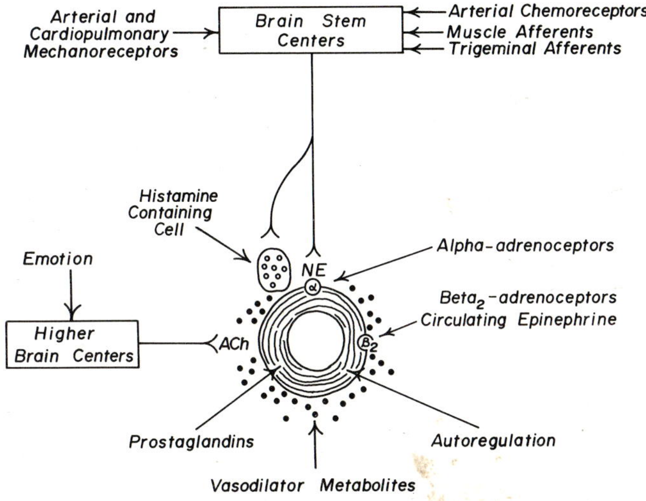

FIG. 6–16. Regulation of the muscle circulation. Products of metabolism, acting directly on the muscle arterioles, provide for the blood flow to meet the changing metabolic needs of the muscles (p. 92). The muscle vessels also are involved in the reflex regulation of arterial blood pressure by participating in the changes in total systemic vascular resistance caused by changes in sympathetic outflow. These changes are governed by the arterial and cardiopulmonary mechanoreceptors (p. 131), the arterial chemoreceptors (p. 140), and afferents from the contracting muscles (p. 149) and from the skin of the face via the trigeminal nerve (p. 165). Other factors which alter muscle flow are emotion, which increases the output of epinephrine from the adrenal medulla (p. 156) to activate the beta$_2$ receptors and also activates cholinergic nerves (p. 156). The muscle vessels are also sensitive to changes in transmural pressure (autoregulation; p. 95). Prostaglandins synthesized in the vessel wall can contribute to vasodilatation (p. 103), and histamine may be liberated from cells in the vicinity of the arterioles (p. 101). ACh = acetylcholine, α = alpha-adrenergic receptor, β_2 = beta-adrenergic receptor. NE = norepinephrine.

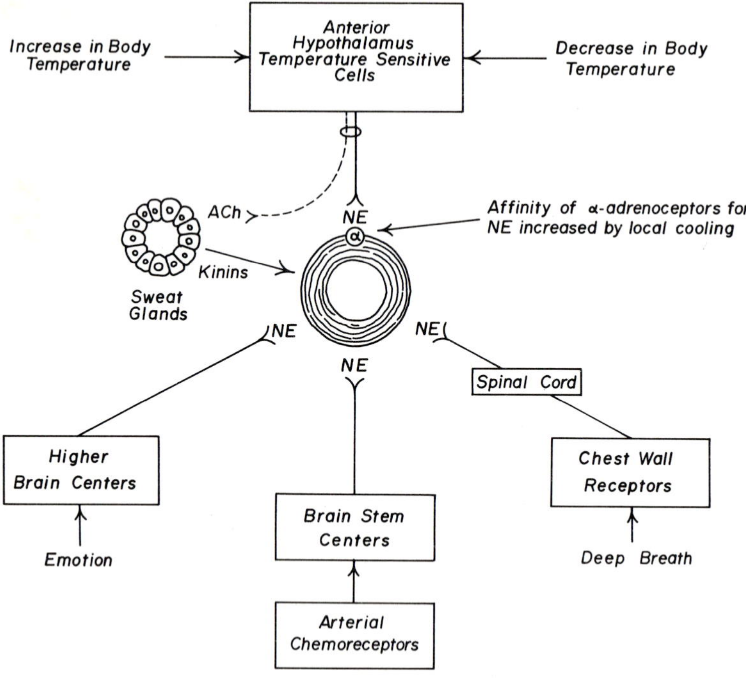

FIG. 6–17. Regulation of skin circulation. Only a small blood flow is required to meet the metabolic requirements of the skin. The major function of the skin vessels is in the regulation of body temperature. Changes in caliber of the skin arterioles and veins are mediated by temperature receptors in the skin and thermosensitive cells in the anterior hypothalamus, which modulate the amount of norepinephrine (NE) released from the sympathetic nerve terminals. The local changes in skin temperature reinforce the nervous-system-mediated effects by altering the affinity of the alpha-adrenoceptors (α) for norepinephrine (p. 99). When the sweat glands are activated, kinins are liberated which increase the blood flow to the glands (p. 102). Other changes in skin flow are caused by emotion (p. 156), respiration (p. 320), stimulation of the arterial chemoreceptors (p. 140), and increases in the levels of circulating vasoactive agents.

the excess adipose tissue. During exercise the relation between changes in cardiac output and oxygen uptake are normal. The oxygen consumption and pulmonary ventilation are almost twice as great as in normal persons performing identical amounts of external work because of the weight of the excess fat.

Isometric Exercise

During moderate rhythmic exercise, there are only modest increases in arterial blood pressure. The rhythmic character of the skeletal muscle contractions allows

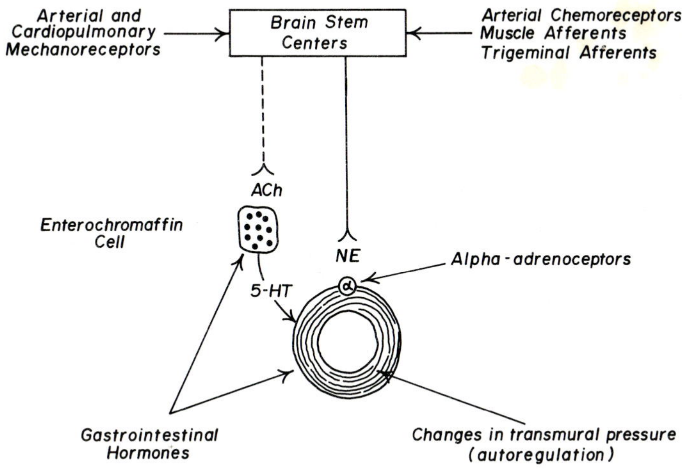

FIG. 6–18. Regulation of the splanchnic circulation. The splanchnic bed has a large flow relative to its oxygen requirements (p. 63), and its resistance and capacitance vessels contribute importantly to the regulation of arterial blood pressure. Reflex changes in splanchnic resistance are accomplished via the arterial and cardiopulmonary mechanoreceptors (p. 131), arterial chemoreceptors (p. 140), afferents from the contracting muscles (p. 149), and the trigeminal afferents (p. 165). During digestion 5-hydroxytryptamine (5-HT) is liberated from enterochromaffin cells and causes dilation of the arterioles in the gastrointestinal tract. The liberation occurs through an action of the gastrointestinal hormones (gastrin, cholecystokinin, secretin) on the enterochromaffin cells and by mechanical squeezing of these cells by intestinal movements. These hormones may also affect the arterioles directly to cause their dilatation (p. 154). NE = norepinephrine.

proper perfusion of the tissue between the contractions (Fig. 4–7). When sustained isometric contractions are performed (static exercise), marked increases in systemic arterial pressure, heart rate, and ventilation occur; these are in excess of those seen during rhythmic exercise that requires a similar increase in oxygen consumption (Fig. 6–8). The increase in arterial pressure tends to counteract the external pressure imposed on the blood vessels by the contracting skeletal muscle cells (p. 98). The blood pressure rises in proportion to the intensity of the contraction reached by the muscle groups involved. The difference in the magnitude of the arterial blood pressure response between isometric and isotonic muscle contractions is unexplained. In part, it relates to the greater mental effort involved in maintaining isometric contractions, the greater activation of receptors in the contracting muscle (Fig. 5–33), and a temporary overriding of the compensating action of the arterial mechanoreceptors. Thus the stress imposed on the cardiovascular system depends not only on the severity of the work but also on the type of exercise performed, with jogging and weight lifting at the two extremes.

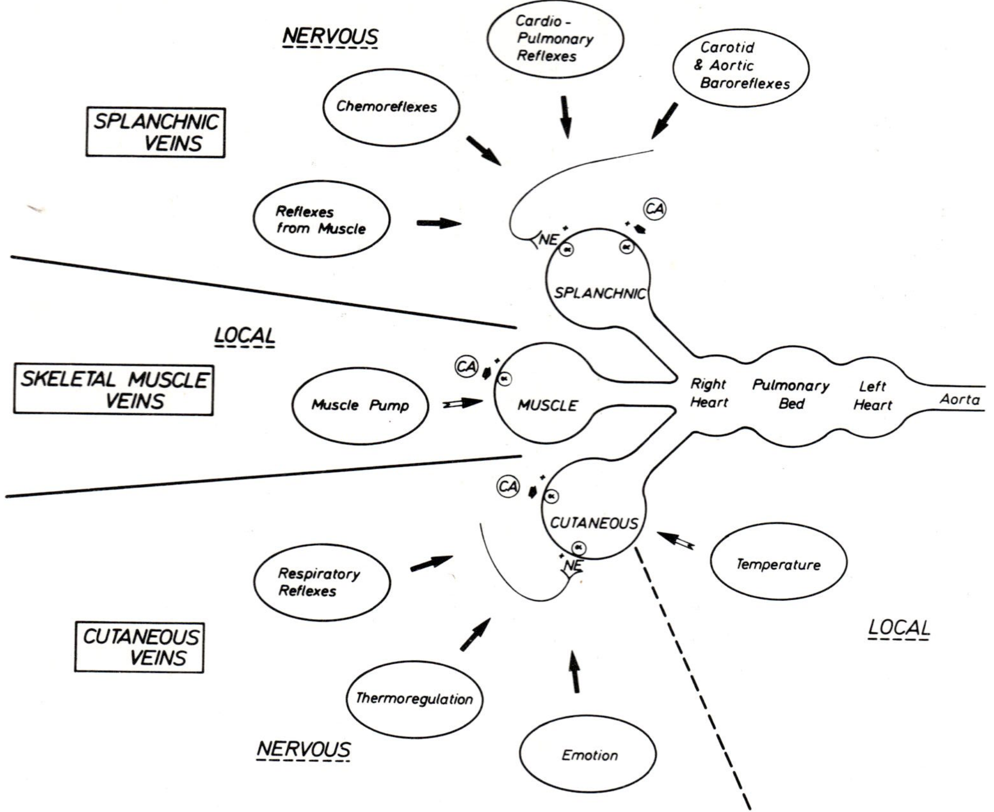

FIG. 6–19. Summary of the neurohumoral and local factors regulating the capacitance vessels. CA = circulating catecholamines. NE = norepinephrine. α = alpha-adrenergic receptor.

CONCLUSION

In normal circumstances when all the peripheral sensors and brain centers affecting the cardiovascular system are operative, the traffic in the nerves to the heart and blood vessels is the final outcome of an elaborate transformation within the nervous system of multiple sensory inputs. To this must be added the effects of local and humoral factors which, together with the nervous system, dictate the final responses of the heart and blood vessels to various stresses. As a consequence of these integrations at the central and local levels, the responses of the various components of the cardiovascular system to a given stress are not uniform, but each has its particular contribution to the functioning of the whole as summarized in Figs. 6–12 to 6–19.

SELECTED REFERENCES

Andersen, H. T. (1966): Physiological adaptation in diving vertebrates. *Physiol. Rev.,* 46:212.

Åstrand, P. O., and Rodahl, K. (1977): *Textbook of Work Physiology,* 2nd ed. McGraw-Hill, New York.

Bevegård, B. S., and Shepherd, J. T. (1967): Regulation of the circulation during exercise in man. *Physiol. Rev.,* 47:178.

Clausen, J. P. (1977): Effect of physical training on cardiovascular adjustments to exercise in man. *Physiol. Rev.,* 57:779.

Daly, M. de B. (1972): Interaction of cardiovascular reflexes. In: *The Scientific Basis of Medicine Annual Reviews, University of London,* p. 307. Athlone Press, London.

Epstein, M. (1978): Renal effects of head-out water immersion in man: Implications for an understanding of volume homeostasis. *Physiol. Rev.,* 58:529.

Fishman, A. P. (1976): Hypoxia on the pulmonary circulation: How and where it acts. *Circ. Res.,* 38:221.

Johnston, R. S., and Dietlein, L. F., editors (1977): *Biomedical Results from Sky Lab.* National Aeronautics and Space Administration, Washington, D.C.

Lind, A. R., and McNicol, G. W. (1967): Circulatory responses to sustained hand-grip contractions performed during other exercise, both rhythmic and static. *J. Physiol. (Lond),* 192:595.

Mitchell, J. H., and Wildenthal, K. (1974): Static (isometric) exercise and the heart: Physiological and clinical considerations. *Annu. Rev. Med.,* 25:369.

Mitchell, J. H., Reardon, W. C., and McCloskey, D. I. (1977): Reflex effects on circulation and respiration from contracting skeletal muscle. *Am. J. Physiol.,* 233:H374.

Rowell, L. B. (1974): Human cardiovascular adjustments to exercise and thermal stress. *Physiol. Rev.,* 54:75.

Sonnenblick, E. H., and Lesch, M., editors (1977): *Exercise and Heart Disease.* Grune & Stratton, New York.

Wolthuis, R. A., Bergman, S. A., and Nicogossian, A. E. (1974): Physiological effects of locally applied reduced pressure in man. *Physiol. Rev.,* 54:566.

Wood, E. H., Nolan, A. C., Donald, D. E., and Cronin, L. (1963): Influence of acceleration on pulmonary physiology. *Fed. Proc.,* 22:1024.

7

Pharmacodynamics

> It is much easier to write upon a disease than upon a remedy. The former is in the hands of nature and a faithful obsever with an eye to tolerable judgment can not fail to delineate a likeness; the latter will ever be subject to the whim, the inaccuracy and the blunder of man.
>
> William Withering (1758)

Pharmacology may be defined as the search for molecules which alter the function of the body cells, in the hope of using them for therapeutic purposes. Pharmacodynamics refers to the understanding of how and why these substances initiate changes in cellular activity. Pharmacokinetics refers to the absorption, distribution, biotransformation, and excretion of drugs, which together with the administered quantity of the drug determines its biological effect. Pharmacotherapeutics refers to the clinical use of the drugs. This chapter aims to serve as a brief pharmacodynamic introduction to the rational use of drugs acting on the cardiovascular system.

Certain substances used for therapeutic purposes compensate for the failure of the body to produce or absorb enough of them. The best examples are: (1) hormonal substitution therapy with insulin in diabetes mellitus and corticosteroids in adrenal insufficiency (Addison's disease), and (2) the administration of vitamins in avitaminosis. Other therapeutic agents are not normally present in the body and are administered to compensate for a deficient function of certain groups of cells by increasing or decreasing their activity. Preferably, the therapeutic agent is "selective"; i.e. it should affect only those cells which are not functioning normally. Unfortunately, most drugs affect all body cells to different degrees, which explains the occurrence of side effects. The more selective the drug, the better is its therapeutic value.

The activity of cardiac and vascular smooth muscle cells is determined by their inherent automaticity, their local environment, and the presence of neurohumoral substances. Hence pharmacological agents can alter cardiovascular function by interfering directly with the effector cells or by altering the production of local regulatory or neurohumoral substances.

DRUGS AFFECTING CARDIAC AND VASCULAR EFFECTOR CELLS

Ultimately every reaction to a drug implies that the cell has recognized a chemical signal. The site of recognition usually is at the cell membrane, although occasionally it is intracellular as is the case for the hormone estrogen (p. 154).

Cell Membrane

Drug–Receptor Interaction

When a substance binds to the cell membrane, the latter not only recognizes the chemical structure of the "ligand" but can transduce it across the membrane to initiate an intracellular signal, which alters the activity of the cell. Certain macromolecular lipoprotein complexes in the cell membrane, because of their steric arrangement and physicochemical properties, act as the specific binding sites for certain molecules. If the binding of a molecule to such a site causes a change in cellular activity, this site is called a "receptor," and the molecule is referred to as an "agonist" (Fig. 7–1).

In many instances the receptor binds not to only one substance but to a number of chemically related compounds (Fig. 7–2). The binding with the latter does not necessarily imply an identical change in the activity of the cell. When a low concentration of a drug initiates a strong response, it is said to act as an agonist with "high intrinsic activity." Although some drugs bind to the receptor sites, they have weak or no intrinsic activity and thus elicit little or no response (Fig. 7–3). The appetite of the receptor for a given molecule (affinity) is not necessarily the same for other molecules with similar structures, which can act as ligands. The affinity of the receptor sites for related molecules bears no relationship with their intrinsic activity. Thus it is possible that if a receptor is presented with molecules of different intrinsic activity, it will preferentially bind to that with the lowest. Hence a molecule with high affinity and low intrinsic activity can occupy the receptor, making the latter inaccessible for a true agonist; such a molecule is called an "antagonist" or "inhibitor." There are two types of specific antagonists. One type binds strongly to the receptor and cannot be displaced regardless of the concentration of the true agonist; these substances are called "noncompetitive" or "unsurmountable" antagonists.

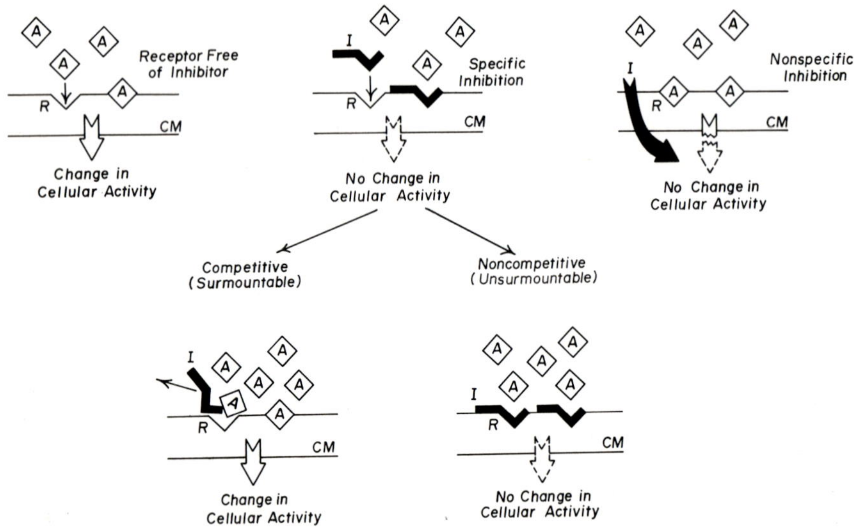

FIG. 7–1. Drug–receptor interaction and specific competitive, specific noncompetitive, and nonspecific inhibition. A = agonist. CM = cell membrane. I = inhibitor or antagonist. R = receptor.

The second type of antagonist can be displaced from the receptors by molecules with lower affinity, provided a high concentration of the latter is present. When such a "competitive" or "surmountable" antagonist is used, it is possible to overcome the inhibition (Figs. 7–1 and 7–4). Nonspecific antagonists do not interfere with the drug–receptor interaction; they depress the response of the effector cells in a noncompetitive way.

The term "drug–receptor interaction" is frequently used when an agonist evokes a change in activity (reaction) of the tissue studied and when this response can be blocked specifically by other pharmacological agents (antagonist). A given drug–receptor interaction can lead to excitatory or inhibitory responses depending on the tissue. An example of this is that acetylcholine inhibits cardiac

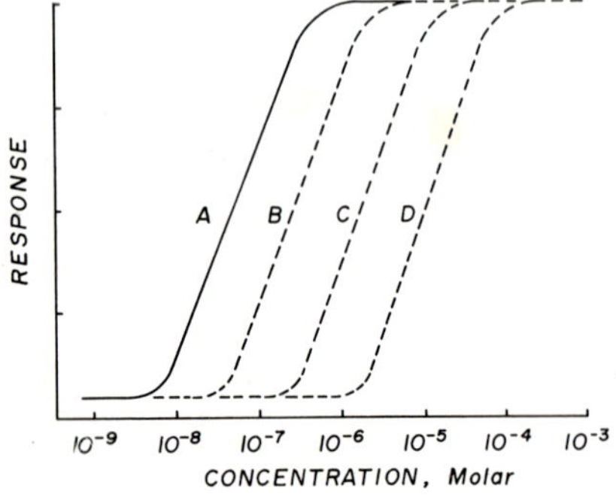

FIG. 7–2. Response of a tissue to various drugs which act on the same receptor. Different concentrations of the compounds ($A < B < C < D$) are needed to initiate a response, indicating the differences in affinity ($A > B > C > D$). The maximal response of the tissue is the same for the four drugs, indicating that they have the same intrinsic activity.

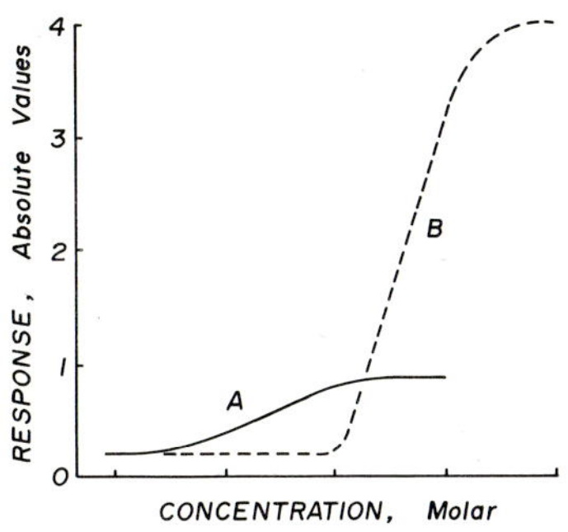

FIG. 7–3. The two drugs A and B act on the same receptor. Lower concentrations of A than of B evoke a response, indicating that A has a higher affinity than B. The maximal response to B is larger than that to A, illustrating that B has higher intrinsic activity.

function and augments gastrointestinal activity, although both effects are specifically prevented by atropine (Fig. 7–5). How the binding of the same agonist to a given receptor can either activate or inhibit cellular activity is unknown. For cardiac and vascular smooth muscle, inhibitory and excitatory drug–receptor interactions ultimately must decrease or increase, respectively, the Ca^{2+} concentration in the vicinity of the contractile proteins.

Adrenergic Receptors

For understanding the pharmacological effects of catecholamines on cardiac and vascular smooth muscle, it is helpful to consider the effects not only of the naturally occurring substances dopamine, epinephrine, and norepinephrine,

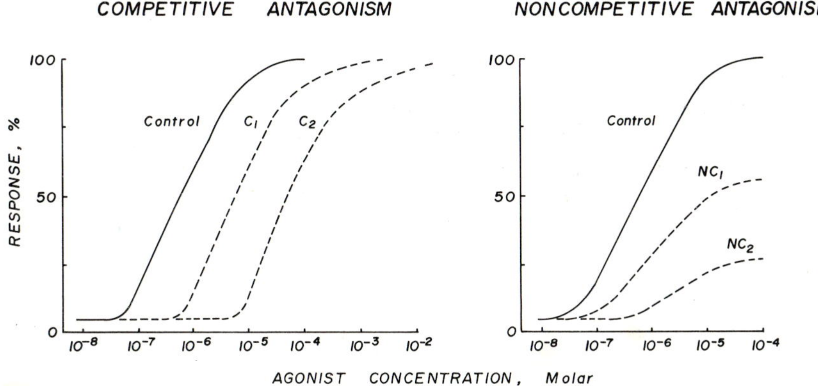

FIG. 7–4. Competitive and noncompetitive antagonism. **Left:** When the specific competitive inhibitor C is given in increasing concentrations ($C_2 > C_1$), more of the agonist *(abscissa)* is required to overcome the blockade and cause the same degree of activity of the tissue *(ordinate)* as in control conditions. Thus the specific competitive antagonist causes a shift to the right of the dose–response curve to the agonist. **Right:** When the noncompetitive antagonist NC is given in increasing concentrations ($NC_2 > NC_1$), augmenting the concentration of the agonist does not overcome the blockade. Thus the dose–response curve to the agonist is displaced to the right, and its maximum is depressed.

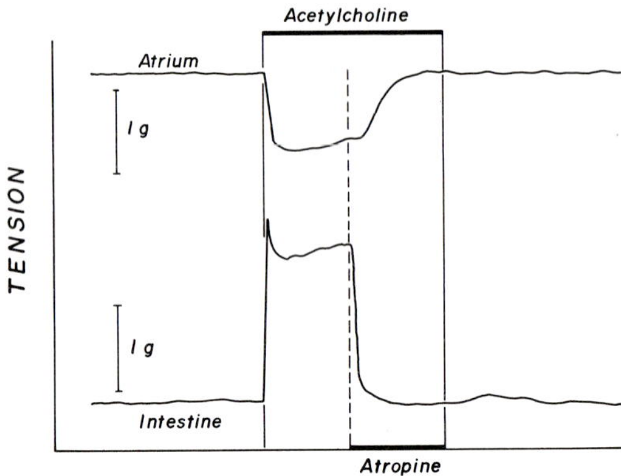

FIG. 7–5. The same "drug–receptor interaction" can have opposite effects in different tissues. In the examples shown, acetylcholine inhibits the spontaneously beating atrium *(upper)* but causes contraction of a segment of ileum *(lower).* In both cases the response is antagonized by the muscarinic inhibitor atropine.

but also their synthetic analogs of which isoproterenol (isopropylnorepinephrine) and phenylephrine are the prototypes (Fig. 7–6). Catecholamines can activate three categories of receptor in the cardiovascular system: alpha-, beta$_1$-, and beta$_2$-adrenergic receptors. This classification rests on the different affinities for catecholamines and adrenergic blocking drugs (Figs. 7–7 and 7–8). The alpha- and beta$_2$-receptors are located mainly in the blood vessel wall, whereas the beta$_1$-receptors are mainly in the heart.

Alpha-adrenergic receptors. The alpha-adrenergic receptor is very sensitive to norepinephrine and phenylephrine, less sensitive to epinephrine, and relatively insensitive to isoproterenol. The interaction between the alpha-adrenergic receptor and its agonists can be competitively inhibited by synthetic drugs such as phentolamine, prazosin, and labetalol or by ergot derivatives; it can be blocked noncompetitively by drugs such as phenoxybenzamine. Alpha-receptors are sparse in the heart but abundant on the cell membrane of all vascular smooth muscle cells, particularly those innervated by sympathetic nerve endings. Alpha-adrenergic activation causes constriction of the resistance vessels throughout the body and of the splanchnic and cutaneous veins. This is due to depolarization of the vascular smooth muscle cells, an increase in cell membrane permeability for Ca^{2+}, and the release of Ca^{2+} from intracellular stores. In the heart alpha-adrenergic activation causes an increase in contractility presumably by increasing the influx of extracellular Ca^{2+} during the plateau phase of the action potential (Fig. 2–23) and its storage by the sarcoplasmic reticulum (Fig. 7–9).

Administration of alpha-adrenergic antagonists disconnects the peripheral blood vessels from sympathetic control. This decreases peripheral vascular resistance and causes venodilation; the filling of the heart, stroke volume, and blood pressure decrease. During standing this may lead to "orthostatic" or "postural"

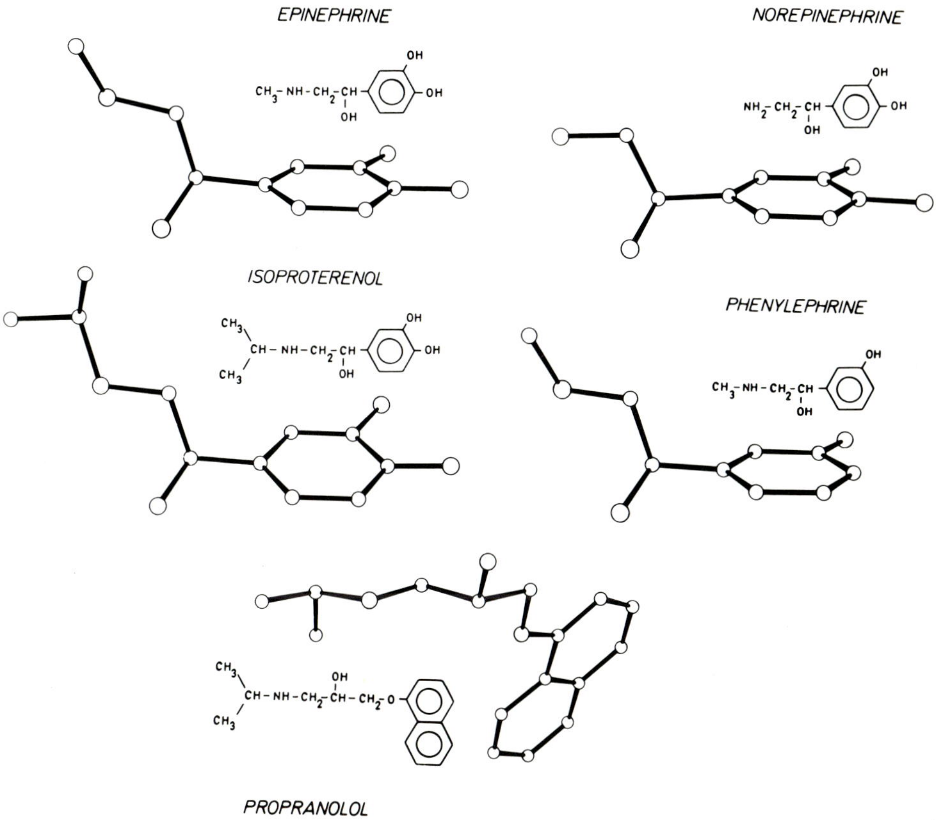

FIG. 7–6. Structure of the naturally occurring catecholamines epinephrine (adrenaline) and norepinephrine (noradrenaline), and of the synthetic alpha-adrenergic agonist phenylephrine and the beta-adrenergic agonist isoproterenol. The term "catecholamine" refers to compounds possessing a catechol (1,2-dihydroxybenzene) ring and a side chain of either ethylamine or ethanolamine. The perspective drawings are derived from X-ray crystallographic data; hydrogen atoms are omitted for the sake of clarity. (Modified from Tollenaere et al.: *Atlas of the Three Dimensional Structure of Drugs.* Elsevier North-Holland, Amsterdam, 1979.)

hypotension. Because of the latter, the use of alpha-adrenergic antagonists should be restricted to competitive drugs, since in case of emergency the injection of large amounts of alpha-adrenergic agonists can overcome the blockade.

Beta$_1$-adrenergic receptors. Beta$_1$-adrenergic receptors are sensitive to isoproterenol, epinephrine, and norepinephrine and insensitive to phenylephrine. The interaction between the beta$_1$-adrenergic receptor and its agonists can be blocked competitively by selective inhibitors such as atenolol and metoprolol, by nonselective inhibitors such as propranolol (which blocks beta$_1$- and beta$_2$-receptors), and by nonspecific adrenergic blockers such as labetalol (which blocks alpha- and beta-adrenergic receptors) (Fig. 7–7).

Beta$_1$-receptors are present in the heart. Their activation causes an increased

RECEPTOR	NAME	STRUCTURE
α	PHENTOLAMINE	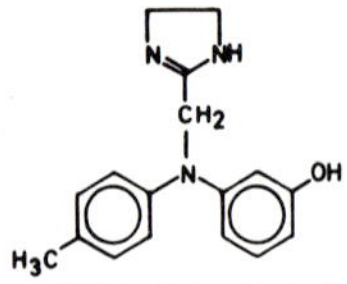 [chemical structure]
α	PRAZOSIN	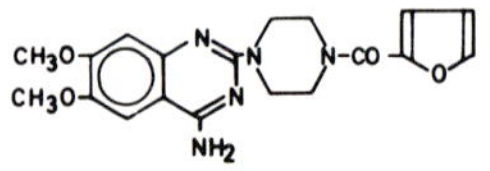 [chemical structure]
β_1	ATENOLOL	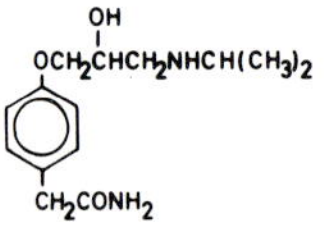 [chemical structure]
β_1	METOPROLOL	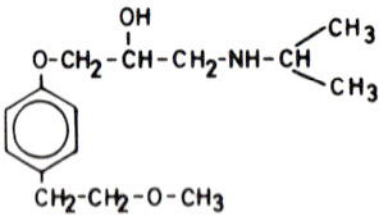 [chemical structure]
$\beta_1 + \beta_2$	PROPRANOLOL	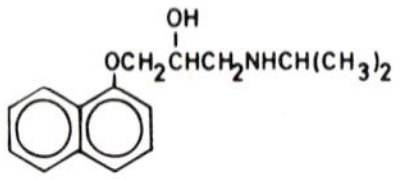 [chemical structure]
$\beta_1 + \beta_2$	TIMOLOL	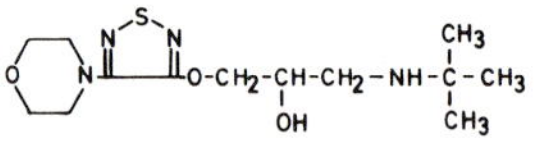 [chemical structure]
$\beta_1 + \beta_2 + \alpha$	LABETALOL	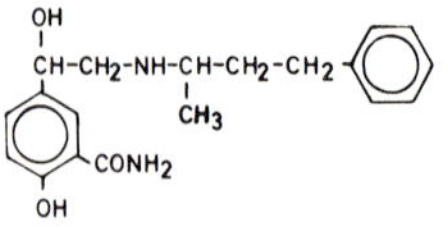 [chemical structure]

FIG. 7–7. Chemical structure of commonly used adrenergic blocking drugs, with an indication of their specificity. α = alpha-adrenergic receptor. β_1 = beta$_1$-adrenergic receptor. β_2 = beta$_2$-adrenergic receptor.

firing rate of the sinus node; an increase in the velocity of conduction in the atria, the atrioventricular node, and the Purkinje system; and an increase in myocardial contractility. Beta$_1$-adrenergic activation by norepinephrine, epinephrine, and isoproterenol thus increases cardiac output. This is due to stimulation of adenyl cyclase in the cell membrane; the consequent increase in cyclic 3′,5′-adenosine monophosphate augments the mobilization of Ca^{2+} and thus the contractility of the muscle (Fig. 7–9). Administration of beta$_1$-antagonists

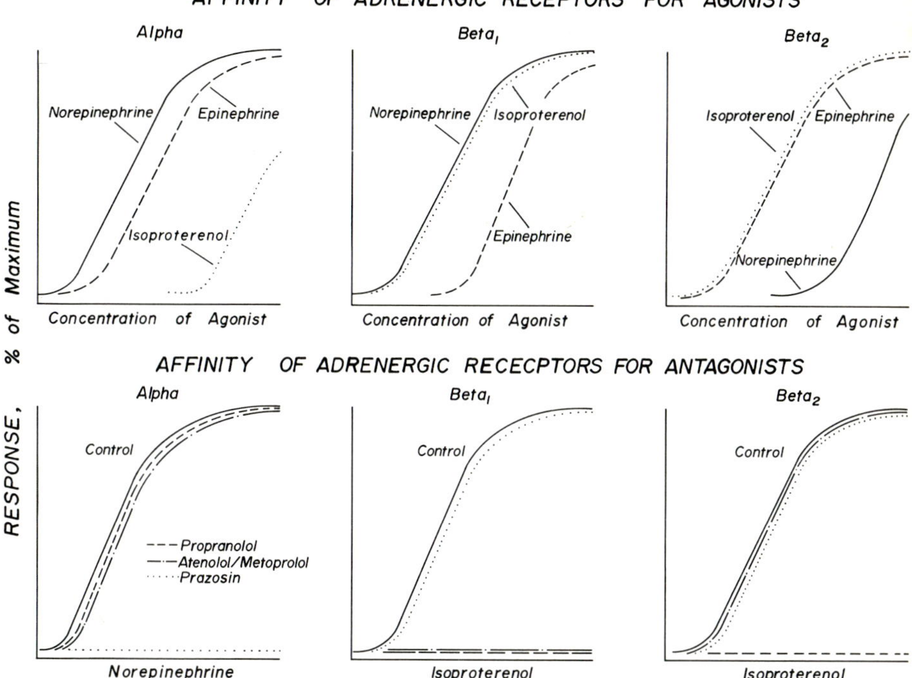

FIG. 7–8. The adrenergic receptors have varying affinities for the agonists epinephrine, isoproterenol, and norepinephrine, as indicated by the concentrations of these compounds needed to elicit their activation *(upper).* In addition, the response of these receptors to their preferred agonist can be antagonized using the appropriate adrenergic blocking agent *(lower).* For example, in the bottom left panel the response to alpha-adrenergic activation by norepinephrine (control) is abolished by the alpha-adrenergic blocking drug prazosin but is unaffected by the beta-adrenergic blocking drugs atenolol, metoprolol, and propranol.

disconnects the heart from sympathetic control and reduces heart rate, cardiac contractility, and cardiac output. Although large doses of beta-blockers have local anesthetic and/or stimulating properties, these properties play little role in the usual clinical dosages.

Beta-adrenergic activation causes coronary vasodilatation. This is due to the increased metabolic activity of the cardiac muscle and to the stimulation of beta-receptors on the coronary smooth muscle cells.

Beta$_2$-adrenergic receptors. Beta$_2$-adrenergic receptors are sensitive to isoproterenol and epinephrine, and insensitive to norepinephrine and phenylephrine; they can be blocked by nonselective beta-blockers such as propranolol and labetalol. Beta$_2$-receptors are present in most but not all vascular smooth muscle cells. They are most abundant in skeletal muscle resistance vessels but are practically absent in kidney, skin, and splanchnic resistance vessels. Beta$_2$-adrenergic agonists cause relaxation of vascular smooth muscle by hyperpolarization of

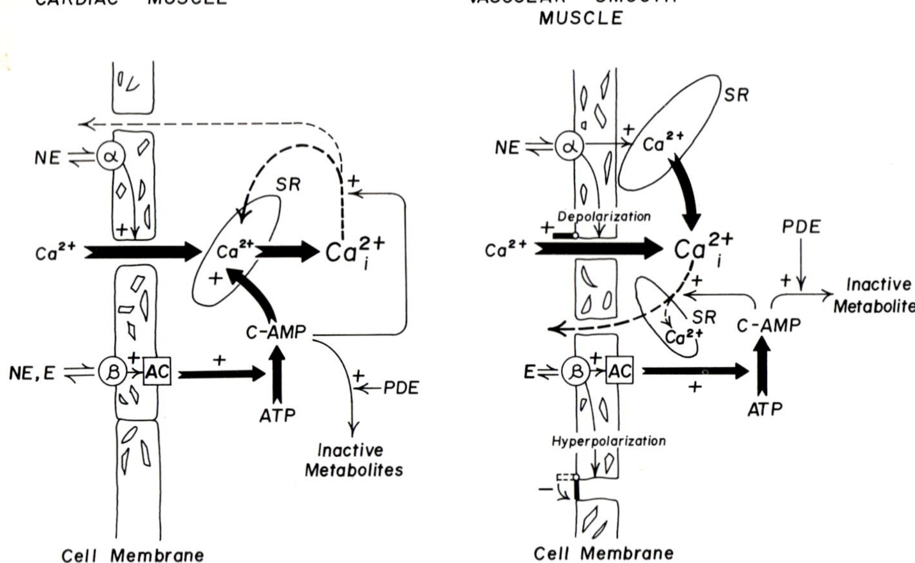

FIG. 7–9. Effects of catecholamines on Ca^{2+} metabolism in cardiac and vascular smooth muscle. **Left:** In the myocardium alpha-adrenergic activation augments the influx of Ca^{2+} from the outside of the cell and its storage in the sarcoplasmic reticulum, making more Ca^{2+} available for subsequent contractions. Beta-receptor stimulation activates adenyl cyclase with increased production of 3′,5′-adenosine monophosphate (cyclic AMP, c-AMP); this in turn facilitates the release of Ca^{2+} from the sarcoplasmic reticulum, increasing the amount of activator Ca^{2+} made available to the contractile proteins and thus augmenting contractility. At the end of the contraction, the cyclic AMP facilitates removal of the ion *(dotted lines),* thus shortening the relaxation. **Right:** In vascular smooth muscle alpha-adrenergic activation causes depolarization, increased influx of extracellular Ca^{2+}, and in some blood vessels release of sarcoplasmic Ca^{2+}. Beta-adrenergic activation causes hyperpolarization, which decreases the Ca^{2+} influx, and activation of cyclic AMP formation, which facilitates removal of activator Ca^{2+} *(dotted lines).* α = alpha-adrenergic. β = beta-adrenergic. CM = cell membrane. AC = adenyl cyclase. E = epinephrine. NE = norepinephrine. SR = sarcoplasmic reticulum. i = intracellular. ATP = adenosine triphosphate. PDE = phosphodiesterase.

the cell membrane, thus decreasing its excitability, and by activation of adenyl cyclase, resulting in increased formation of cyclic 3′,5′-adenosine monophosphate. The latter accelerates the removal of Ca^{2+} from the cytoplasm. In the intact organism only circulating epinephrine stimulates vascular beta$_2$-receptors. The alpha-adrenergic effect of the hormone predominates in most resistance vessels and in the veins, but the resistance vessels of the skeletal muscle dilate when the levels of epinephrine are increased (Fig. 7–10). Acute administration of nonselective beta-blockers (e.g., propranolol) prevents the skeletal muscle vasodilator effect of circulating epinephrine and may cause an acute increase in peripheral resistance. Paradoxically, prolonged treatment with beta-blockers sometimes decreases peripheral resistance, for unknown reasons.

Renin release from the juxtaglomerular cells induced by sympathetic nerve

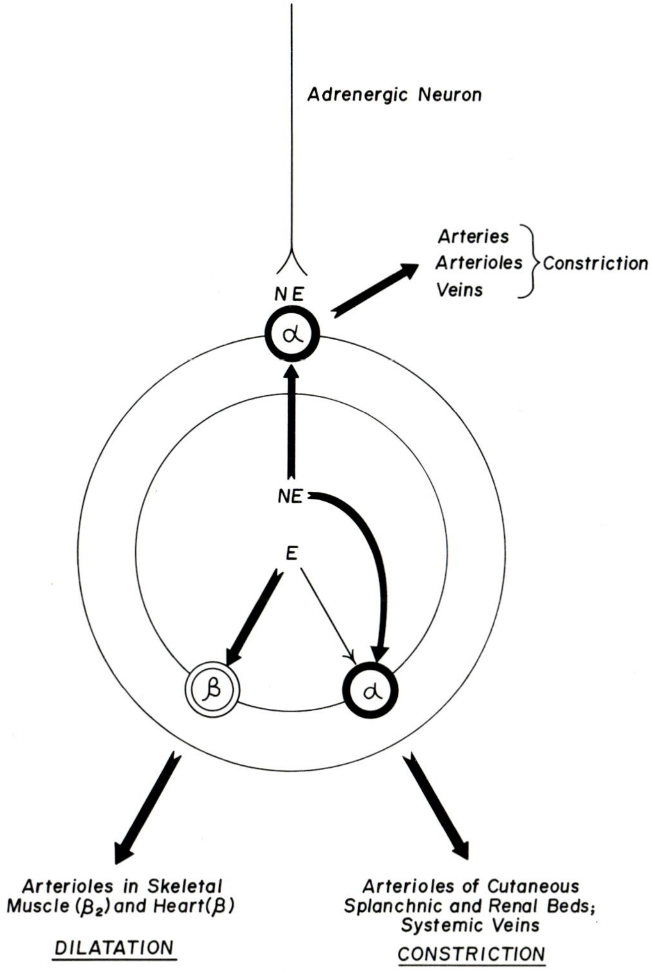

FIG. 7–10. Effects of catecholamines on blood vessels. Norepinephrine released from sympathetic nerves causes constriction throughout the vascular tree by activation of alpha-adrenergic receptors. Circulating epinephrine can activate alpha- and beta-adrenergic receptors of the vascular smooth muscle cells. The latter is of particular importance in skeletal muscle and the heart, where the beta-adrenergic inhibitory effect of the catecholamine predominates. In other resistance vessels and veins epinephrine causes mainly alpha-adrenergic activation. α = alpha-adrenergic receptor. β = beta-adrenergic receptor. β_2 = beta$_2$-adrenergic receptor. E = epinephrine. NE = norepinephrine.

activity is mediated by beta-receptors (p. 121). The exact nature of the receptor involved (beta$_1$ or beta$_2$) is debated. Beta-blockers thus disconnect the juxtaglomerular apparatus from sympathetic control and reduce renin release when the latter is neurogenically increased.

Combined effects. When the sympathetic outflow increases or norepinephrine is infused, $beta_1$-adrenergic receptors in the heart and alpha-adrenergic receptors in the blood vessels are activated. The resulting increase in systemic vascular resistance, the decrease in capacity of the systemic veins, and the increase in cardiac contractility combine to elevate systolic, diastolic, and mean arterial blood pressure (Fig. 5–9). When epinephrine is liberated from the adrenal medulla or is given intravenously, the total systemic vascular resistance decreases because the dilatation in the skeletal muscle ($beta_2$-adrenergic effect) exceeds the constriction in the other vascular beds (alpha-adrenergic effect); the constriction of the systemic veins (alpha-adrenergic) leads to maintained or increased filling of the heart. The $beta_1$-adrenergic effect of epinephrine on the heart increases its rate and force, leading to an increase in cardiac output. These various effects result in a higher systolic and a lower diastolic pressure but an unchanged mean arterial pressure (Fig. 5–10). The other naturally occurring catecholamine dopamine also stimulates the adrenergic receptors but, in addition, dilates the kidney blood vessels by combining with specific dopaminergic receptors; its administration increases cardiac output in excess of the decrease in peripheral resistance, so the blood pressure increases (Fig. 7–11).

When synthetic alpha-adrenergic agonists (e.g., phenylephrine) are infused, the increase in total systemic vascular resistance due to the widespread arteriolar constriction increases blood pressure; constriction of the systemic veins increases cardiac filling and hence the stroke volume. With synthetic beta-adrenergic agonists such as isoproterenol, the heart rate and contractility increase ($beta_1$ effect) and the systemic vascular resistance decreases particularly in skeletal muscle ($beta_2$ effect). Since the dilatation is not offset by an alpha-adrenergically mediated constriction in other vascular beds, as is the case with epinephrine, the reduction in resistance markedly decreases the diastolic pressure and the mean blood pressure is lowered despite the increase in systolic pressure, which reflects the activation of the heart.

When any of these drugs is given intravenously, the changes in blood pressure it causes by its direct effect on heart and blood vessels is sensed by the arterial and left ventricular mechanoreceptors. This may lead to changes in autonomic outflow in a compensatory direction. For example, during infusion of norepinephrine and phenylephrine, the vagal tone to the heart increases reflexly and the heart slows (Fig. 5–9).

Cholinergic Receptors

There are two types of cholinergic receptor. The first has a high affinity for acetylcholine and muscarine, is blocked competitively by atropine and atropine-like substances, and is called a muscarinic receptor (Figs. 7–5 and 7–12). The second has a high affinity for acetylcholine and nicotine, is blocked competitively by muscle relaxant drugs or drugs blocking transmission at the autonomic ganglia (p. 205), and is called a nicotinic receptor. The cholinergic receptors of the

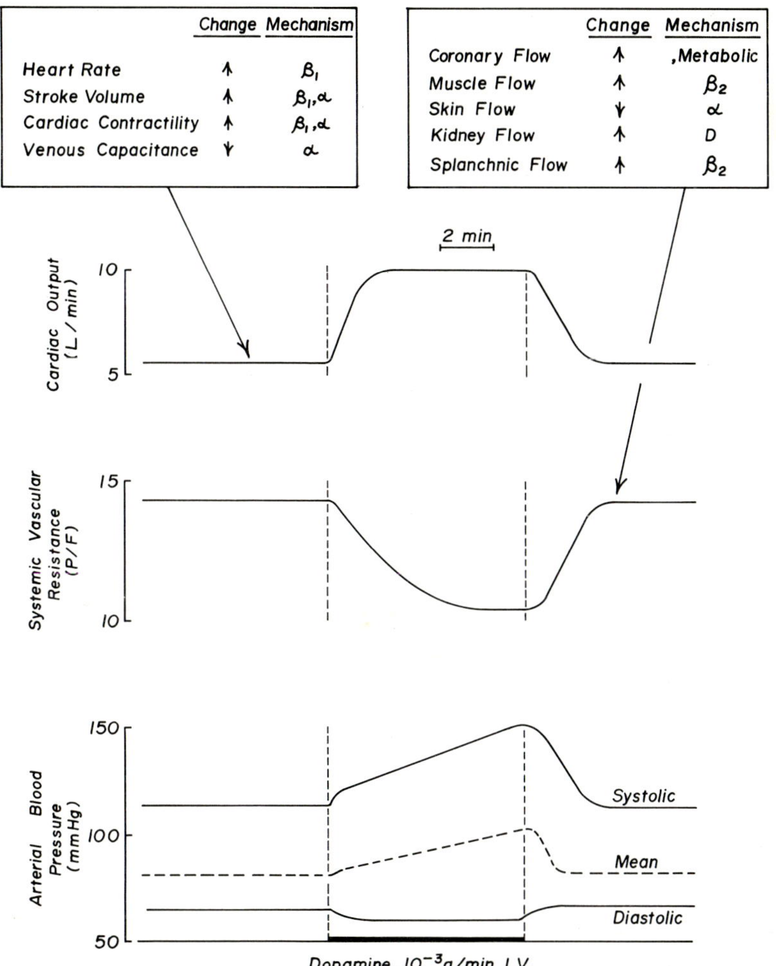

FIG. 7–11. The hemodynamic effects of dopamine consist of: (1) stimulation of alpha-receptors (α) in cutaneous vessels causing their constriction, (2) stimulation of beta$_2$-receptors (β_2) in vessels of skeletal muscle and splanchnic area causing their dilatation, (3) stimulation of dopaminergic receptors (D) in kidney vessels causing their dilatation, (4) activation of beta$_1$-receptors (β_1) in the heart resulting in increases in heart rate and contractility, and (5) activation of alpha-receptors in the heart causing an increase in contractility. The latter effect probably is common to all catecholamines. P = pressure, F = flow.

myocardial and vascular smooth muscle cells are muscarinic in nature. Acetylcholine inhibits the activity of the sinus and atrioventricular nodes, and depresses the other atrial cells, thus slowing the heart. It has little effect on the ventricular myocardium. The inhibitory effect of acetylcholine on the sinus node is due to hyperpolarization and an increased potassium permeability which delays the

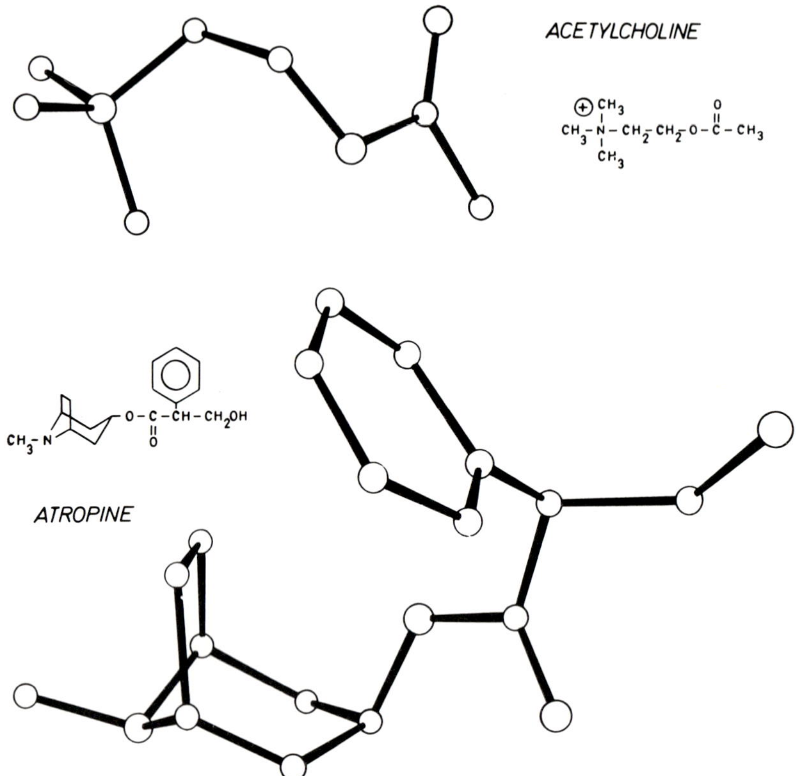

FIG. 7–12. Perspective drawing of the structure of acetylcholine and atropine derived from X-ray crystallographic data; hydrogen atoms are omitted for the sake of clarity. (Modified from Tollenaere, et al.: *Atlas of the Three Dimensional Structure of Drugs.* Elsevier North-Holland, Amsterdam, 1979.)

diastolic pacemaker potential (Fig. 5–16); in the other atrial cells acetylcholine also increases the potassium efflux, shortening the action potential and thus the duration of the actin–myosin interaction. In resistance vessels acetylcholine causes dilation (p. 127). Atropine and other muscarinic antagonists prevent the action of the vagus on the heart, thus permitting the unopposed action of the sympathetic nerves with a resultant increase in heart rate. In resting conditions the cholinergic fibers to the resistance vessels are not activated.

Angiotensin II Receptors

Angiotensin II causes a marked elevation in blood pressure owing to the powerful constriction of the resistance vessels. The capacitance vessels are much less sensitive to the peptide. Angiotensin II does not cause an increase in cardiac

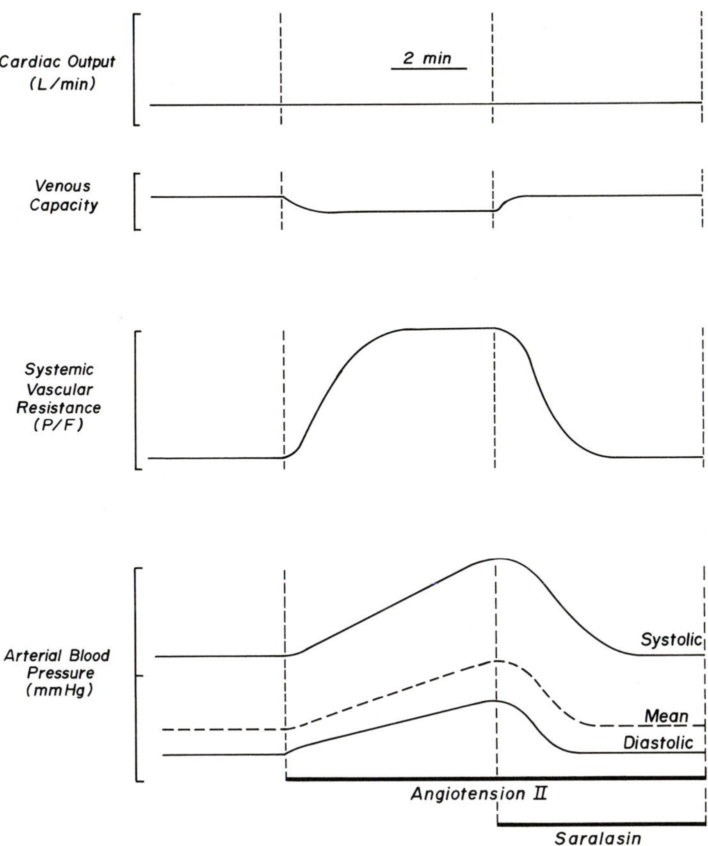

FIG. 7–13. Hemodynamic effects of angiotensin II and their inhibition by saralasin. Angiotensin II acts mainly on the resistance vessels. The small decrease in venous capacity is due to passive mobilization of blood (p. 72). P = pressure, F = flow. Angiotensin II: Asp-Arg-Val-Tyr-Ile-His-Pro-Phe. Saralasin: Sar-Arg-Val-Tyr-Ile-His-Pro-Ala.

output (Fig. 7–13). The constrictor effect of angiotensin II on the vascular smooth muscle cells of the resistance vessels can be competitively antagonized by analogs of the hormone, e.g., saralasin (Fig. 7–13). Hence in conditions of increased production of angiotensin II, saralasin decreases blood pressure.

Na^+,K^+ Exchanges

Withering stated in his monograph *An Account of the Foxglove* (1785) that digitalis (Fig. 7–14) "has a power over the motion of the heart to a degree yet unobserved in any other medicine, and this power may be converted to salutary ends." Although they have been the subject of intensive research and

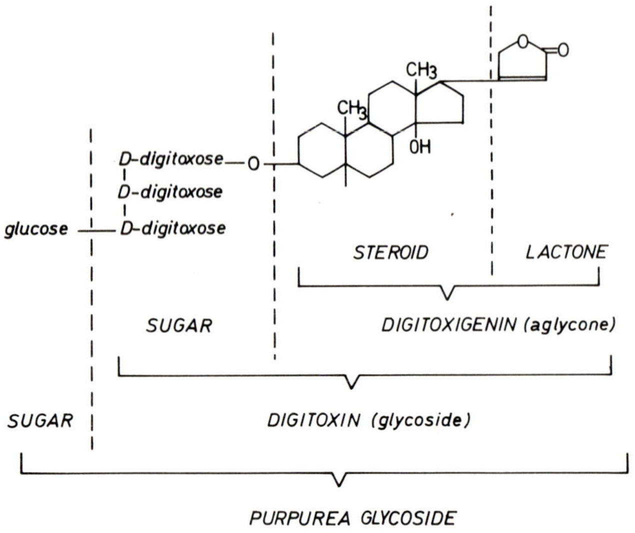

CH_3
CH_3
D-digitoxose—O
D-digitoxose
glucose — D-digitoxose
OH
STEROID
LACTONE
SUGAR
DIGITOXIGENIN (aglycone)
SUGAR
DIGITOXIN (glycoside)
PURPUREA GLYCOSIDE

FIG. 7–14. Chemical structure of digitoxin, one of the cardiac glycosides. The active component of the molecule (genin, aglycone) consists of the steroid nucleus with an unsaturated lactone in the C-17 position. Sugars specific for each glycoside are attached to the C-3 position. The attachment of sugars determines the physicochemical properties of the molecule and thus its pharmacokinetic properties.

are among the most frequently prescribed of all drugs, the exact mechanism of action of the cardiac glycosides is still unknown. These agents are potent inhibitors of the enzyme Na^+,K^+-ATPase, which is located in the cell membrane. The resulting inhibition of the Na^+,K^+ pump increases the intracellular Na^+ concentration, followed by an increase in the intracellular Ca^{2+} concentration. The latter has been explained either by the trapping in the cytoplasm of Ca^{2+} (which normally is removed in exchange for Na^+) because the high intracellular Na^+ concentration makes the calcium–sodium exchange difficult, or activation by the high intracellular Na^+ level of an electroneutral carrier system which exchanges intracellular Na^+ for extracellular Ca^{2+}. The increase in cytoplasmic Ca^{2+} explains the positive inotropic effects of cardiac glycosides on the myocardium as well as their stimulating effect on vascular muscle cells of the arterioles and the veins.

When cardiac glycosides are administered to patients with heart failure (p. 261), the stroke volume and cardiac output increase (cardiotonic effect). The direct effect of these drugs on the myocardium is aided by constriction of the systemic veins, which augments the filling pressure of the heart. The higher blood pressure activates the arterial mechanoreceptors, the sensitivity of which is augmented by the drug. As a consequence the vagal tone to the heart is augmented and the sympathetic outflow to the resistance vessels decreased, which offsets the local effects of the drug on the latter.

Because of their direct action and the increased vagal tone, the cardiac glycosides cause slowing of the sinus pacemaker. By their direct effect they lengthen the refractory period, decrease the conduction velocity, and slightly augment the automaticity of atrial muscle; the increase in vagal tone caused by the glycosides usually predominates, shortens the refractory period, increases the conduction velocity, and decreases the spontaneous firing of ectopic atrial pacemakers if they are present. In the atrioventricular node and the His bundle, the direct and the indirect vagal effects of cardiac glycosides concur to lengthen the refractory period and decrease conduction velocity. The drugs shorten the refractory period and markedly augment the automaticity of Purkinje fibers and the ventricle; part of this effect is due to the facilitation of adrenergic neurotransmission (p. 202) (Fig. 7–15). These complex actions explain why in the individual patient

		EFFECTS OF GLYCOSIDES			
	PARAMETER	DIRECT	INDIRECT		COMBINED
			ORIGIN	EFFECT	
SYSTEMIC VEINS	CAPACITY	↓	NE-release ↑	↓	↓
HEART					
SINUS NODE	RATE	↓	vagus ↑	↓	↓
ATRIAL MUSCLE	CONTRACTILITY	↑	vagus ↑	↓	↑
	REFRACTORY PERIOD	↑	vagus ↑	↓	↓
	CONDUCTION VELOCITY	↓	vagus ↑	↑	↑
	AUTOMATICITY	↑			↑
ATRIOVENTRICULAR NODE	REFRACTORY PERIOD	↑	vagus ↑	↑	↑
	CONDUCTION VELOCITY	↓	vagus ↑	↓	↓
PURKINJE FIBERS	REFRACTORY PERIOD	↓	NE-release ↑	↓	↓
	AUTOMATICITY	↑	NE-release ↑	↑	↑
VENTRICULAR MUSCLE	CONTRACTILITY	↑	NE-release ↑	↑	↑
	REFRACTORY PERIOD	↓	NE-release ↑	↓	↓
	AUTOMATICITY	↑	NE-release ↑	↑	↑
RESISTANCE VESSELS	RESISTANCE	↑	sympathetic tone ↓	↓	≈

FIG. 7–15. Direct and indirect effects of cardiac glycosides on the cardiovascular system. In normal subjects most of the direct effects are offset by the reflex changes they generate mainly through the arterial mechanoreceptors. In patients with cardiac failure the direct effect predominates. With an overdose of cardiac glycosides the effects on the atria tend to cause atrial tachycardia, those on the atrioventricular conduction cause heart block, and those on Purkinje fibers and ventricular myocardium cause extrasystoles, ventricular tachycardia, and even fibrillation (p. 251). NE = norepinephrine. ACh = acetylcholine. + = facilitatory effect. − = inhibitory effect. ↑ = augmented/lengthened. ↓ = decreased/shortened. ≈ = no change in steady-state conditions.

it is important to titrate the dose of digitalis derivatives to avoid the toxic effects (Fig. 7–16).

Because the cardiac glycosides act by inhibiting Na^+,K^+-ATPase, and because this enzyme is activated when the K^+ concentration is low and inhibited when it is high digitalis derivatives are more effective in patients with lowered serum K^+ (hypokalemia) and relatively ineffective in those with increased serum K^+ levels (hyperkalemia).

Production of Cyclic Nucleotides

The hormone glucagon (p. 155) activates adenyl cyclase, has positive inotropic properties, and can be used as a cardiotonic agent. Unlike catecholamines and cardiac glycosides, it little affects cardiac rhythm and excitability.

Local Anesthetic Effect

A number of pharmacological agents can stabilize the cell membrane and decrease its excitability. These include propranolol (Fig. 7–7), quinidine, procainamide, lidocaine, and diphenylhydantoin (Fig. 7–17). They act by reducing the membrane permeability for Na^+ and increasing it for K^+. The amplitude and slope of the pacemaker potentials decreases, the threshold for stimulation augments, and spike electrogenesis is inhibited. This explains their antiarrhythmic properties, particularly the antagonism of abnormal pacemaker activity (p. 254). They also cause relaxation of vascular smooth muscle and thus induce dilation when injected locally; in some commercial preparations this effect is counteracted by the addition of alpha-adrenergic agonists.

Inhibition of Ca^{2+} Influx

Certain substances can reduce the transmembrane inward movement of Ca^{2+}. Of these agents, verapamil (iproveratril) is particularly effective in the heart, where it slows the pacemaker activity of the sinus node, depresses conduction in the atrioventricular node, and has a negative inotropic effect. In vascular smooth muscle drugs such as cinnarizine, flunarizine, and lidoflazine inhibit the influx of Ca^{2+} and cause vasodilation (Fig. 7–18).

Intracellular Effects

Inhibitors of Phosphodiesterase

Phosphodiesterase, the enzyme catalyzing the breakdown of cyclic 3′,5′-adenosine monophosphate (Fig. 2–30), can be inhibited by drugs such as the methylxanthines (e.g., theophylline) (Fig. 7–19). These substances increase the intracellular levels of cyclic 3′,5′-adenosine monophosphate and have opposite

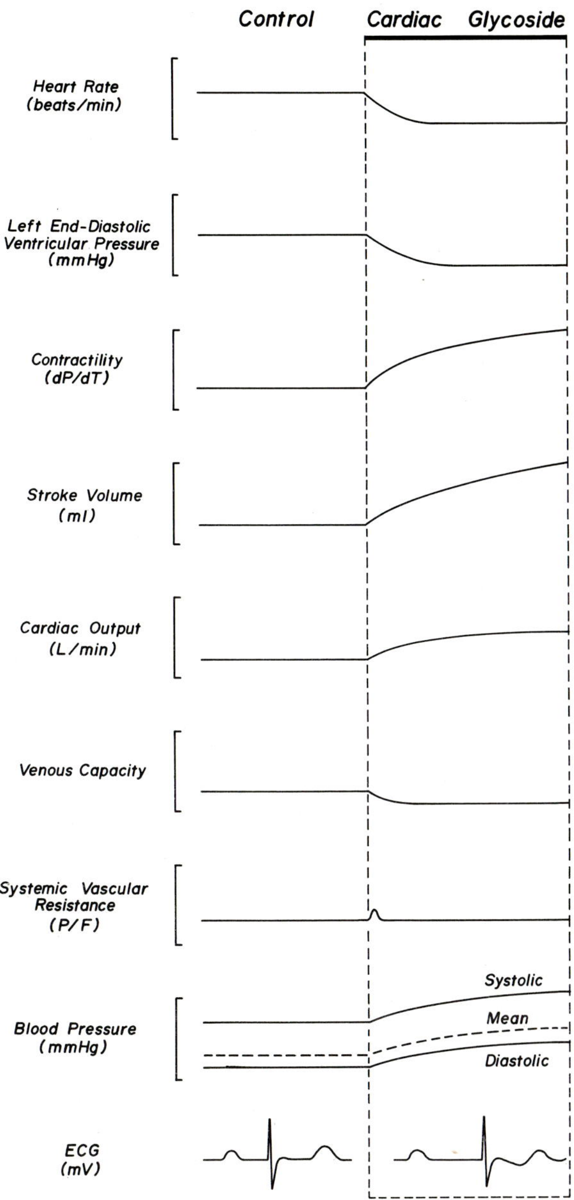

FIG. 7–16. Hemodynamic effects of cardiac glycosides in patients with congestive heart failure. The main electrocardiographic consequences are prolongation of the P–R interval, shortening of the Q–T interval, depression of the S–T segment, and depression or inversion of the T-wave. F = flow, T = time, P = pressure.

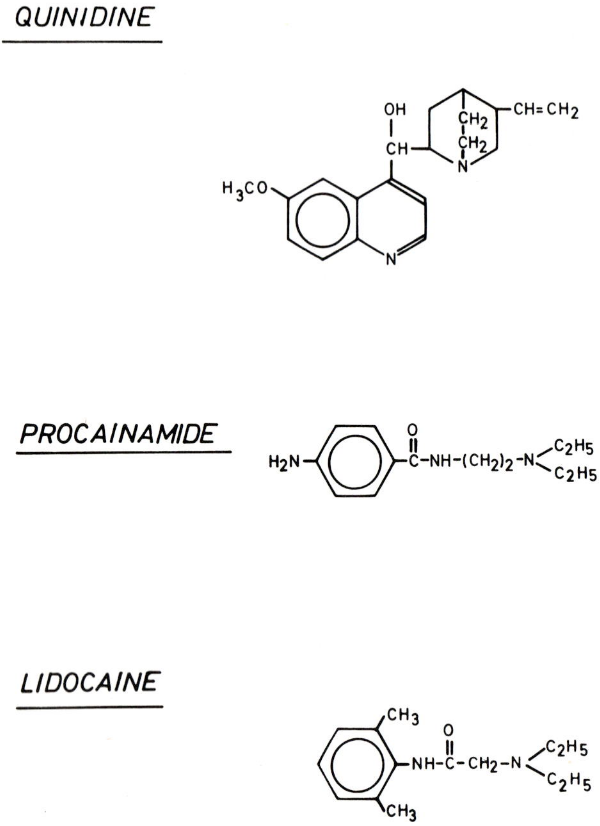

QUINIDINE

PROCAINAMIDE

LIDOCAINE

FIG. 7–17. Chemical structure of commonly used antiarrhythmic drugs which have the property of stabilizing the cell membrane.

effects on cardiac and vascular smooth muscle, increasing cardiac contractility but causing peripheral vasodilatation (p. 188). Other vasodilators (e.g., papaverine and dipyridamole, Fig. 17–9) also inhibit phosphodiesterase, which partly explains their effect.

Nonspecific Vascular Relaxants

Substances such as diazoxide, furosemide, nitrates, sodium nitroprusside, and hydralazine (Fig. 7–20) are potent relaxers of vascular smooth muscle. Their mechanism of action is unknown. Furosemide, nitrates, and in particular sodium nitroprusside decrease the oxygen requirements of the failing heart by reducing its preload and its afterload. By causing venodilatation they permit more blood to accumulate in the systemic venous bed, reduce the congestion of the pulmonary circulation, decrease the end-diastolic intravascular pressure, and thus shift the

VERAPAMIL

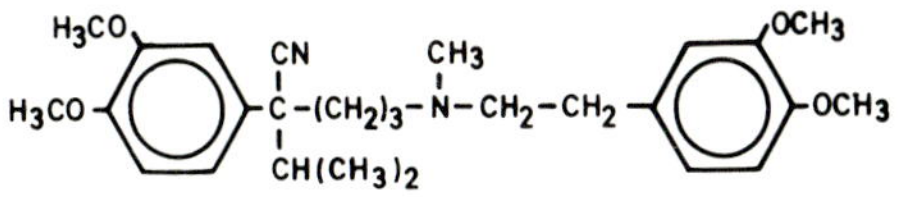

FLUNARIZINE

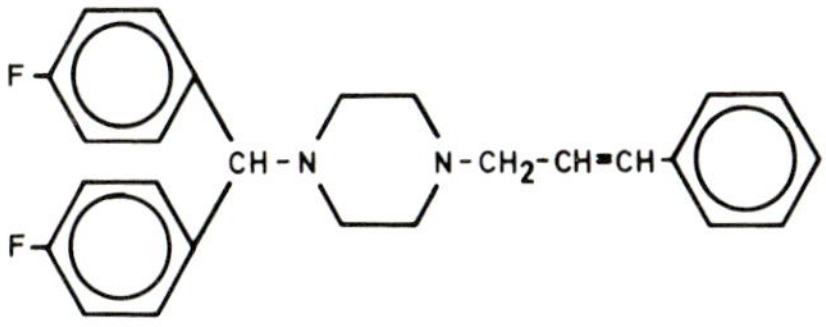

LIDOFLAZINE

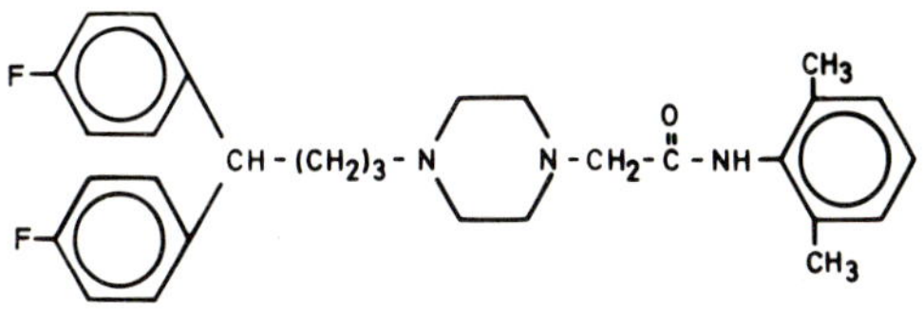

FIG. 7–18. Structures of inhibitors of Ca^{2+} influx: verapamil, flunarizine, and lidoflazine.

myocardium to a more optimal point of its length–tension relationship (p. 70). By dilating the resistance vessels they decrease the diastolic pressure and the work of the heart. Diazoxide and hydralazine are nonspecific depressants of vascular smooth muscle reactivity which affect mainly the resistance vessels; hydralazine depresses the formation of collagen fibers by the vascular smooth muscle cells (p. 214).

DRUGS AFFECTING THE PRODUCTION OF LOCAL REGULATORY SUBSTANCES

Interference with the local production of vasoactive substances can affect blood vessel diameter (Fig. 7–21). Thus part of the beneficial effect that substances such as aspirin and indomethacin have on the inflammation process can be explained by the vasoconstriction resulting from the decreased production of

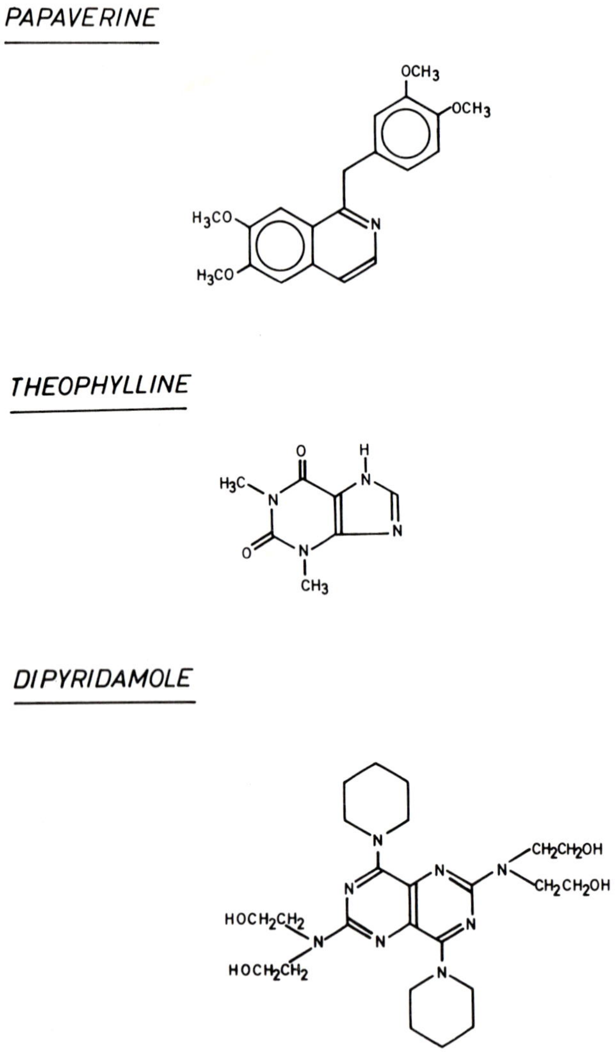

PAPAVERINE

THEOPHYLLINE

DIPYRIDAMOLE

FIG. 7–19. Structures of vasodilator drugs that inhibit phosphodiesterase: papaverine, theophylline, and dipyridamole.

vasodilator prostaglandins (p. 103). Inhibitors of converting enzymes (e.g., captopril) decrease blood pressure presumably by inhibiting the formation of angiotensin II, although part of their effect may be due to decreased breakdown of bradykinin (p. 102). Dipyridamole and lidoflazine cause coronary vasodilatation in part because they inhibit the breakdown of the endogenous vasodilator metabolite adenosine (p. 92). Dipyridamole also antagonizes platelet aggregation, thus reducing the liberation of vasoconstrictor agents such as 5-hydroxytryptamine (p. 23).

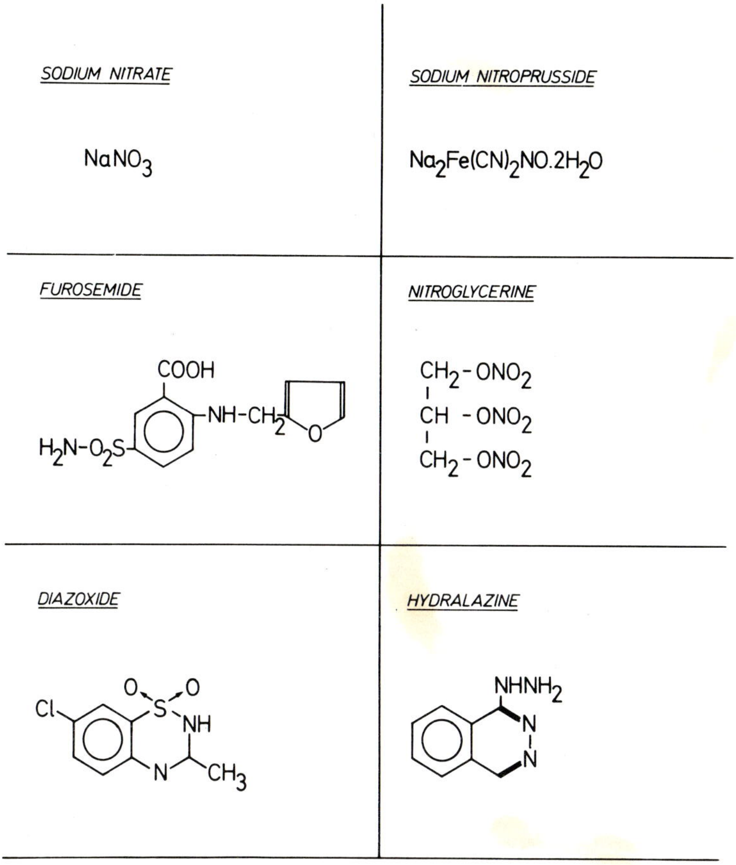
SODIUM NITRATE
NaNO3
SODIUM NITROPRUSSIDE
Na2Fe(CN)2NO.2H2O
FUROSEMIDE
COOH
H2N-O2S-
-NH-CH2
O
NITROGLYCERINE
CH2-ONO2
CH -ONO2
CH2-ONO2
DIAZOXIDE
Cl
O
S
O
NH
N
CH3
HYDRALAZINE
NHNH2
N
N

FIG. 7–20. Structure of nonspecific vasodilator drugs.

DRUGS AFFECTING THE RELEASE OF AUTONOMIC NEUROTRANSMITTERS

Sympathetic Nerves

Neuroeffector Interaction

Substances such as tyramine, amphetamine, or ephredrine stimulate cardiac function and cause constriction of resistance and capacitance vessels by displacing norepinephrine from the storage sites in the adrenergic nerve endings into the junctional cleft (indirect sympathomimetic effect) (Fig. 7–22). However, because they do so not only in the cardiovascular system but throughout the body, these drugs cause a multiplicity of side effects and should not be used. Cardiac

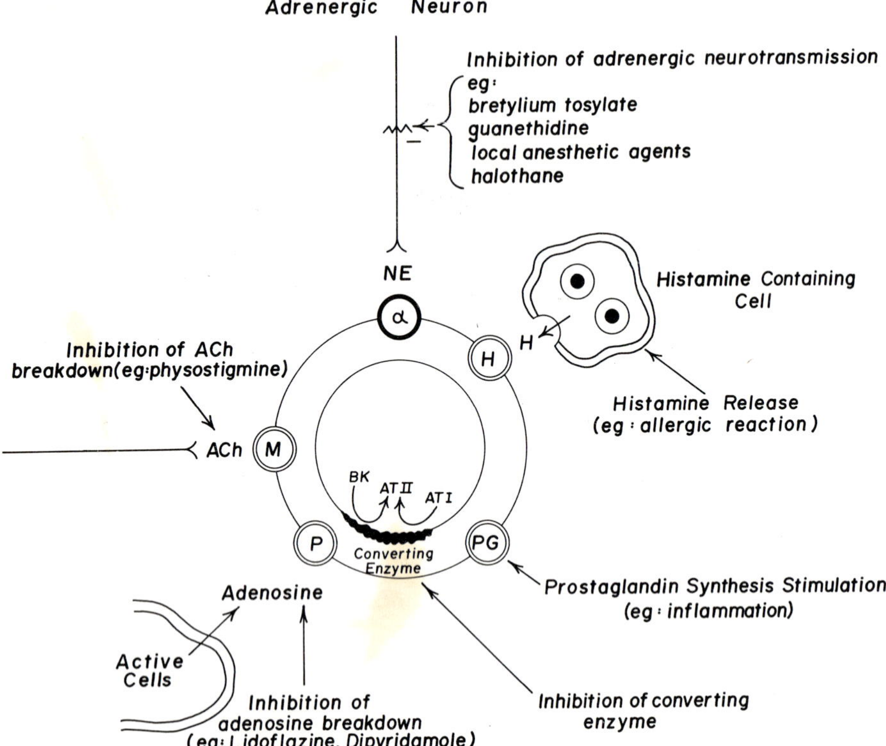

FIG. 7–21. Drugs causing vasodilation by altering the local concentration of vasoactive substances. *Open circles:* vasodilator responses. *Full circles:* vasoconstrictor responses. α = alpha-adrenergic receptor. ACh = acetylcholine. AT = angiotensin. BK = bradykinin. H = histamine receptor. M = muscarinic receptor. P = purinergic receptors, PG = prostaglandin-like substances. (Modified from Van Nueten: In: *Mechanisms of Vasodilatation,* edited by Vanhoutte and Leusen, p. 137. Karger, Basel, 1978.)

glycosides also facilitate the release of norepinephrine from adrenergic endings, which reinforces their direct effect on the cardiac and vascular effector cells (Fig. 7–15).

Reserpine inhibits the uptake of norepinephrine in nerve endings and storage vesicles, and causes depletion of catecholamines, thereby rendering the sympathetic nervous system ineffective (Fig. 7–23). However, its central nervous system effects, including a suicidal tendency, restrict its use.

Guanethidine inhibits peripheral adrenergic neurotransmission. It must be taken up by the nerve endings, which explains why drugs which inhibit neuronal uptake (e.g., cocaine, tricyclic antidepressants) antagonize its effect. It has reserpine-like action, causing norepinephrine depletion, and it prevents the release of norepinephrine (Fig. 7–23). As with reserpine, peripheral resistance decreases, the veins dilate, the heart slows, cardiac output falls, and blood pressure decreases. Guanethidine interferes with reflex adjustments, in particular those

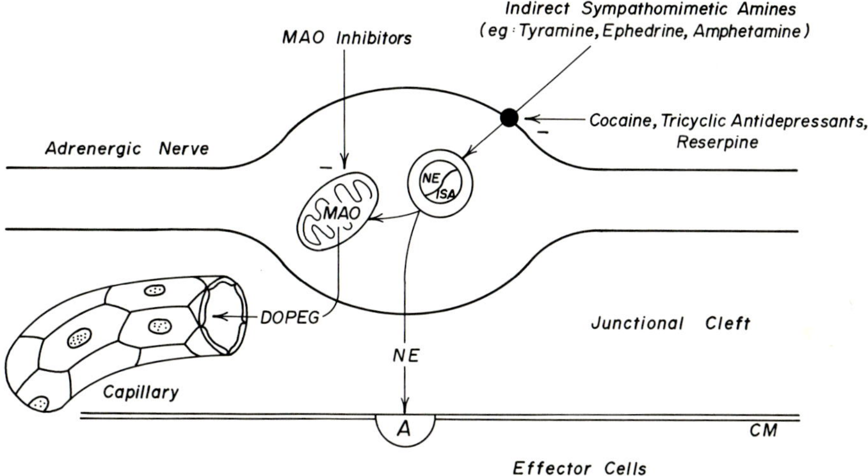

FIG. 7–22. Action of drugs which cause displacement of norepinephrine (NE) from the adrenergic nerve endings (indirect sympathomimetic amines; ISA). Since these drugs are taken up actively by the neuronal cell membrane, their effect can be antagonized by inhibitors of neuronal uptake, e.g., cocaine or tricyclic antidepressant drugs. The indirect sympathomimetic amines displace the norepinephrine from its storage sites. Part of the norepinephrine reaches the synaptic cleft unchanged, and part is metabolized by mitochondrial monoamine oxidase (MAO) to 3,4-dihydroxyphenylglycol (DOPEG). Drugs which inhibit this enzyme potentiate the effect of indirect sympathomimetic amines. — = inhibitory effect. ● = active carrier. A = adrenergic receptor.

during exercise and changes in body posture, and thus may decrease exercise tolerance and cause postural hypotension. As is true for all denervated tissues, the cardiac and vascular smooth muscle cells become more sensitive to the transmitter (p. 219). Hence patients treated with guanethidine are supersensitive to injected catecholamines. This cellular supersensitivity is aided by the fact that guanethidine occupies the carrier system for the uptake of transmitter by the sympathetic nerve endings, thus allowing norepinephrine to remain longer in the vicinity of the adrenergic receptors. The side effects of guanethidine are those common to all agents which interfere in a nonspecific way with adrenergic mechanisms throughout the body (e.g., diarrhea, impotence).

Alpha-methyldopa inhibits decarboxylation of DOPA (Fig. 5–4), resulting in the reduced synthesis of norepinephrine. In the process, alpha-methylnorepinephrine is formed, which is stored by the adrenergic storage vesicles and is liberated upon nerve activation. The intrinsic activity of alpha-methylnorepinephrine is less than that of norepinephrine, so it acts as a "false transmitter" (Fig. 7–23). The cardiovascular effects of alpha-methyldopa are similar to those of guanethidine.

Certain drugs act by interfering with prejunctional modulation of norepinephrine release (Fig. 5–6). The prejunctional alpha-adrenergic receptors, which are located on the adrenergic nerve endings and mediate feedback inhibition

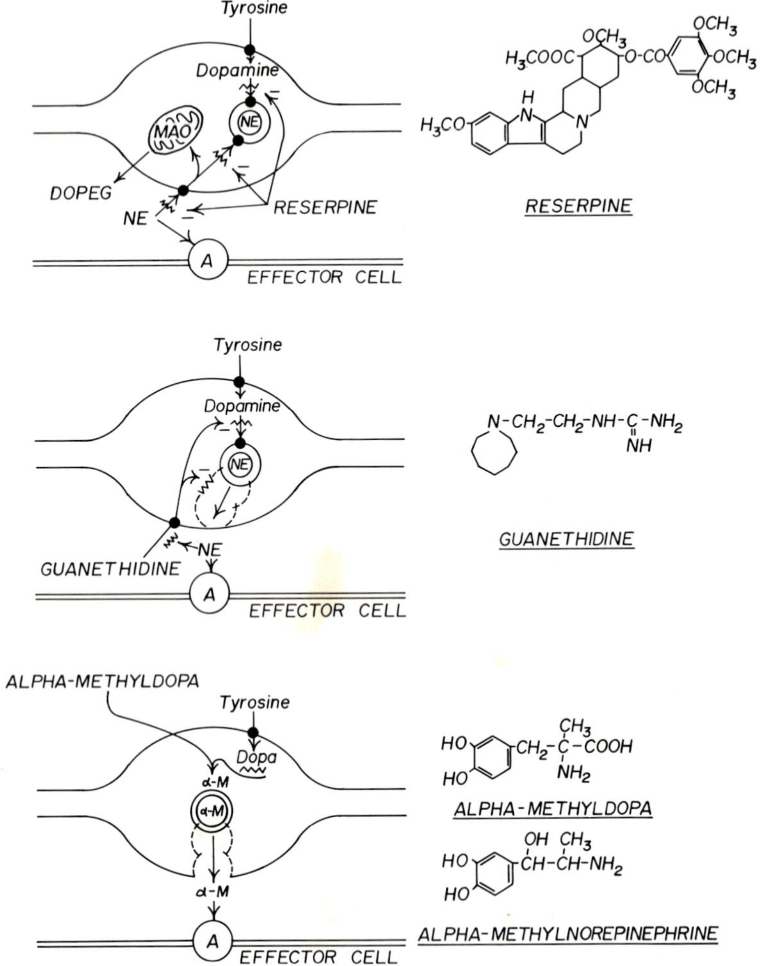

FIG. 7–23. Structure of reserpine, guanethidine, and alpha-methyldopa and mechanism of action at the adrenergic neuroeffector junction. Reserpine causes depletion of norepinephrine (NE). In addition to depletion, guanethidine inhibits the exocytotic process. Alpha-methyldopa inhibits the synthesis of norepinephrine and acts as a false transmitter. NE = norepinephrine. MAO = monoamine oxidase. A = adrenergic receptor. α-M = alpha-methylnorepinephrine. – = inhibitory effect.

of adrenergic neurotransmission, are activated by naturally occurring catecholamines and synthetic agonists such as clonidine (Fig. 7–24) and inhibited by certain alpha-adrenolytic drugs (e.g., yohimbine, phentolamine, antidepressant drugs). The latter cause a marked increase in the liberation of norepinephrine during activation of the sympathetic nerves, which in the heart results in tachycardia, and in the blood vessel wall may offset their inhibitory effect on the smooth muscle cells. Therefore when alpha-adrenolytic agents are used, prefer-

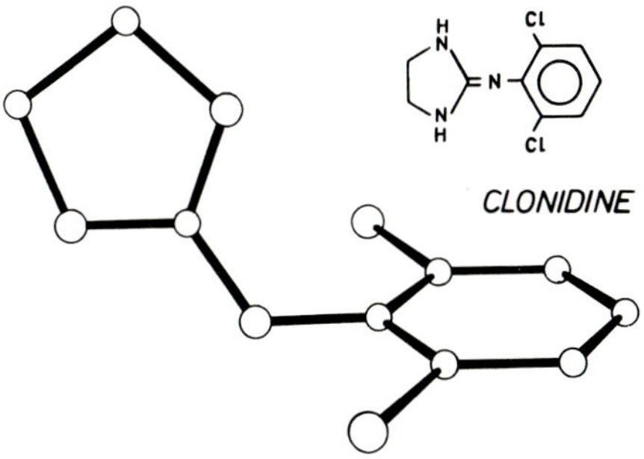

CLONIDINE

FIG. 7–24. Perspective drawing of the structure of clonidine derived from X-ray crystallographic data; hydrogen atoms are omitted for the sake of clarity. (Modified from Tollenaere et al.: *Atlas of the Three Dimensional Structure of Drugs.* Elsevier North-Holland, Amsterdam, 1979.)

ence should be given to drugs such as prazosin and labetalol, which have little affinity for the prejunctional alpha-adrenergic receptors. Likewise, part of the cardiac acceleration and of the increase in plasma catecholamine concentration caused by muscarinic antagonists (e.g., atropine, gallamine, pancuronium bromide) is due to withdrawal of the prejunctional inhibition of adrenergic neurotransmission caused by acetylcholine released from the cholinergic nerves.

Ganglionic Transmission

Ganglionic blocking agents, which act by inhibiting the nicotinic receptors on ganglionic cells, are powerful hypotensive and vasodilator drugs. However, they block all autonomic neurogenic control systems, resulting in a variety of side effects, and are no longer used for therapeutic purposes.

Centrally Acting Agents

There are three ways by which therapeutic agents decrease the central sympathetic outflow to the cardiovascular system and cause a fall in blood pressure (Fig. 7–25).

1. Decreasing the drive which higher centers exert via the hypothalamus on the medullary centers. This explains the beneficial effects that tranquilizers, sedatives, and beta-adrenergic blocking drugs have in patients with high blood pressure in whom stress and emotion increase sympathetic outflow. The beneficial effect of morphine in lung edema is explained by venodilation due to withdrawal of sympathetic tone.

2. Binding to central alpha-adrenergic receptors with resulting inhibition of the cardiovascular centers. In normal conditions these receptors are controlled by a series of adrenergic neurons which impinge on many centers of the brain and modify their activity for reasons yet unknown (p. 129). When weak alpha-adrenergic agonists such as clonidine (Fig. 7–24) or alpha-methylnorepinephrine bind to these receptors, the sympathetic outflow is reduced.

3. Inhibiting the stimulating effect of angiotensin II on the cardiovascular

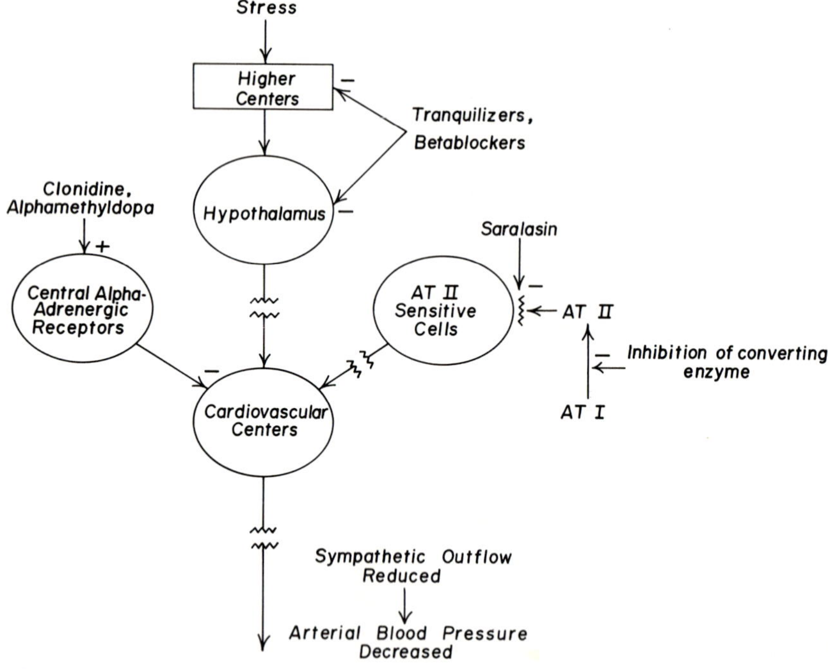

FIG. 7–25. Central action of drugs causing reduction in arterial blood pressure. + = activation. − = inhibition. AT = angiotensin. ≈ = reduced nerve traffic.

centers (p. 122) by the administration of angiotensin II antagonists (saralasin) or inhibitors of converting enzymes (captopril).

Cholinergic Nerves

Part of the increase in vagal tone seen with cardiac glycosides is due to direct facilitation of the cholinergic neurotransmission by the agents. Likewise, inhibition of cholinesterase by drugs such as physostigmine prolongs and exaggerates the effects of cholinergic nerve stimulation in the heart and the blood vessels (Fig. 7–21).

DIURETICS

The Na^+ and water content of the body determine the blood volume and hence contribute to the filling of the heart. In addition, excess Na^+ may cause water-logging in the blood vessel wall. This is of particular importance in the arterioles where the thickening of the wall reduces the diameter, increases the resistance to blood flow, and thus augments blood pressure (p. 214). Diuretics, in particular the benzothiazides, augment Na^+ and water excretion in the kidney, which results in less plasma volume, less extracellular fluid, and less waterlogging of the vessel wall. In addition, certain diuretics (e.g., diazoxide, furosemide) have a direct inhibitory effect on vascular smooth muscle (p. 198).

SELECTED REFERENCES

Ahlquist, R. P. (1976): Present state of alpha- and beta-adrenergic drugs. *Am. Heart J.,* 92:661, 804; 93:117.

Amsterdam, E. A., Awan, N. A., DeMaria, A. N., and Mason, D. T. (1978): Vasodilators in myocardial infarction: Rationale and current status. *Drugs,* 16:506.

Beeler, G. W. (1977): Ionic currents in cardiac muscle: A framework for glycoside action. *Fed. Proc.,* 36:2209.

Brody, T. M., and Akera, T. (1977): Relations among Na^+,K^+-ATPase activity, sodium pump activity, transmembrane sodium movement, and cardiac contractility. *Fed. Proc.,* 36:2219.

Brogden, R. N., Heel, R. C., Speight, T. M., and Avery, G. S. (1978): Labetalol: A review of its pharmacology and therapeutic use in hypertension. *Drugs,* 15:251.

Cambridge, D., Davey, M. J., and Massingham, R. (1977): The pharmacology of antihypertensive drugs with special reference to vasodilators, α-adrenergic blocking agents and prazosin. *Med. J. Aust. (Suppl 2),* p. 2.

Cohn, J. N., and Franciosa, J. A. (1977): Vasodilator therapy of cardiac failure (first of two parts). *N. Engl. J. Med.,* 297:27.

Godfraind, T., and Morel, N. (1978): Inhibitors of calcium influx. In: *Mechanisms of Vasodilatation,* edited by P. M. Vanhoutte and I. Leusen, p. 144. Karger, Basel.

Haber, E., and Wrenn, S. (1976): Problems in identification of the beta-adrenergic receptor. *Physiol. Rev.,* 56:317.

Koch-Weser, J. (1976): Drug therapy: Diazoxide. *N. Engl. J. Med.,* 294:1271.

Koch-Weser, J. (1976): Drug therapy: Hydralazine. *N. Engl. J. Med.,* 295:320.

Kreye, V. A. W. (1978): Organic nitrates, sodium nitroprusside, and vasodilation. In: *Mechanisms of Vasodilatation,* edited by P. M. Vanhoutte and I. Leusen, p. 158. Karger, Basel.

Langer, G. A. (1977): Relationship between myocardial contractility and the effects of digitalis on ionic exchange. *Fed. Proc.,* 36:2231.

Mikulic, E., Cohn, J. N., and Franciosa, J. A. (1977): Comparative hemodynamic effects of inotropic and vasodilator drugs in severe heart failure. *Circulation,* 56:528.

Palmer, R. F., and Lasseter, K. C. (1975): Drug therapy: Sodium nitroprusside. *N. Engl. J. Med.,* 292:294.

Rosen, R., and Hoffman, B. F. (1973): Mechanism of action of antiarrhythmic drugs. *Circ. Res.,* 32:1.

Ross, G. (1976): Adrenergic responses of the coronary vessels. *Circ. Res.,* 39:461.

Schnaar, R. L., and Sparks, H. V. (1972): Response of large and small coronary arteries to nitroglycerin, $NaNO_2$, and adenosine. *Am. J. Physiol.,* 223:223.

Schwartz, A., and Allen, J. C. (1977): Newer aspects of cardiac glycoside action. *Fed. Proc.,* 36:2207.

Smith, T. W. (1973): Digitalis. *N. Engl. J. Med.,* 21:1125.

Stoclet, J-C., and Lugnier, C. (1978): Inhibitors of cyclic AMP breakdown. In: *Mechanisms of Vasodilatation,* edited by P. M. Vanhoutte and I. Leusen, p. 152. Karger, Basel.

Van Nueten, J. M. (1978): Vasodilatation or inhibition of peripheral vasoconstriction? In: *Mechanisms of Vasodilatation,* edited by P. M. Vanhoutte and I. Leusen, p. 137. Karger, Basel.

Zimmerman, B. G. (1978): Action of angiotensin on adrenergic nerve endings. *Fed. Proc.,* 37:199.

8

Hypertension and Hyperreactivity of the Cardiovascular System

The hemodynamic consequences of the many and complex types of disease that can affect the cardiovascular system can be deduced from the knowledge of its normal functioning on the one hand, and from the primary changes causing the disease process on the other. From the functional point of view, cardiovascular diseases can be classified into those in which the system is hyperactive (this chapter), those in which it fails (Chapters 9 and 10), and those where a congenital abnormality causes the dysfunction (Chapter 11).

HIGH BLOOD PRESSURE

In healthy subjects the systemic arterial blood pressure is lowest during sleep and highest during emotional and physical stresses. In most people the systolic arterial blood pressure increases throughout life, but the increase in mean pressure usually is less than 20 mm Hg from youth to old age (Fig. 8–1). In most countries, and particularly in the Western world, the blood pressure in about 15% of the adult population is increased persistently above the normal range. Such prolonged elevation increases morbidity and mortality. Since high blood pressure in the absence of complications causes no symptoms, a large number of people are unaware they are hypertensive unless their blood pressure is measured at intervals. Resting systolic pressures of less than 140 mm Hg and diastolic

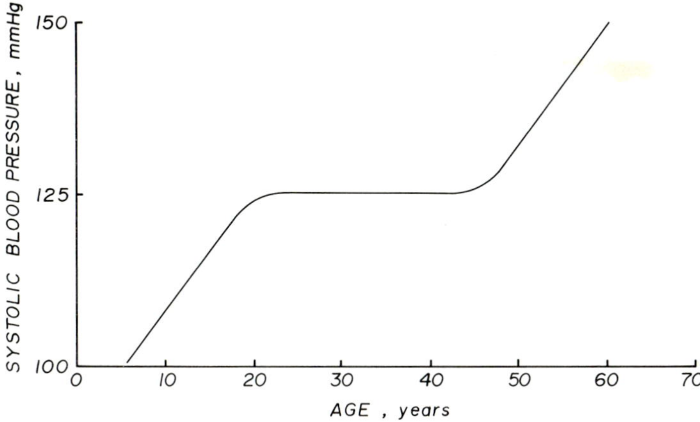

FIG. 8–1. Changes in systolic arterial blood pressure with age. The increase in older adults reflects mainly the decreased elasticity of the aorta and large arteries.

pressures of less than 90 mm Hg are said to be normal. Adults with values which persistently exceed 160 and 95 mm Hg, respectively, are said to be hypertensive. Those with pressures which frequently lie between the normal and the hypertensive groups are said to have "borderline" hypertension and are at an increased risk of developing sustained hypertension. A persistent elevation of arterial blood pressure implies that the control systems, in particular the arterial mechanoreceptors, are no longer able to maintain the blood pressure within a normal range.

Essential Arterial Hypertension

In the great majority of patients with hypertension the cause of the abnormal increase in blood pressure is unknown (essential hypertension). The word essential was coined from an erroneous translation of the German word *essentiele,* which means idiopathic or of unknown origin.

Possible Mechanisms

About 30% of the subjects with borderline hypertension have an elevated cardiac output although their systemic vascular resistance is near normal; however, if the cardiac output is lowered by using a combination of atropine and beta-blockers, the peripheral vascular resistance increases and the same borderline hypertensive blood pressure level is maintained. In the remaining 70% and in patients with long-established hypertension, the cardiac output and the viscosity of the blood are normal; the blood pressure is raised owing to an abnormal narrowing of the systemic resistance vessels.

From the large number of studies that have been conducted in animals and man to determine the cause of the increased systemic vascular resistance in essential hypertension, it is evident that no single derangement can be held accountable (Fig. 8–2). Studies of families, including identical and fraternal twins, have demonstrated that genetic factors are important in the distribution of blood pressure in the population. The onset of the hypertensive process is symptomless. Therefore at the time it is detected the initiating factors may be obscured by adaptations secondary to the prolonged increase in pressure.

Adrenergic System

In most patients with essential hypertension the resting plasma levels of catecholamines are elevated, and there is a significant relationship between resting plasma norepinephrine levels and systolic and diastolic blood pressure. The plasma concentration of dopamine-β-hydroxylase, the enzyme released together with norepinephrine from the adrenergic nerves (p. 113), usually also is increased

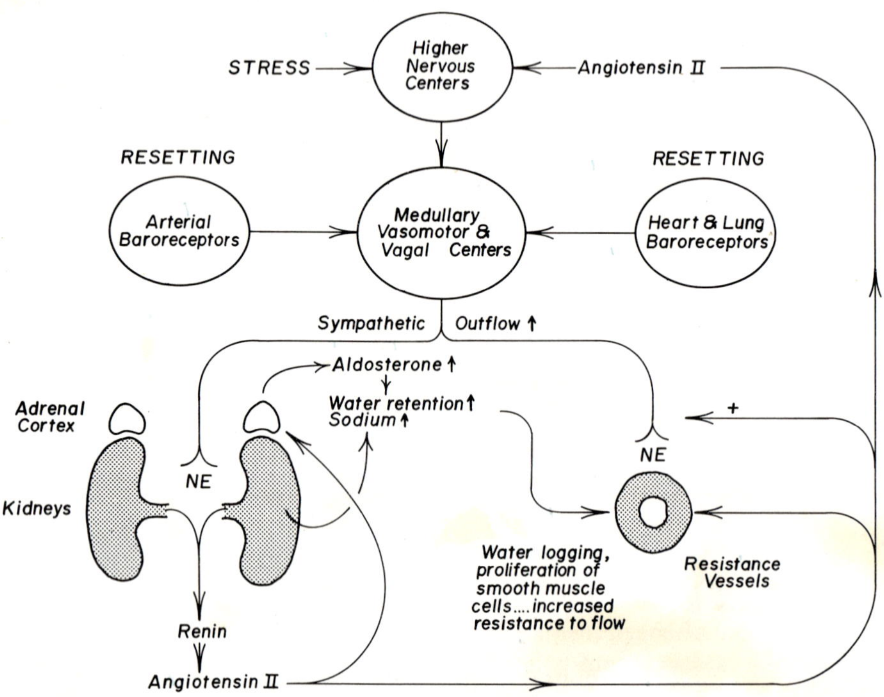

FIG. 8–2. Factors which may be involved in the genesis of essential hypertension. In addition, for each level of sympathetic nerve activity, the adrenergic nerve terminals may liberate more norepinephrine than normal, and the alpha-receptors of the vascular smooth muscle cells may be more sensitive to the transmitter. BP = arterial blood pressure. CO = cardiac output, NE = norepinephrine, PR = peripheral resistance, ↑ = increase, + = facilitation.

in these patients. This implies that in many instances excess sympathetic activity contributes to the increase in blood pressure. However, other patients have plasma levels of norepinephrine and dopamine-β-hydroxylase within the normal range.

The high level of norepinephrine and dopamine-β-hydroxylase can be due to an increased activity of any of the components of the reflex arcs controlling blood pressure:

1. The carotid and aortic baroreceptors may be "reset" in hypertension and the threshold pressure at which they start to fire increased (Fig. 8–3). This leads to an increase in peripheral sympathetic nervous activity and a diminution of vagal tone. Whether the resetting is due to an altered sensitivity of the sensors or to an altered structure of the blood vessel wall which becomes more resistant to stretch is unknown.
2. The neurons in the central nervous system which control the autonomic outflow may be overactive because of genetic factors, circulating agents (e.g., angiotensin II), or continued emotional stress.
3. At the adrenergic neuroeffector junction, more norepinephrine may be liberated per impulse or less taken back into the nerve (p. 113).
4. The sensitivity for norepinephrine of the alpha-adrenergic receptors on the vascular smooth muscle cells of the resistance vessels may be increased, so for each amount of norepinephrine released a stronger vasoconstriction is obtained (Fig. 8–4).

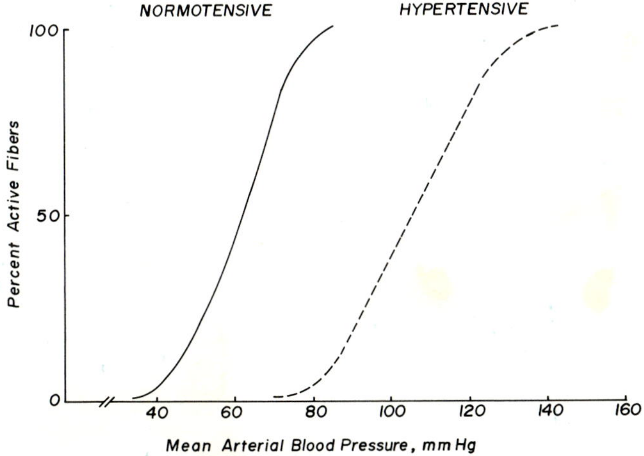

FIG. 8–3. Resetting of the arterial mechanoreceptors in experimental hypertension. In Normotensive and hypertensive animals the firing of the aortic baroreceptors increases as the arterial pressure rises. However, the pressure–response curve in the hypertensive animals is displaced to the right, indicating that the receptors function normally but at a higher set point. (Modified from Jones and Thorén: *Acta Physiol. Scand.,* 101:286, 1977.)

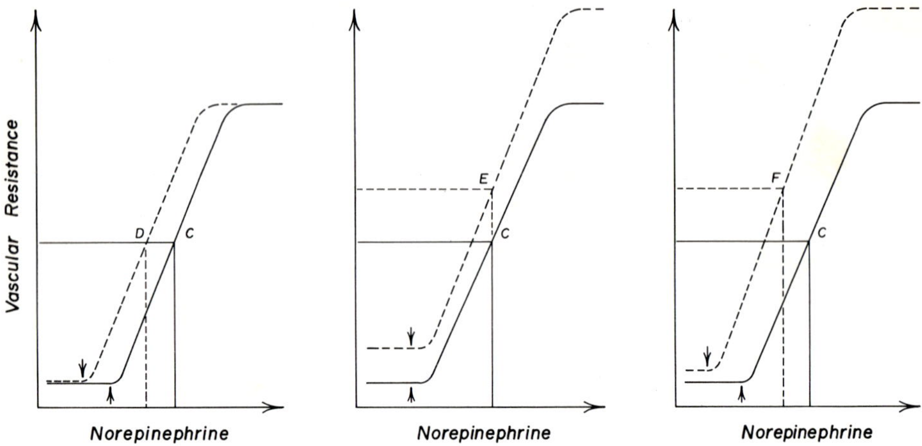

FIG. 8–4. Mechanisms of augmentation of vascular resistance in hypertension. **Left:** An increase in vascular resistance *(ordinate)* can be caused by increasing the amount of norepinephrine *(abscissa)* liberated by the sympathetic nerve endings; this increased release can be due either to an increased sympathetic outflow or to an augmented release per nerve impulse. If the sensitivity of the smooth muscle cell is not augmented, the response follows the normal pattern (C). If the affinity of the alpha-adrenergic receptors is augmented, smaller amounts of norepinephrine initiate constriction *(arrow)* and the dose–response curve is shifted to the left, as illustrated by the shift in the concentration which causes half-maximal constriction (Effective dose$_{50}$ (ED$_{50}$) as indicated by vertical lines). The maximal response is unaltered (D). **Middle:** If the wall of the arteriole thickens, the wall-to-lumen ratio increases and the diameter decreases. In such vessels the resistance to flow is higher even when the smooth muscle cells are inactive (Fig. 1–6). If the sensitivity of these cells is normal, they respond to the same concentration of norepinephrine as normal vessels *(arrow),* but at each concentration of the transmitter the amplitude of the response is greater; the ED$_{50}$ is unaltered (E). **Right:** In arterioles of hypertensive subjects, wall thickening (water-logging, proliferation of smooth muscle, increased collagen) usually is combined with hyperreactivity of the smooth muscle cells. The dose–response curve to norepinephrine is shifted upward and to the left. The ED$_{50}$ is smaller and the maximal response larger (F).

Renin–Angiotensin–Aldosterone Axis

The juxtaglomerular cells of the kidney can release renin when the activity in the renal sympathetic nerves is increased, the distending pressure in the afferent arterioles is lowered, or the amount of sodium delivered to the macula densa is reduced (p. 119). The resulting formation of angiotensin II, which in turn stimulates the synthesis and release of aldosterone, makes the renin–angiotensin–aldosterone axis potentially important in causing abnormal elevations of blood pressure. Angiotensin II can activate central and peripheral neurons, causing increased sympathetic outflow, increasing the concentration of norepinephrine in the synaptic cleft, sensitizing the alpha-adrenergic receptors of the vascular smooth muscle to the sympathetic neurotransmitter, and causing direct constriction of the resistance blood vessels (Fig. 8–2). Aldosterone causes retention of sodium, expansion of the extracellular fluid volume, and water-logging of the blood vessels, which further decreases their caliber. The role of angiotensin II and aldosterone in the genesis or maintenance of essential hypertension is uncertain. About 20% of patients with essential hypertension have high levels of plasma renin, about 50% have normal levels, and in 30% the levels are subnormal.

Sodium Retention and Blood Volume

If, because of disease, the kidneys lose their ability to excrete the normal daily load of salt and water, the level of the systemic arterial blood pressure increases. In hypertension due to disease of the renal parenchyma, sodium retention may be the prime cause of the pressure elevation. The resultant increase in extracellular fluid and intravascular volume could increase the filling pressure of the heart and lead to an increased cardiac output. The increased perfusion of the systemic organs and tissues without a concomitant increase in their metabolism might evoke local constriction of the vessels in order to adjust the flow to the actual needs of the tissues (autoregulation). The blood pressure might be maintained at the higher level because of the continued increase in vascular resistance due to the excess sodium content of the vascular wall, causing water-logging (Fig. 8–4). An alternative explanation is to assume that the increased blood volume initiates the secretion of "natriuretic hormone(s)," which inhibits Na^+,K^+ATPase throughout the body. This might cause increased responsiveness of cardiac and vascular smooth muscle cells to normal stimuli. The increased arteriolar resistance, combined with the decreased venous capacity and the increased cardiac contractility, might cause the hypertension. The normal Na^+ and water content of the body could be explained by inhibition of the Na^+K^+ exchanges in the kidney.

Epidemiological studies have demonstrated a relationship between the prevalence of hypertension and the amount of salt intake. Hypertension is not found in populations still unexposed to modern civilization, nor does blood pressure rise in these groups with age if salt is not added to their diet. It has been postulated that in many instances of essential hypertension a genetic defect results in lowered sodium excretion at normal glomerular hydrostatic pressures. In this case augmenting kidney perfusion by increasing the arterial pressure would facilitate sodium and water excretion. If this view is correct, hypertension will occur in an individual's life as soon as an imbalance becomes manifest between the intake of sodium and the ability of the kidney to excrete it. Thus in populations exposed to the stress of modern life, the genetic background of the individual and in particular the ability to balance intake and output of salt may determine the susceptibility to develop essential hypertension.

Adaptive Changes in the Blood Vessel Wall

When the vascular smooth muscle cells of a given vascular bed are completely relaxed, the resistance to flow is greater in a hypertensive subject than in a normotensive individual because of structural narrowing of the arterioles. In such vessels the same increase in sympathetic activity will cause a greater increase in resistance even if the sensitivity of the smooth muscle cells is normal (Fig. 8–4). The increased thickening of the vessel wall is due not only to water-logging but also to proliferation of the smooth muscle cells and their increased production of collagen fibers. The proliferation is secondary to the increase in intravascular pressure and is facilitated by catecholamines. Once there is more collagen in the vascular wall, it becomes difficult to reverse the hypertensive process.

In addition to the morphological changes, the vascular smooth muscle cells are more sensitive to vasoconstrictor agents. Thus the vessels become more reactive to the customary stimuli and the increase in systemic vascular resistance, however initiated, will be sustained (Fig. 8–4).

Similar structural changes reduce the distensibility of the walls of the carotid sinus and aortic arch, and could account, at least in part, for the resetting of the carotid and aortic baroreceptors.

The involvement of the systemic veins in the hypertension process is uncertain. Decreases in venous wall distensibility have been reported in hypertensive animals and man. If this were to occur in the early stages of hypertension, the decreased venous compliance could shift blood from the systemic veins to the central circulation. If the cardiopulmonary mechanoreceptors did not cause a sufficient compensatory decrease in total blood volume, the filling pressure of the heart would increase. This could cause an augmented cardiac output, which in turn might initiate the hypertensive process by causing autoregulatory increases in resistance throughout the body.

Consequences

The increased afterload due to the rise in arterial pressure leads to a gradual hypertrophy of the muscle of the left ventricle (p. 258). Eventually the heart fails when the energy required to maintain the high blood pressure exceeds the ability of the coronary vessels to provide the hypertrophied myocardium with enough blood for its metabolism (p. 91). In addition to heart failure, the high blood pressure predisposes to atherosclerosis and its associated complications (p. 224). If untreated, hypertension eventually causes death, usually from heart or kidney failure, or cerebral hemorrhage (stroke).

In some patients the arterial blood pressure rises rapidly, reaching levels of 200 mm Hg or more systolic and 140 mm Hg or more diastolic. Such malignant hypertension (hypertensive crisis) can occur early or after prolonged periods of moderate hypertension. These high pressures cause acute necrotic changes in the arterioles, especially in brain and kidney. This leads to brain dysfunction (hypertensive encephalopathy, papilledema) and acute renal failure. The plasma levels of renin and aldosterone are augmented and contribute to the accelerated increase in blood pressure. The increased renin secretion presumably is secondary to the kidney damage.

Principles of Treatment

The blood pressure can be decreased in the following ways (Fig. 8–5):

1. Reducing the sympathetic outflow to the periphery by decreasing the activity of the vasomotor centers. This is done most typically by drugs such as clonidine and alpha-methyldopa but can also be achieved with beta-blockers (p. 186).

2. Interrupting ganglionic transmission (ganglion blocking drugs); this form of treatment is no longer used.

3. Reducing the release of norepinephrine by adrenergic nerve endings with drugs such as guanethidine and alpha-methyldopa.

4. Disconnecting the heart from sympathetic control and thus reducing cardiac output by using cardioselective beta-blockers.

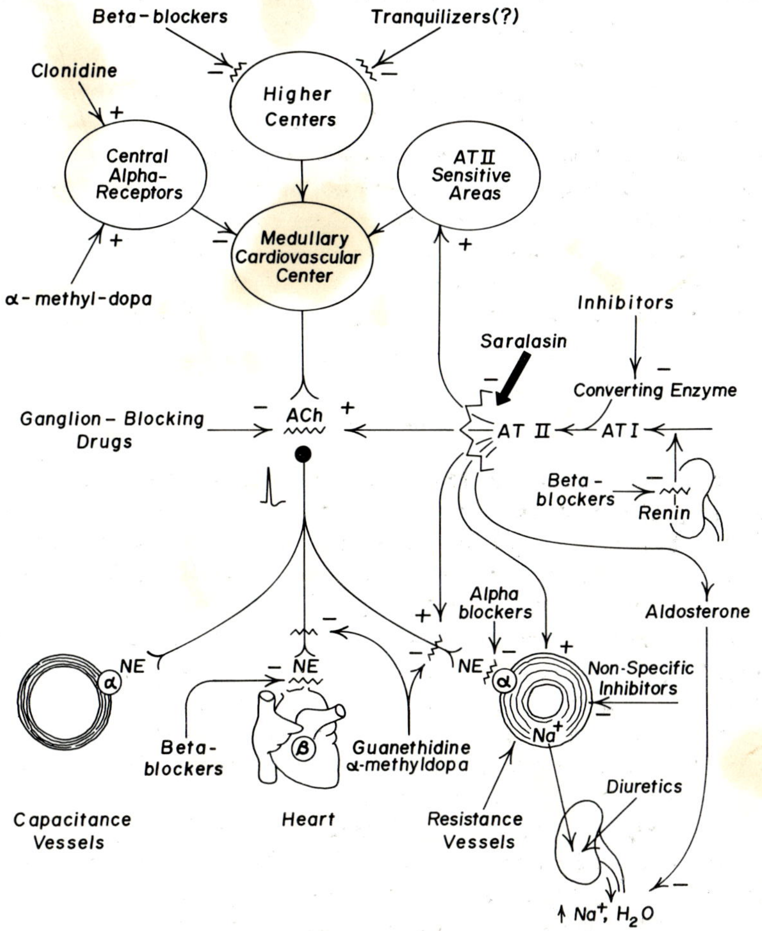

FIG. 8–5. Principles of treatment in hypertension. AT = angiotensin ||. NE = norepinephrine. α = alpha-adrenergic. β = beta-adrenergic. −, +, = inhibition. ⌒⌒ = activation.

5. Disconnecting the vascular smooth muscle cells from sympathetic control by using alpha-adrenergic blocking drugs. Drugs such as prazosin affect arteriolar resistance vessels more than the systemic veins so orthostatic hypotension is infrequent.

6. Combining beta-adrenergic and alpha-adrenergic blockade, with drugs such as labetalol.

7. Using an inhibitor of converting enzyme or specific antagonists to block the receptors for angiotensin II when the plasma levels of this hormone are elevated. Beta-adrenergic blockers reduce the release of renin when this is increased.

8. Using nonspecific inhibitors of vascular smooth muscle activity such as hydralazine.

9. Decreasing the water-logging of the vascular wall by lowering the total body content of salt. This can be done by using diuretics and/or decreasing salt intake.

In practice, combinations of these approaches are used most commonly. Whatever the cause of the hypertension, the pressure can be controlled by appropriate treatment. Since established hypertension is due to an increase in systemic vascular resistance, treatment of the process should reduce the latter. If only the cardiac output is decreased, the resulting fall in blood pressure may avoid the complications of hypertension but at the same time this creates conditions in which most tissues are underperfused.

High Blood Pressure Associated with Specific Lesions

Renovascular Hypertension

Decreasing the blood supply to one kidney by partial occlusion of the renal artery and leaving the contralateral kidney undisturbed causes persistent hypertension in animals. This mimics the changes seen in humans when one renal artery is stenosed. The augmented release of renin from this kidney helps initiate the hypertensive process; how much it contributes to its maintenance is debated. The hypertension is cured by surgical relief of the stenosis or removal of the kidney, although in longstanding cases when the blood vessels have undergone structural changes the pressure may not return to normal.

Renal Failure

Renal diseases such as glomerulonephritis are accompanied by hypertension. In acute conditions this is probably due to the decreased excretion of sodium chloride by the diseased renal parenchyma in combination with augmented renin release as the sodium delivery to the macula densa decreases. In chronic renal disease, when the parenchyma and the juxtaglomerular cells are destroyed, the insufficient excretion of sodium and the secondary morphological changes of the arteriolar wall are the main causes of the persistent hypertension.

Pheochromocytoma

Pheochromocytoma is a rare tumor of the adrenal medulla. It may also occur at other sites which contain chromaffin tissue. The tumor, which has no nerve supply, secretes large amounts of norepinephrine, epinephrine, or most commonly a mixture of both into the circulation. The secretion may occur intermittently or continuously and causes paroxysmal or sustained hypertension owing to peripheral arteriolar vasoconstriction, peripheral venoconstriction, and cardiac stimulation. The increased plasma level of catecholamines also causes excessive sweating, headache, anxiety, and tremors. The defect which results in the enhanced synthesis and release of catecholamines is unknown. The urinary excretion of catecholamines and their metabolites is greatly increased. The sudden removal of the tumor may precipitate severe hypotension requiring temporary substitution by intravenous norepinephrine to maintain blood pressure.

Adrenal Hyperplasia

Hypertension is a feature of a variety of adrenal cortical abnormalities. In primary aldosteronism caused by an adrenal tumor, the increased secretion of aldosterone causes initial sodium retention by stimulating the renal tubular absorption of sodium in exchange for potassium. The extracellular fluid volume and the blood volume increase. The potassium depletion (hypokalemia) persists as long as the levels of mineralocorticoids are high. After some days the sodium retention becomes limited, because by an unknown mechanism the proximal tubules of the kidney reabsorb progressively less of the ion while more escapes in the urine. The stimulation of the cardiopulmonary mechanoreceptors by the increase in blood volume temporarily reduces the sympathetic outflow to the kidneys. This, together with the relatively high levels of Na^+ reaching the macula densa, inhibits the release of renin. In the vessel wall the increase in the Na^+/K^+ ratio is accompanied by water-logging. The high levels of mineralocorticoids delay the disposition of catecholamines by inhibiting their extraneuronal uptake (p. 154). Thus the smooth muscle cells react more forcefully to normal levels of sympathetic activity. Together these changes cause hypertension.

Excess plasma levels of glucocorticosteriods (Cushing's syndrome) can be due to hypothalamic–pituitary dysfunction, an adrenal tumor, or excessive administration of medications containing corticosteriods. This may cause hypertension because in high concentrations these hormones have mineralocorticoid properties and delay the disposition of norepinephrine.

Toxemia of Pregnancy

In a number of pregnant women the increased levels of estrogen and progesterone have mineralocorticoid effects which result in Na^+ and water retention, hypervolemia, and mild hypertension (preeclampsia). In certain of these hypertensive women, the placenta becomes hypoxic and liberates vasoactive polypeptides, which cause constriction of the brain and kidney vessels. The secretion of renin is augmented. The high levels of the vasopressor polypeptides and angiotensin II cause constriction of the resistance vessels and severe acute hypertension (eclampsia). The constriction of the brain vessels results in cerebral hypoxia, causing convulsions and coma. The constriction of the placental vessels eventually causes anoxia and death of the fetus. These symptoms disappear when the placenta is removed.

IDIOPATHIC PULMONARY HYPERTENSION

In idiopathic pulmonary hypertension the pulmonary vascular resistance and the pulmonary artery pressure are markedly increased and the pulmonary venous pressure is normal. In these patients there is no evidence of other circulatory abnormalities. The cause of the disease is unknown; it occurs at sea level in contrast to the pulmonary hypertension present in dwellers at high altitude (p. 162). The changes in the pulmonary vessels include progressive hypertrophy of the media and fibrous intimal proliferation. The increased resistance augments the work of the right ventricle, which hypertrophies and eventually fails (p. 255). In the early stages of the disease pulmonary vasoconstriction plays a subsidiary role, and an infusion of acetylcholine results in a small decrease in pulmonary vascular resistance. When such patients exercise, loss of consciousness is common because acute failure of the right ventricle causes a marked decrease in cardiac output and arterial blood pressure.

SPASTIC VASCULAR DISEASE

In certain subjects the blood vessels are hyperreactive to normal stimuli, resulting in their excessive and prolonged constriction. The most typical examples are the following.

Raynaud's Disease

Raynaud's disease, most common in young females, is characterized by prolonged constriction (spasm) of the digital arteries of the hands when they are exposed to a cold stimulus, particularly when the subjects are emotionally upset. During an attack there is complete interruption of blood flow and the finger becomes waxy white. As the spasm slowly wanes and blood trickles in, its passage through the capillaries is delayed, oxygen desaturation occurs, and the color changes to blue (cyanosis). Before returning to normal, the finger becomes pink because of reactive hyperemia.

The vasospasm is attributed to a local fault in the vessels, which are most sensitive to temperatures in the 12° to 15°C range. One explanation for this phenomenon is the absence of beta-receptors in the digital vascular smooth

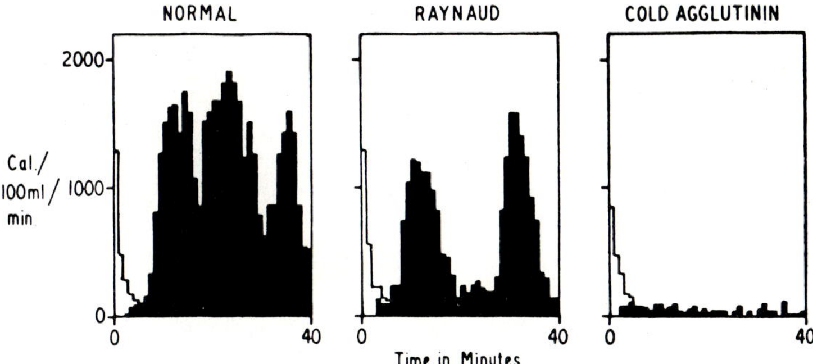

FIG. 8–6. In patients with Raynaud's disease, finger blood vessels exposed to water at 2°C respond normally with the sequence of constriction, cold vasodilatation, and the hunting phenomenon (p. 101). By contrast, in patients with cold agglutinins the decrease in blood flow seen upon exposure to cold is sustained because of the mechanical obstruction created by the aggregating erythrocytes. The blood flow is estimated from the heat elimination by the finger. (From Marshall et al.: *Clin. Sci.,* 12:255, 1953.)

muscle of these patients; in normal subjects the sensitivity of the beta-adrenergic receptors increases with cooling, which partly offsets the facilitating effect on alpha-adrenergic receptors (p. 99). The digital vessels in patients with Raynaud's disease dilate normally when exposed to temperatures lower than 10°C (cold vasodilatation) (Fig. 8–6). In chronic cases structural changes occur which reduce the ability of the vessels to dilate. Repeated attacks can lead to trophic lesions such as skin ulcers and bone necrosis.

Occasionally cervical sympathectomy is performed to prevent reflex constriction of the vessels. The blood flow immediately after the operation is increased but decreases over the next 2 to 3 weeks as tone returns to the denervated vessels. The reason for the return of tone is unknown. One possibility is denervation supersensitivity, which renders denervated smooth muscle more reactive to circulating catecholamines, in part because the latter are not taken up by the adrenergic nerve endings (p. 114). In a cool environment the temperature of the digits is higher than in control subjects because the sympathectomy eliminates reflex constriction.

The obstruction caused by the exaggerated spasm of the vascular wall upon cooling can be contrasted with the mechanical obstruction of the blood flow caused by agglutination of red cells in the capillaries. This occurs in sickle cell anemia or when substances are present in the plasma which when exposed to cold induce aggregation of the erythrocytes (cold agglutinins). When the hands of such patients are cooled, the blood trapped in the capillaries is desaturated below normal, and the part exposed to cooling becomes cyanotic; the blue color does not disappear when pressure is applied to the tissues (Fig. 8–6). Similar obstruction on exposure to cold occurs in patients with high circulating levels of abnormal proteins (cryoglobulinemia).

Coronary Vasospasm

Spasms of the large coronary arteries can be induced experimentally after beta-adrenergic blockade by the administration or release of norepinephrine in the coronaries. It also may occur during catheterization (coronary arteriography; p. 311) due to direct mechanical stimulation of the coronary smooth muscle. A number of patients without evident abnormalities of the coronary circulation develop the typical symptoms of angina pectoris at rest (variant angina, Prinzmetal angina). These episodes are due to coronary arterial spasm and result in myocardial ischemia. The mechanism is unknown. In such patients the attacks can be elicited by the injection of ergonovine maleate, an ergot alkaloid with alpha-adrenergic agonistic properties. Spasms, possibly caused by 5-hydroxytryptamine released from aggregating platelets, may precipitate myocardial infarction in patients with atherosclerosis of the coronary arteries. These spasms can be alleviated by nitrates, Ca^{2+} antagonists, and alpha-adrenergic blocking agents.

Cerebral Vasospasm

Radiographic studies of patients with brain infarction demonstrate spasm of the large arteries of the brain. Some transient neurological disorders can also be attributed to such spasms. One example is migraine in which the symptoms range from visual disturbances to mental confusion; the spasm is followed by cerebral vasodilation, which causes headache, nausea, and vomiting. The cause of migraine is unknown. Alpha-adrenolytic ergot derivatives (e.g., dihydroergotamine) and certain 5-hydroxytryptamine antagonists (e.g., methysergide) reduce the severity of the attacks.

THYROTOXICOSIS

Thyroid hormone augments the metabolism of the body cells and facilitates the effect of catecholamines. The circulatory consequences of thyrotoxicosis include: (1) Increase in heart rate, cardiac contractility, and cardiac output. The chronic increase in volume load, together with the uncoupling of oxidative metabolism leads to heart failure. (2) Decrease in total systemic vascular resistance secondary to increased metabolism, the facilitation of beta-adrenergic vasodilatation in skeletal muscle caused by circulating epinephrine, and skin vasodilatation to compensate for the increased heat production. (3) Dilatation of the cutaneous veins because of the thermoregulatory demands.

SELECTED REFERENCES

Brody, M. J., and Zimmerman, B. G. (1976): Peripheral circulation in arterial hypertension. *Prog. Cardiovasc. Dis.,* 18:323.

Davis, J. O. (1977): The pathogenesis of chronic renovascular hypertension. *Circ. Res.,* 40:439.

Dustan, H. P. (1976): Evaluation and therapy of hypertension. *Mod. Concepts Cardiovasc. Dis.,* 45:97.

Ferrario, C. M., and Page, I. H. (1978): Current views concerning cardiac output in the genesis of experimental hypertension. *Circ. Res.,* 43:821.

Folkow, B. (1978): Cardiovascular structural adaptation; its role in the initiation and maintenance of primary hypertension. *Clin. Sci. Mol. Med.,* 55:3s.

Freis, E. D. (1975): Salt, volume and the prevention of hypertension. *Circulation,* 53:589.

Frohlich, E. D. (1977): Hemodynamics of hypertension. In: *Hypertension,* edited by J. Genest, E. Koiw, and O. Kuchel, p. 15. McGraw-Hill, New York.

Genest, J., Nowaczynski, W., Kuchel, O., Boucher, R., Rojo-Ortega, J. M., Constantopoulos, G., Ganten, D., and Messerli, F. (1976): The adrenal cortex and essential hypertension. *Recent Prog. Horm. Res.,* 32:377.

Guyton, A. C., Coleman, T. G., Cowley, A. W., Jr., Manning, R. D., Jr., Norman, R. A., and Ferguson, J. D. (1974): A systems analysis approach to understanding long-range arterial blood pressure control and hypertension. *Circ. Res.,* 35:159.

Haddy, F. J., and Overbeck, H. W. (1976): The role of humoral agents in volume expanded hypertension. *Life Sci.,* 19:935.

Hillis, D. L., and Braunwald, E. (1978): Coronary-artery spasm. *N. Engl. J. Med.,* 299:695.

Julius, S., Pascual, A. V., Sannerstedt, R., and Mitchell, C. (1971): Relationship between cardiac output and peripheral resistance in borderline hypertension. *Circulation,* 43:382.

Korner, P. I., and Fletcher, P. J. (1977): Role of the heart in causing and maintaining hypertension. *Cardiovasc. Med.,* 2:139.

Mancia, G., Ludbrook, J., Ferrari, A., Gregorini, L., and Zanchetti, A. (1978): Baroreceptor reflexes in human hypertension. *Circ. Res.,* 43:170.

Manger, W. M., and Gifford, R. W., Jr. (1977): *Pheochromocytoma.* Springer-Verlag, New York.

Maseri, A., Parodi, O., Severi, S., and Pesola, A. (1976): Transient transmural reduction of myocardial blood flow, demonstrated by thallium-201 scintigraphy, as a cause of variant angina. *Circulation,* 54:280.

Zanchetti, A., and Bartorelli, C. (1977): Central nervous mechanisms in arterial hypertension: experimental and clinical evidence. In: *Hypertension,* edited by J. Genest, E. Koiw, and O. Kuchel, p. 59. McGraw-Hill, New York.

9

Diseases of the Endothelium and the Supporting Structures

When considering the conditions that can impair the function of the cardiovascular system and lead to its failure, it is convenient to classify them according to the component where the disturbance originates. The present chapter deals with the passive components of the cardiac and vascular walls.

ABNORMAL FUNCTION OF THE LINING

Atherosclerosis

With hypertension, of which it can be a complication, atherosclerosis is the major cause of death and disability. Together they account for about 50% of the diseases which afflict mankind. The term atherosclerosis is derived from the Greek word αθερος meaning gruel. This describes the consistency of the lesions, which are present in the wall of the affected blood vessel.

Origin

Atherosclerosis is a disease primarily caused by a lesion of the endothelium which ultimately leads to the formation of an atherosclerotic plaque by initiating the following series of events (Fig. 9–1):

1. No prostacyclin is produced at the sites of endothelial injury (p. 103), and platelets aggregate and adhere to the exposed subendothelial connective tissue since collagen is a potent activator of platelet aggregation.

2. The aggregated platelets release substances, probably peptides, which permeate through the intima to the media. The smooth muscle cells of the media migrate to the intima and undergo mitosis as a consequence of the production of a peptide (mitogenic factor or growth factor) by the aggregating platelets and the permeation of low-density lipoproteins from the plasma to the suben-

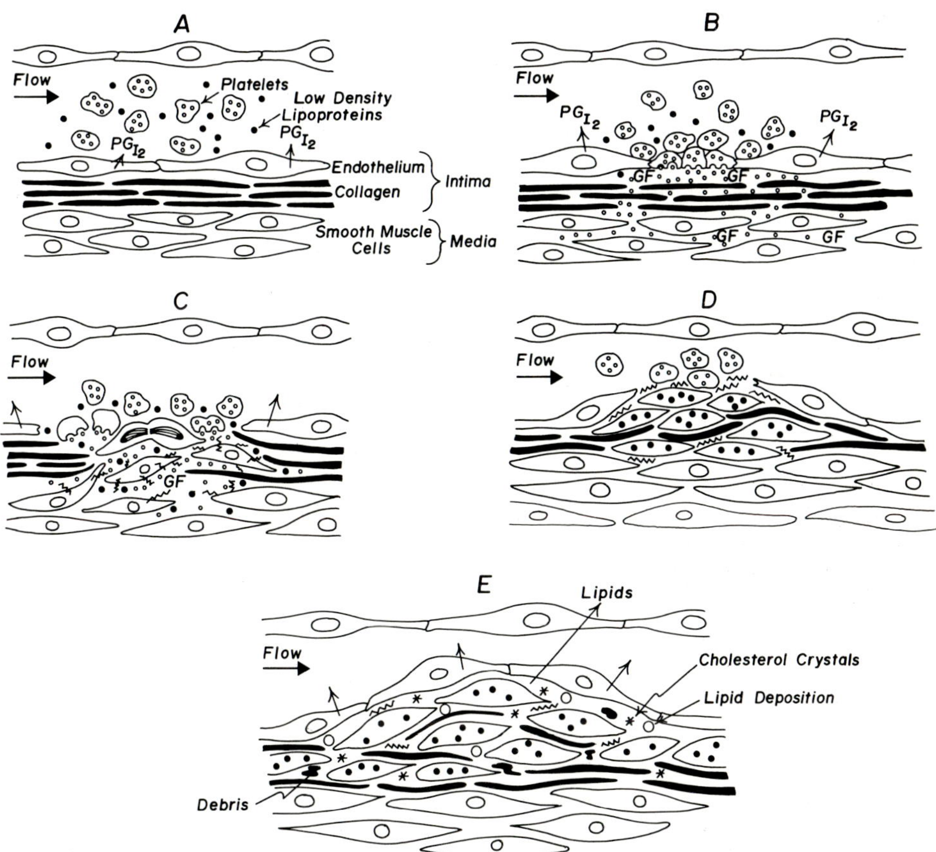

FIG. 9–1. Origin of the atherosclerotic plaque. **A:** Under normal conditions the endothelium prevents the adhesion and aggregation of platelets by secreting prostacyclin (PGI_2). **B:** With endothelial injury the platelets adhere because they are exposed to von Willebrand's factor, and they aggregate because they are exposed to collagen. The aggregating platelets produce growth factor (GF). **C:** Growth factor promotes migration of the smooth muscle cells from the media to the intima and their mitosis. Those phenomena are accelerated by the presence of low-density lipoproteins and thrombin. **D:** The smooth muscle cells secrete large amounts of connective material (~) and further accumulate lipids. **E:** When the endothelial integrity is restored, the process ceases but the atherosclerotic plaque causes obstruction to flow.

dothelial layers. The local formation of thrombin facilitates the production of growth factor.

3. The muscle cells infiltrating the intima produce large amounts of collagen, tissue matrix, elastic fiber, proteins, and glycosaminoglycans.

4. Plasma constituents and particularly lipids pass through the lesion to the intima and accumulate in the smooth muscle cells and the surrounding connective tissue. The cholesterol in atherosclerotic lesions is derived from plasma cholesterol which has been modified by the proliferating smooth muscle cells (Figs. 9–2 and 9–3).

Thus atherosclerotic plaques contain many smooth muscle cells and large amounts of dense connective tissue, consisting largely of collagen fibers; lipoproteins and sometimes cholesterol crystals can be found both intra- and extracellularly. Fatty debris from dead and dying cells is present. Such lesions are found mainly in the coronary vessels, aortic arch, cerebral vessels, kidney vessels, lower parts of the aorta, and arteries of the lower limbs.

The major pathogenic factors believed to play a role in the atherosclerotic process are:

1. Greater mechanical stress, which leads to endothelial damage. This would explain why hypertension predisposes to this condition. It also may help explain why arteries are particularly susceptible at their branching points.

2. Genetic predisposition, of which the best example is provided by patients with type I hyperlipidemia. In these subjects the low density lipoproteins predominate, and vascular lesions occur early in life, presumably because the hydrolytic enzyme systems of the lysosomes in the cells of the blood vessel wall are overwhelmed and cannot degrade the lipoproteins at a rate sufficient to prevent their accumulation (Fig. 9–3). For unknown reasons the presence of high density lipoproteins protects against the development of the lesions. Thus the familial incidence of atherosclerosis can be related to the ratio between the high and low density lipoproteins, which is determined by genetic factors (amount of high density lipoproteins) and dietary habits (amount of low density lipoproteins). The plasma level of cholesterol, which is a normal constituent of the body and serves as a precursor for many hormones, reflects the rate of lipid turnover (Fig. 9–2). When excessively high, it may indicate an increased risk to develop or accelerate the atherosclerotic process.

3. Toxic factors (e.g., nicotine or homocystine), which induce necrosis of the endothelial cells.

4. Factors facilitating the adhesion and aggregation of platelets, e.g., increased levels of catecholamines. Atherosclerotic lesions cannot be evoked by a fatty diet in pigs with a defect in platelet adhesion (von Willebrand's disease), although it induces the lesions in normal animals.

5. Sex differences. Until menopause women have a much lower incidence of atherosclerosis than men, presumably due to the protective effects of the female sex hormones.

6. Increased turnover of fat, as seen in diabetes mellitus, with a resultant

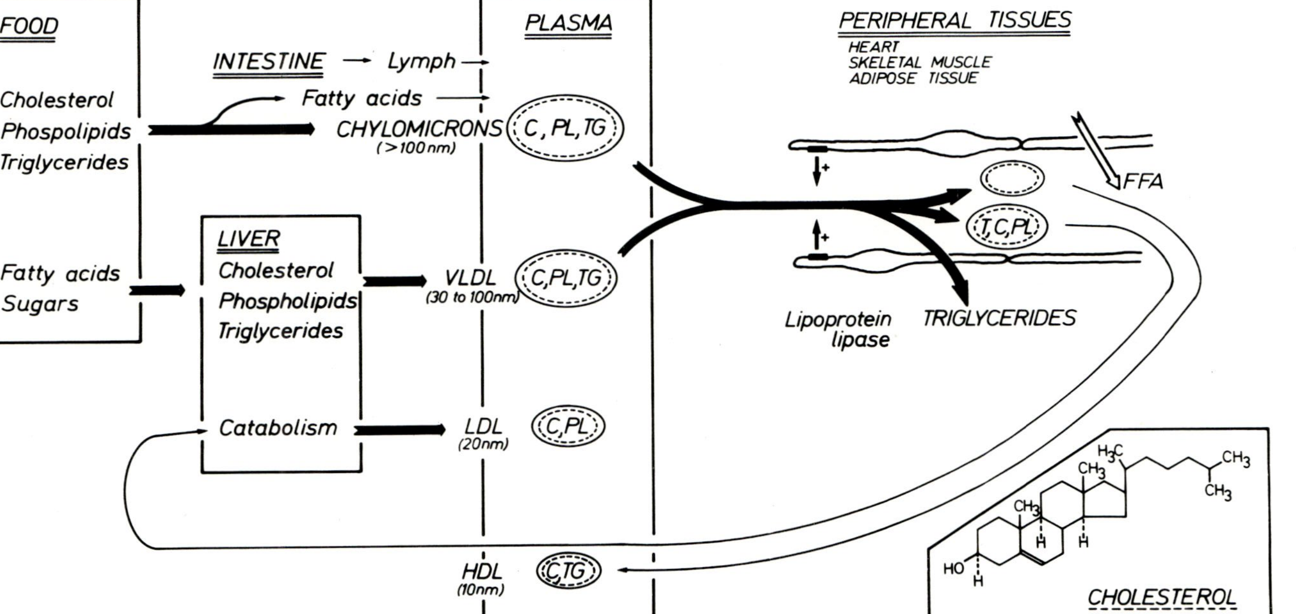

FIG. 9–2. Summary of lipid turnover in man. Cholesterol (C), phospholipids (PL), and triglycerides (TG) are transported in the plasma as a complex with proteins (lipoprotein complexes, ⋯); free fatty acids bind to albumin. The lipoprotein complexes differ in composition, size (given in nanometers, nm), and electrophoretic mobility. Exogenous lipids are either broken down by the intestinal mucosa to free fatty acids or transported by the lymph to the general circulation as large lipoprotein complexes, the chylomicrons (no electrophoretic mobility). The lipids (cholesterol, phospholipids, triglycerides) synthesized by the body cells, in particular by the liver, are transported as very low density lipoproteins (VLDL; pre-β). When the large lipoprotein complexes reach the sites of utilization (in particular muscle and fat cells), they are acted on by the endothelial enzyme lipoprotein lipase, which removes most of the triglycerides. In the hydrolysis process two smaller lipoproteins are formed. The smallest are the high density lipoproteins (HDL; α_1), which contain mainly cholesterol and phospholipids. The remnant particle, which contains triglycerides, cholesterol, and phospholipids, is metabolized in the liver to form the low density lipoprotein (LDL; β), which contains mainly cholesterol and phospholipids. The cholesterol level of the plasma reflects the rate of lipid turnover. **Insert:** Structure of cholesterol.

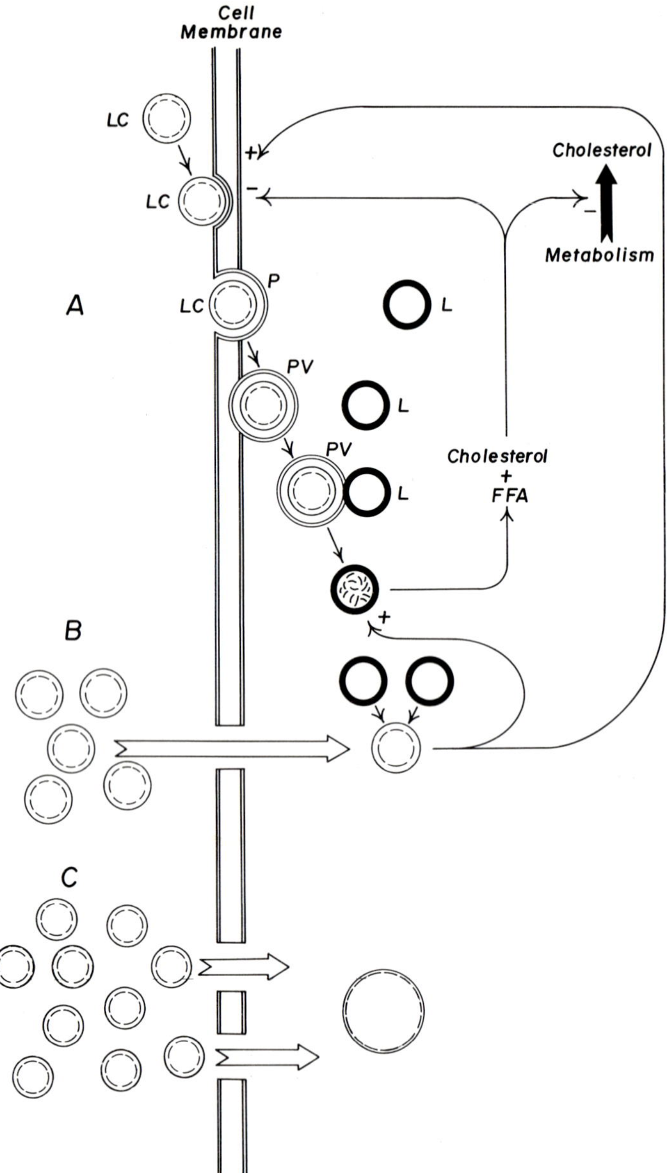

FIG. 9–3. In normal conditions **(A)** the vascular smooth muscle cells actively take up the limited amounts of lipoproteins (LC) using a specific pinocytotic carrier transport system (P). The pinocytotic vesicles fuse with lysosomes (L). The lysosomal enzymes hydrolyze the lipoprotein into cholesterol (C), free fatty acids (FFA), and protein. The cholesterol released by the lysosomes inhibits the synthesis of cholesterol by the cell and exerts a negative feedback on the active uptake process. If the levels of lipoproteins are higher **(B),** they permeate the cell membrane by diffusion. The presence of "free" lipoprotein complexes in the cell activates the carrier process, and the production of lysosomes is augmented. However, the ability of the cell to manage lipoproteins is limited; and if the external concentration is too large **(C),** the lipids permeate the cell membrane and massive intracellular accumulation occurs. This ultimately leads to cell death, in which case the lipids remain in the extracellular space (Fig. 9–1).

increase in plasma levels of free fatty acids, cholesterol, and low density lipoproteins, as well as acceleration of the atherosclerotic process (diabetic macroangiopathy.)

Consequences

The hemodynamic consequences of atherosclerotic lesions are related to the degree of obstruction. When complete occlusion occurs, it usually results from the formation of a thrombus over a superficial defect in an atherosclerotic plaque. The obstruction results in progressive hypoxia of the tissues and thus impairs their function. When the obstruction is complete, the degree of nourishment of the tissues subserved by the occluded artery depends on the presence of anastomotic channels between the pre- and postocclusion part of the vascular bed. If this collateral circulation is insufficient, infarction occurs, most commonly in the heart and brain. The factors controlling the number of collaterals in each tissue, and their development when the latter becomes hypoxic, are unknown.

Similar hemodynamic changes occur in any situation where a mechanical impediment of the circulation is present (e.g., emboli, thrombosis, external compression).

Angina Pectoris and Myocardial Infarction

When the coronary arteries are narrowed by the atherosclerotic process, the blood supply to the myocardium, sufficient at rest, may become inadequate when the work of the heart increases (Fig. 9–4). The accumulation of metabolites in the hypoxic muscle activates afferent nerve fibers which travel with the sympathetic nerves to the central nervous system. This causes the typical precordial pain (angina pectoris) which is relieved by rest (Fig. 9–5). Occasionally recurrent episodes of angina pectoris occur at rest and in the absence of any change in heart rate, blood pressure, or ventricular contractility. These episodes are due to prolonged constriction of a coronary artery (vasospasm; p. 220). When a coronary artery is completely occluded (myocardial infarction), pain is usually continuous. Such occlusion has immediate and delayed consequences (Fig. 9–5), as follows.

Heart rate. Changes in heart rate are frequent. Tachycardia can result from increased adrenergic activation of the sinus node as a consequence of the emotional stress or as part of the reflex response to the fall in blood pressure. Bradycardia can result from reflex activation of the vagus (p. 126). The complications responsible for most deaths during the early hours after myocardial infarction are ventricular fibrillation or cardiac arrest (p. 252).

Cardiac performance. Acute or chronic heart failure may result from the inability of the infarcted heart to maintain proper pumping because of damage to the conducting system or necrosis of myocardial fibers. During the ventricular

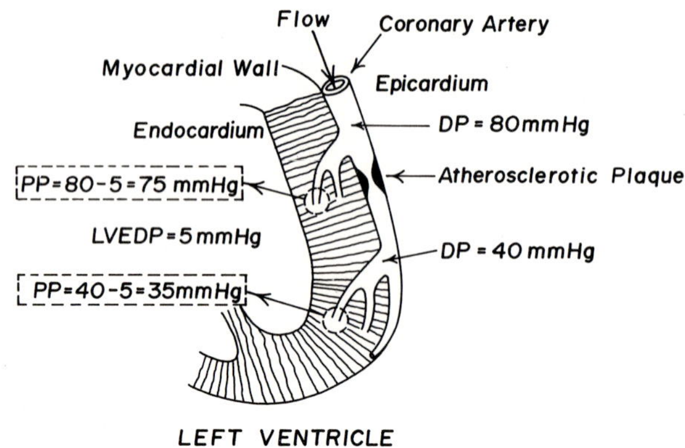

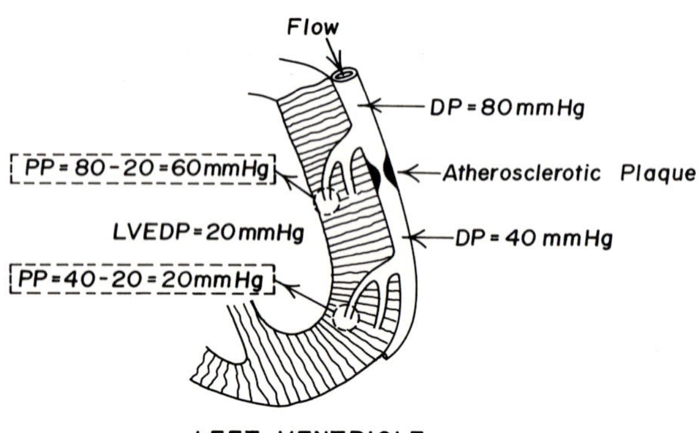

FIG. 9–4. Influence of obstruction of the coronary artery on blood supply to the myocardium. Since the major flow to the myocardium occurs during diastole, the perfusion pressure (PP) in the small coronary vessels equals the diastolic coronary pressure (DP) minus the left ventricular end-diastolic pressure (LVEDP). Downstream to the atherosclerotic plaque, the diastolic pressure, and hence the perfusion pressure, is reduced. If heart failure occurs **(bottom)** and LVEDP increases, the perfusion pressure distal to the occlusion is decreased further. This endangers the blood supply to the heart and in particular that to the endocardial layers (Fig. 4–6). The tissue hypoxia results in swelling of myocardial cells, which causes progressive compression of the small blood vessels within the myocardium and hence further impairs its perfusion.

contraction the infarcted area bulges since the anoxic parts cannot contract. The damaged muscle eventually is replaced by fibrous tissue. The arterial mechanoreceptors cannot maintain an appropriate perfusion pressure to the tissues, including the heart itself, not only because of the failure of the heart to maintain an adequate output but also because the reflex constriction of the systemic resistance vessels and veins is attenuated. The latter is due to inhibition of the

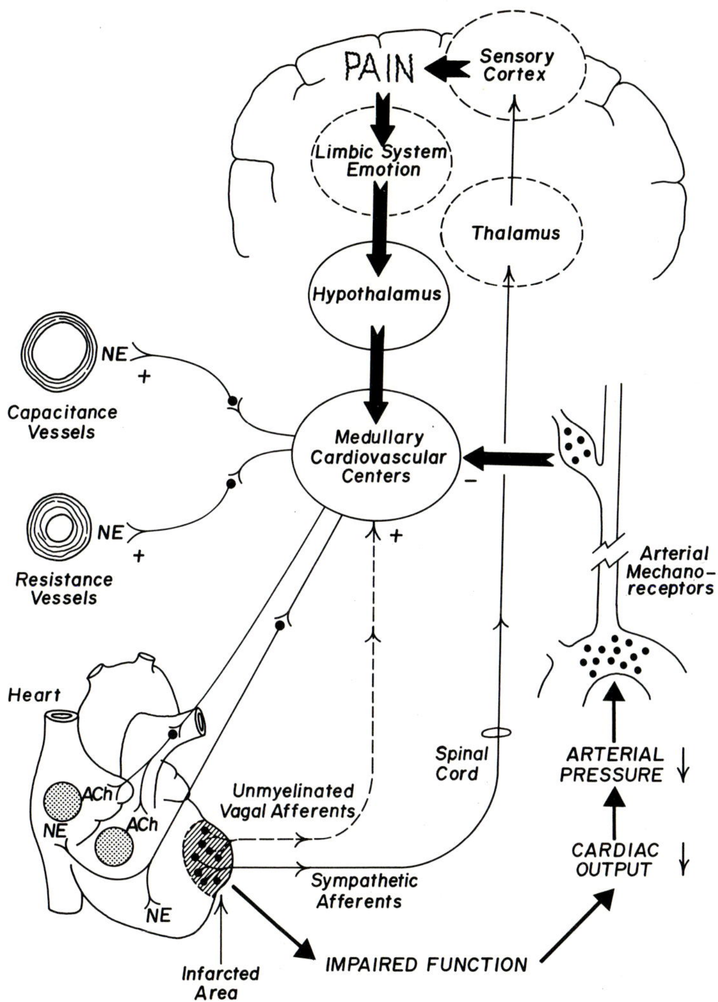

FIG. 9–5. Factors involved in the cardiovascular response to myocardial infarction. Ach = acetylcholine, NE = norepinephrine, + = activation.

cardiovascular centers resulting from activation of mechanoreceptors in the hypoxic myocardium as it bulges with each systole (p. 136) (Fig. 9–5).

Other complications. Other complications include: (1) formation of a thrombus at the site of infarction with subsequent embolization of other vessels, in particular those of the brain; (2) ventricular aneurysm due to continued bulging of the fibrotic myocardium; (3) heart block due to impairment of the blood supply to the conducting tissues; and (4) rupture of the interventricular septum, causing a ventricular septal defect and heart failure as a consequence of the large shunting of blood from the left ventricle into the right (Fig. 9–6).

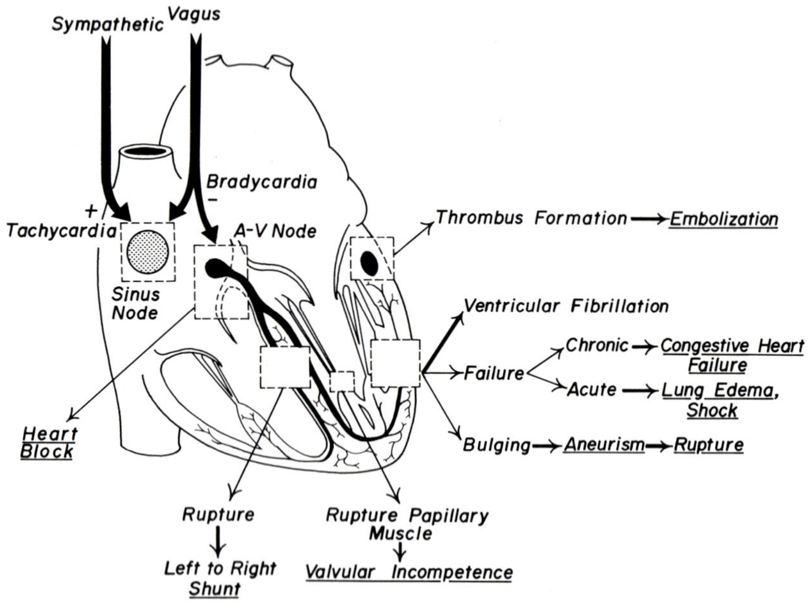

FIG. 9–6. Major complications of myocardial infarction.

Stroke

When an atherosclerotic plaque, a thrombus, or an embolism interrupts the blood suppy to a part of the brain, the resulting damage and the symptomatology depend on the area involved (stroke).

Kidney Failure

If atherosclerosis of the renal artery impairs the blood flow to the kidney, it causes increased renin production, kidney dysfunction, and hypertension, (p. 216).

Intermittent Claudication

Interruption of the blood supply to the lower limbs usually occurs in the iliac, common femoral, or popliteal arteries. The classic symptom is intermittent claudication, from the Latin *claudicare,* which means "to limp." When such patients walk, the accumulation of metabolites in the ischemic skeletal muscle results in dull pain and weakness. The patient is forced to stop until the pain

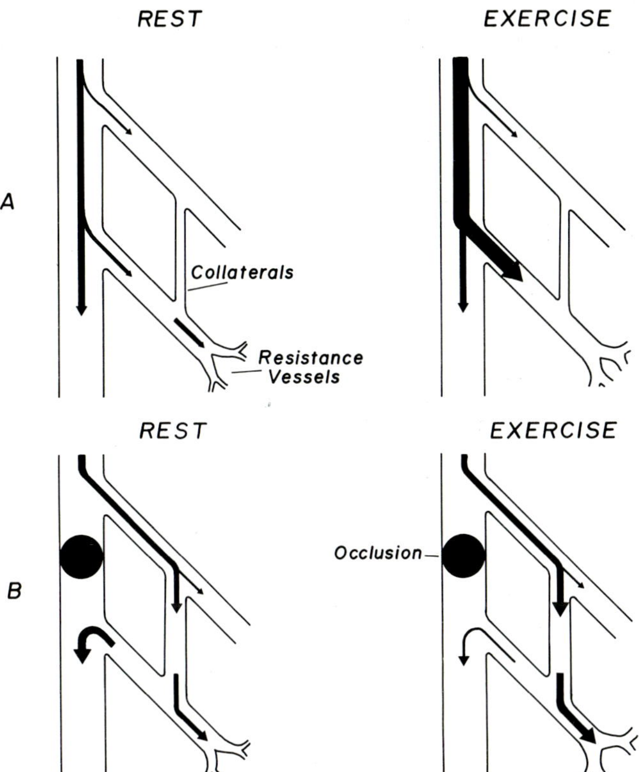

FIG. 9–7. A: Blood flow through a main limb artery at rest and during exercise. Exercise causes dilatation of the muscle resistance vessels and increased blood flow to the muscles. Because of the low resistance to flow through the main artery, the increased muscle flow can occur without impairment of the blood supply to the more distal parts of the limb. **B:** In the presence of an arterial occlusion the high resistance to flow through the collateral vessels limits the increase in blood flow to the exercising muscle; the inflow to the more distal parts of the limb is decreased because the dilated arterioles in the exercising muscle form a low-resistance channel which "steals" the available blood.

subsides. On starting exercise again the process is repeated. Hence the use of the word "intermittent" is the description. In most cases the flow at rest is normal because the collaterals can provide the necessary flow, and pulsations may still be felt in the more distal arteries (Fig. 9–7). More information on the functional capacity of the arterial tree can be obtained from the measurement of hyperemic flow immediately after either exercise or arterial occlusion (Fig. 9–8). With exercise the pulses disappear in patients with severe obstruction, and the flow to the feet decreases as the limited amount of blood that the collateral vessels can carry is diverted to the more proximal parts of the limb (steal phenomenon). Patients with obstruction of the arteries to the lower limbs tend to keep their legs dependent with occasional muscle movements to reduce

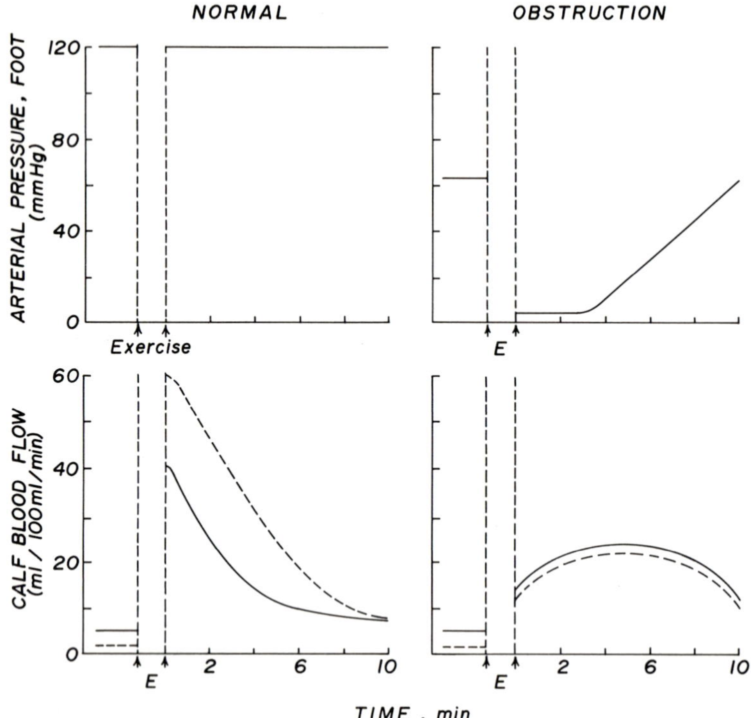

FIG. 9–8. Changes in blood flow and arterial pressure in the foot after exercise in legs with a normal **(left)** and an occluded **(right)** main artery. In the normal leg, there is a marked increase in blood flow with exercise which rapidly subsides; if the exercise is repeated during arrest of the circulation by means of an occlusion cuff *(dotted line),* and if the cuff is released at the time the exercise ceases, the increase in blood flow is much larger, indicating the vascular reserve of the limb. In a patient with major obstruction of the arterial inflow, the arterial pressure in the foot is lower than normal and drops after the muscular contraction to return slowly to pre-exercise values. The blood flow is only moderately augmented at the end of the exercise but increases further for several minutes before slowly decaying toward control values. Performing the same exercise with the occlusion cuff on does not change the response, indicating that prior to occlusion the patient is already using up the total vascular reserve of the limb. The further increase in flow after cessation of the exercise illustrates that blood is first diverted to more proximal parts of the limb (steal phenomenon) before the needs of the calf can be fulfilled.

the increased hydrostatic pressure in the veins; this improves the perfusion of the tissues (p. 87). With severe obstruction, gangrene may develop.

Principles of Treatment

When the blood supply to a tissue is insufficient, the following therapeutic steps may be taken:

1. Surgical bypassing of the obstruction. This applies for peripheral arteries as well as for the coronaries (coronary bypass).

2. Decreasing the activity of the tissue. This can be achieved for the myocardium by either (a) decreasing the preload and afterload by dilating resistance and capacitance vessels, e.g., with the administration of nitrates; (b) interrupting sympathetic control by giving a cardioselective beta-blocker; (c) decreasing the contractile force of the heart by giving an inhibitor of Ca^{2+} influx, e.g., verapamil.

3. Since the arterioles can dilate normally, little benefit is to be expected from arteriolar vasodilation, either with drugs or sympathectomy. If spasm of the arteries complicates the mechanical obstruction (p. 220) vasodilator substances may be used.

4. The long-range therapeutic goal is to prevent the occlusive process. So far, this prevention is limited to elimination of proved and potential risk factors, in particular by reduction of saturated fat intake, elimination of smoking, appropriate treatment of hypertension, and physical activity. As knowledge of the chain of events causing the atherosclerotic lesions increases, it may be possible to cause their regression and to limit their extension by appropriate therapy, e.g., by preventing platelet aggregation.

Thromboangiitis Obliterans

Thromboangiitis obliterans is an uncommon disease of the blood vessels which affects young males (Buerger's disease); it is of unknown etiology. The small arteries of the hands and feet are involved in an inflammatory process leading to thrombosis and occlusion. The peripheral veins may also be affected. The tissue ischemia results in ulceration and may lead to gangrene. Tobacco smoking appears to be a precipitating factor.

Edema

Edema is an abnormal increase in the amount of extracellular fluid in the interstitial spaces of the tissues or the body cavities. It can be localized or generalized (anasarca, dropsy). If fluid accumulates in the pleural cavities it is called pleural effusion (hydrothorax). In the abdominal cavity it is called ascites. All cases of edema can be explained by an alteration in the equilibrium between the forces which govern fluid movements at the capillary level (Fig. 9–9) (p. 83). The fluid accumulates more easily in those parts of the body where the connective tissue structure is relatively loose (e.g., periorbital region). Large amounts of fluid may accumulate before clinical signs become evident. In the edematous tissues diffusion from the capillary to the tissue cells is impaired because of the greater distance to be bridged.

Increased Capillary Permeability

When the capillary permeability increases abnormally, more proteins cross the endothelial barrier. The augmented tissue colloid osmotic pressure attracts

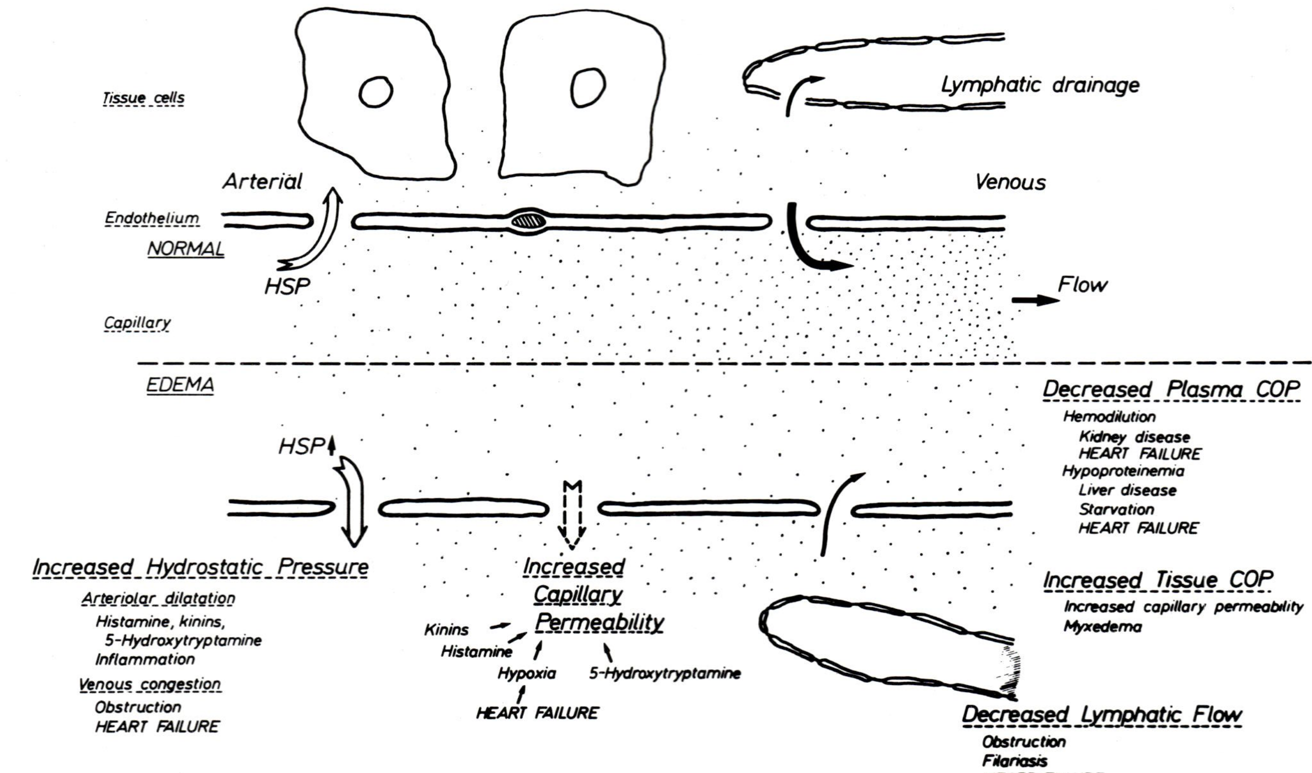

FIG. 9–9. Major factors leading to edema. HSP = hydrostatic pressure. COP = colloid osmotic pressure. *Dots* = proteins and other colloids.

fluid into the interstitial space. This usually is a localized phenomenon caused by substances such as histamine, 5-hydroxytryptamine, and kinins, which are liberated when tissues are damaged (trauma, infection, bites). Such liberation in the skin causes the "triple response," which consists, in succession, of: (1) the red reaction due to localized vasodilation; (2) the wheal, caused by the localized edema of the area; and (3) the flare, an irregular area of warm skin surrounding the wheal due to dilatation of the surrounding arterioles.

Increased Hydrostatic Pressure

Increases in hydrostatic pressures can cause either localized or generalized edema. The former can be due to: (1) Arteriolar vasodilatation, resulting in increased capillary pressure. An example of this is the excess quantity of fluid which leaves the capillaries in exercising muscle. An increase in capillary pressure contributes to the edema caused by substances such as histamine and kinins, which are arteriolar dilators. (2) Local increases in venous pressure due to mechanical obstruction of the venous outflow. Among the common causes are thrombosis of the veins, liver cirrhosis causing obstruction of the portal venous system and thus ascites, external pressure as may occur during late stages of pregnancy when the gravid uterus compresses the pelvic veins, and augmented hydrostatic pressure resulting in edema can be seen in heart failure, when an imbalance exists between the right and the left heart. If the right heart fails first, systemic edema occurs; if the left heart is primarily involved, pulmonary edema ensues.

Decreased Plasma Colloid Osmotic Pressure

A decrease in the plasma protein concentration from the normal of about 7 g/100 ml to less than 5 g/100 ml causes generalized edema. This can be due to: (1) *Hemodilution:* When the total amount of plasma proteins is normal, augmentation of the fluid volume leads to an abnormally low plasma protein concentration. This occurs mainly in conditions when the kidney cannot excrete the Na^+ and water necessary to maintain the fluid balance of the body. This is the case when glomerular filtration is decreased in kidney disease, or in heart failure because of insufficient perfusion. Increased levels of steroid hormones, as seen in pregnancy or Cushing's disease, may cause exaggerated reabsorption of Na^+ and water by the kidney. (2) *Hypoproteinemia:* An absolute decrease in plasma proteins causes a decrease in colloid osmotic pressure. Decreased production of plasma proteins by the liver occurs in cirrhosis, hepatitis, starvation, or severe heart failure. Augmented loss of plasma proteins occurs in the nephrotic syndrome because of abnormal permeability of the glomeruli of the kidney.

Increased Tissue Colloid Osmotic Pressure

The tissue colloid osmotic pressure can increase because the capillary permeability is augmented or because abnormal protein-like material is present in the interstitial space. The latter occurs locally with infection and generally in hypothyroidism where the deposition of proteins, polysaccharides, hyaluronic acid, and chondroitin sulfate in the interstitial fluid leads to water retention (myxedema).

Lymphatic Obstruction

Lymphedema occurs when the lymphatics are absent or obstructed. The former can be congenital or a consequence of surgery. The latter is caused by mechanical obstructions (e.g., tumor) or local inflammation (lymphangitis). In tropical regions worms (filaria) can invade the lymphatics and obstruct them; filariasis can lead to elephantiasis when extensive obstruction occurs. An increase in central venous pressure, as in heart failure, also provides a hindrance to lymphatic drainage.

Diabetic Microangiopathy

Diabetes mellitus is characterized by a thickening of the basal membrane throughout the body, in particular at the capillary level. The reason for it is unknown; presumably it involves the deposition of abnormal glycoproteins, the formation of which is catalyzed by the enzyme glycosyl-galactosyl-hydroxylysine transferase, which normally is inhibited by insulin. The thickening of the basal membrane is accompanied by an increased permeability and propensity to abnormal filtration. The edema resulting from it is particularly obvious in the eye (diabetic retinopathy) and the glomeruli of the kidney (diabetic nephropathy). These events may endanger proper oxygenation of the tissues and hence their function.

DISEASES OF CONNECTIVE TISSUE

Valvular Disease

Normal cardiac valves offer little resistance to the forward flow of blood, and there is almost no pressure gradient across them when they are open. When the valve orifice becomes narrowed, the pressure in the proximal heart chamber increases, the quantity of blood across the valve decreases, or both changes occur. If the valves become leaky (insufficient), blood regurgitates into the upstream chamber. Each type of valvular disease causes typical murmurs. Valvular heart disease usually is due to rheumatic fever or congenital anomalies; the mitral and aortic valves are most commonly affected.

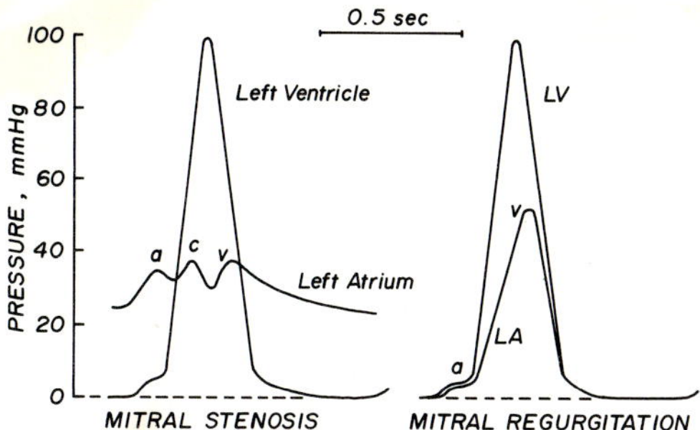

FIG. 9–10. Mitral stenosis and mitral regurgitation. In mitral stenosis there is a pressure gradient between the left atrium and the left ventricle during ventricular diastole, and the atrial pressure decreases relatively slowly because of the obstruction caused by the narrowed mitral orifice. In mitral regurgitation there is little or no pressure gradient during diastole, but the left atrial pressure rises steeply during ventricular systole owing to the stream of blood regurgitating from the left ventricle (v wave). A = atrial contraction. C = mitral valve closure. V = atrial filling.

Mitral Stenosis

Narrowing of the mitral valve impairs emptying of the left atrium into the left ventricle during diastole. In normal adults the cross-sectional area of the mitral valve is about 5 cm^2, and few symptoms occur until the area is reduced to 2.5 cm^2, at which time the pressure increases in the left atrium, pulmonary veins, pulmonary capillaries, and pulmonary artery. Usually the adjustment to the stenosis consists of an increase in the pressure gradient across the valve and a decrease in blood flow. When the stenosis is mild, an abnormal pressure gradient is present during the phase of rapid ventricular filling immediately after the mitral valve opens as well as during atrial contraction. When the stenosis is severe, the pressure gradient across the valve is augmented throughout diastole (Fig. 9–10).

The increased left atrial pressure is transmitted to the pulmonary circulation. When the pressure in the capillaries rises above 25 to 35 mm Hg, it exceeds the colloid osmotic pressure of the blood, resulting in exudation of fluid into the alveoli. If this fluid cannot be removed simultaneously by the lymph vessels, pulmonary edema occurs. In some patients with longstanding stenosis, there is augmented resistance to blood flow through the precapillary pulmonary vessels due to hypertrophy of their walls. This further increases pulmonary artery pressure and the load on the right ventricle.

When patients with mitral stenosis exercise, the pressure gradient between left atrium and ventricle increases as the cardiac output augments. The ability to increase the cardiac output is limited, and the capacity for exercise is diminished. The systemic blood pressure is maintained, in spite of the vasodilatation in the active muscles, by an exaggerated constriction of the resistance vessels in the splanchnic bed (Fig. 6–8), kidneys, and muscles not involved in the exercise (p. 168).

Aortic Stenosis

Aortic stenosis usually develops slowly. The resting cardiac output is normal until the late stage of the disease because the left ventricle hypertrophies and can generate systolic pressures of up to 300 mm Hg (pressure overload). The left atrium also undergoes hypertrophy, and its strong contraction makes an important contribution to ventricular filling. If atrial fibrillation (p. 250) is associated with the aortic stenosis, the atrium does not contract in a coordinated way, its contribution to ventricular filling is lost, and the cardiac output decreases. During systole there is a marked pressure gradient across the aortic valve. Because of the slowing of ejection of blood from the left ventricle, the upstroke of the aortic systolic pulse is slow, and the characteristic differences between the aortic and peripheral arterial pressure pulses disappear (p. 79) (Fig. 9–11).

With exercise, the cardiac output cannot increase normally. The aortic blood pressure decreases because the resistance vessels dilate in the active muscles. Unlike normal subjects, in patients with aortic stenosis the sympathetic outflow to other vascular beds is reflexly decreased because of the activation of ventricular mechanoreceptors by the forcefully contracting myocardium (p. 136). This may precipitate fainting (p. 266).

The high wall tensions generated in the left ventricle and the decreased aortic pressure greatly impede the coronary circulation. Eventually the left ventricle fails; the left ventricular end-diastolic pressure increases, which causes an increase in upstream pressures and pulmonary edema.

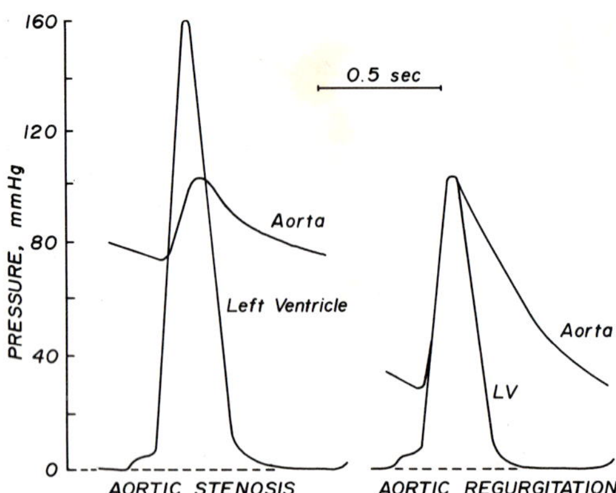

FIG. 9–11. Aortic stenosis and aortic regurgitation. In aortic stenosis there is a pressure gradient between the left ventricle and the aorta during peak systolic pressure in the left ventricle. The pulse pressure in the aorta is less than normal. In aortic regurgitation the systolic pressures in the left ventricle and aorta are similar; the aortic pressure decreases sharply during diastole because of regurgitation of blood into the left ventricle, and the aortic pulse pressure is wide.

Mitral Regurgitation

Mitral regurgitation (insufficiency) may result from dilation of the valve annulus during the course of cardiac failure or from disease of the valve cusps or their attachments. The failure of the mitral valve to close permits backflow of blood from the left ventricle into the left atrium during ventricular systole. The left atrial pressure rises. Although the ventricular stroke volume is increased, the flow into the aorta is reduced. The regurgitant flow is returned to the left ventricle during diastole together with the normal flow from the lungs. The flow across the mitral valve is very large during diastole, and the end-diastolic ventricular pressure and volume are augmented (volume overload; p. 76). The ventricle undergoes dilatation and hypertrophy. The dilatation permits accomodation of the large volume of blood that must be pumped with each heart beat. The hypertrophy helps the heart meet the increased work load. The regurgitation causes a prominent "v" wave in the left atrial pressure pulse, which is also transmitted to the pulmonary circulation (Fig. 9–10).

Aortic Regurgitation

If the aortic valve becomes incompetent, blood flows from the aorta into the left ventricle during ventricular diastole. The aortic diastolic pressure is reduced and the aortic pulse pressure augmented, which accounts for the characteristic collapsing pulse in the peripheral arteries. The left ventricle must pump out the blood that enters normally from the left atrium together with that which regurgitates from the aorta. The resulting increase in stroke volume causes an increase in aortic systolic pressure. Because of the wide pressure gradient between the aorta and the left ventricle during early diastole, large volumes of blood may regurgitate into the ventricle within a short period of time and the values for stroke volume may be two to three times as high as the forward flow (Fig. 9–11).

With the progressive increase in stroke volume, the left ventricle dilates and hypertrophies (p. 258). When it begins to fail, the mitral valve ring dilates, mitral regurgitation occurs, and there is an increase in pressure in the left atrium and pulmonary veins leading to pulmonary congestion and edema. Commonly, patients develop episodes of pulmonary edema when sleeping, because in the supine position the intrathoracic blood volume is larger than when sitting or standing. These episodes are characterized by dyspnea (cardiac asthma). The patient struggles to sit up with his legs dependent, thereby permitting more blood to be accommodated in the leg veins and the volume of blood in the chest to decrease.

Combined Lesions

Combined stenosis and insufficiency of the mitral and aortic valves also occurs, and the hemodynamic changes depend on the relative predominance of each.

Tricuspid Valve

Tricuspid valve disease is uncommon and usually coexists with rheumatic lesions of other valves, particularly the mitral valve. Tricuspid regurgitation, caused by dilatation of the valve ring, is common in congestive heart failure.

Pericardium

Pericardial Effusion

The normal pericardial sac contains 5 to 30 ml of clear serous fluid, but up to 100 ml of additional fluid may accumulate without embarrassment to the heart. Further rapid increases cause compression of the heart (acute tamponade) with augmented venous, atrial, and pulmonary vascular pressures; the cardiac output and the systemic blood pressure are decreased. If the fluid accumulates more slowly, the pericardium distends and much larger amounts may be present without causing tamponade. The pressures in the atria increase during inspiration, which is reflected in the veins of the neck.

Constrictive Pericarditis

Constrictive pericarditis occurs when adequate diastolic filling of the ventricles is hampered by the thickening of the pericardium during the course of a chronic inflammation. The venous pressures increase in the pulmonary and systemic circulations.

Aneurysms and Poststenotic Dilation

Any disease process that weakens the arterial wall may result in aneurysmal dilation of the vessel. Hypertension precipitates such aneurysms. In certain cases a hematoma develops and progresses along the media (dissecting aneurysm). Aneurysms occur more frequently in the convex part of the ascending aorta because of the larger wall tension (Laplace's law). They impair the function of the tissues by compressing them or by occluding the origin of the arteries supplying them. Whey they rupture, internal hemorrhage ensues.

Aneurysms can also be initiated when external compression of the arteries causes turbulence since the sonic vibrations generated weaken the connective tissue of the vessel (poststenotic dilatation). Once the dilatation is initiated, the process is enhanced because the velocity of flow decreases and the lateral pressure augments (Bernouilli's principle; Figs. 1–4 and 3–2).

Varicose Veins

Varicose veins are due to abnormal distensibility of the connective tissue in the vein wall. All limb veins from patients with varicosities are more distensible

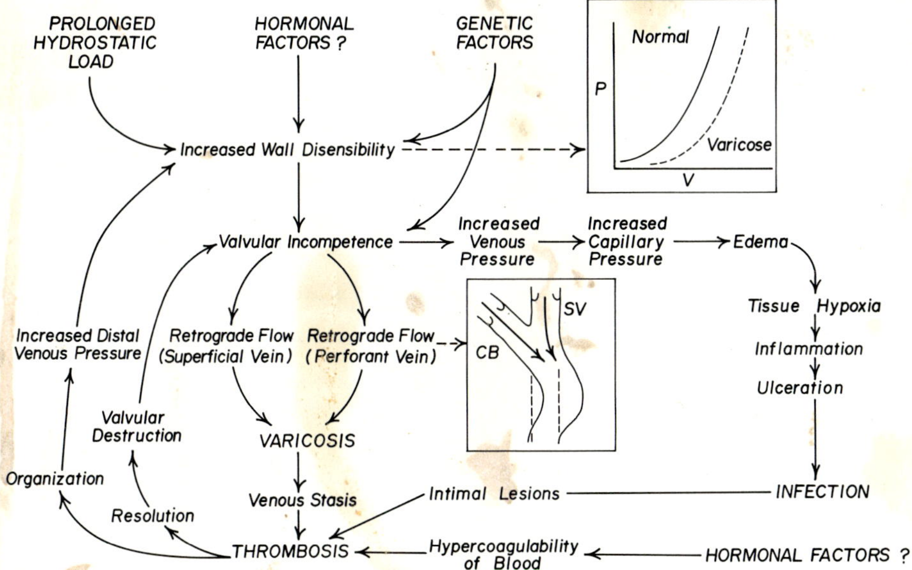

FIG. 9–12. Sequence of events in the development of varicose veins and venous thrombosis. The distensibility of the wall of veins from patients with varicose veins is greater than normal, and for each increase in hydrostatic pressure (P) the veins accommodate a larger volume of blood (V; **upper inset**). The increased distention causes the incompetence of the venous valves of the superficial veins (SV) and the communicating branches (CB) with the deep veins **(lower inset).** The retrograde flows cause the tortuous pattern of the varicose veins. (Modified from Shepherd and Vanhoutte: *Veins and Their Control.* Saunders, London, 1975.)

than normal, indicating the genetic basis for the abnormality. The fact that they occur in the legs illustrates that increased hydrostatic pressure is the major external factor precipitating their occurrence.

The varicosities usually start in the superficial veins at the points where the communicating veins originate. The increased distensibility of the wall renders the valves incompetent, which causes the backflow of blood. The combination of the retrograde flow in the superficial veins and in the communicating branches causes the typical tortuous pattern of the varicosities. The increased transmural pressure in the postcapillary vessels favors exudation of fluid and edema formation. The poor tissue drainage causes ischemia, which favors inflammation, infection, thrombosis, and tissue damage (ulcer). The valvular incompetence associated with varicose veins renders the muscle pump less effective, and, as in the rare cases of congenital absence of the valves, impairs the increase in stroke volume during upright exercise (Fig. 9–12).

SELECTED REFERENCES

Braunwald, E. (1971): Control of myocardial oxygen consumption: Physiologic and clinical considerations. *Am. J. Cardiol.,* 27:416.

Frame, L. H., and Powell, W. J. (1976): Progressive perfusion impairment during prolonged low flow myocardial ischemia in dogs. *Clin. Res.,* 39:269.

Gregg, D. E. (1974): The natural history of coronary collateral development. *Circ. Res.,* 35:335.

Hoffman, J. I. E. (1978): Determinants and prediction of transmural myocardial perfusion. *Circulation,* 58:381.

Marshall, R. J., and Shepherd, J. T. (1968): *Cardiac Function in Health and Disease.* Saunders, Philadelphia.

Maseri, A., Pesola, A., Marzilli, M., Severi, S., Parodi, O., L'Abbate, A., Ballestra, A. M., Maltinti, G., De Nes, D. M., and Biagini, A. (1977): Coronary vasospasm in angina pectoris. *Lancet,* 1:713.

Pantridge, J. F., Adgey, A. A. J., Geddes, J. S., and Webb, S. W. (1975): *The Acute Coronary Attack.* Grune & Stratton, New York.

Ross, R., and Glomset, J. A. (1976): The pathogenesis of atherosclerosis. *N. Engl. J. Med.,* 295:369, 420.

Shepherd, J. T., and Vanhoutte, P. M. (1975): *Veins and Their Control.* Saunders, London.

10

Diseases of the Active Components of the Cardiac and Vascular Walls

Cardiovascular function may become impaired in a variety of circumstances, including primary and secondary diseases of the heart muscle, disturbance of cardiac rhythm, or interference with the nervous control. If the heart fails to pump effectively, the whole cardiovascular system begins to fail and the blood pressure cannot be maintained.

CARDIOMYOPATHIES

The primary diseases of the heart muscle may be classified into three groups.

Hypertrophic Cardiomyopathy

Hypertrophic cardiomyopathy, whose cause is unknown, is manifested by an obstruction to the egress of blood from the left ventricle into the aorta. It is due to hypertrophy of the interventricular septum, particularly at its upper portion adjacent to the anterior cusp of the mitral valve. It has been referred to as subvalvular stenosis, muscular subaortic stenosis, obstructive cardiomyopathy, or idiopathic hypertrophic subaortic stenosis. When the left ventricle contracts there is a rapid ejection of an initial volume of blood. Contraction of the hypertrophied muscle then limits further ejection. In the majority of cases the hypertrophied septum causes reopening of the anterior leaflet of the mitral valve in midsystole, which contributes to the obstruction and causes mitral regurgitation. Normal subjects eject about 60% of their stroke volume during

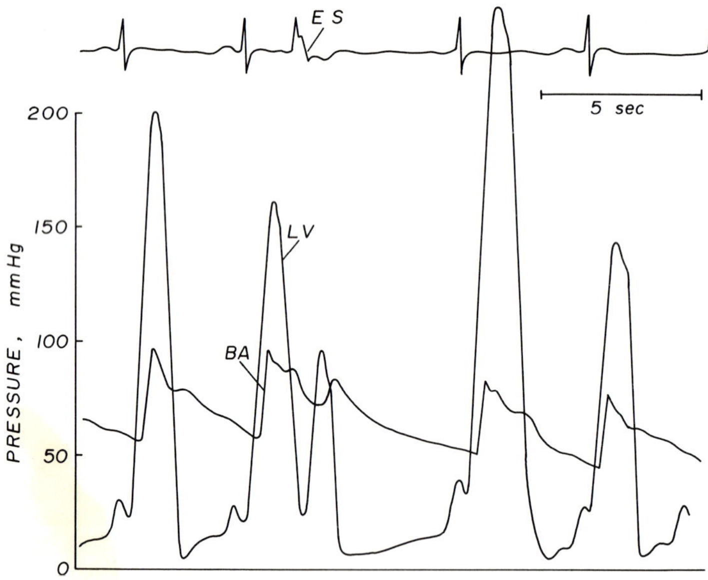

Fig. 10–1. Pressures from left ventricle (LV) and brachial artery (BA) in a patient with obstructive cardiomyopathy. Note the marked systolic pressure difference between the left ventricle and the brachial artery. During the recording the patient exhibited a ventricular premature contraction (extrasystole, ES) during which the pressure generated in the left ventricle was not sufficient to open the aortic valve. In the following postextrasystolic beat the systolic pressure in the left ventricle was greater than that during normal sinus rhythm, but the arterial systolic pressure was less. This is in contrast to subjects without obstructive cardiomyopathy, where both pressures are increased in a postextrasystolic beat. The explanation of the pressure divergence is that the enhanced myocardial contractility following the extrasystole increases the force of contraction of the hypertrophied muscle, thereby rendering the obstruction more complete. A similar diminution in the arterial pressure pulse is seen during the administration of drugs with positive inotropic effects, e.g., cardiac glycosides or beta-adrenergic agents; conversely, the arterial pressure pulse augments with drugs which decrease cardiac contractility, e.g., beta-adrenergic blocking agents. (From Braunwald et al.: *Circulation (Suppl IV),* 30:3, 1964, by permission of the American Heart Association.)

the first half of systole, whereas patients with obstructive cardiomyopathy eject 70 to 85% during the same period. As a result the peripheral arterial pulse is characteristically sharp. Once the outflow tract is closed, the left intraventricular pressure continues to rise throughout systole, and the peripheral arterial pressure starts to fall. This dissociation is exaggerated when the contractility of the myocardium is augmented (Fig. 10–1).

Cardiomyopathies Causing Congestive Failure

In certain diseases the myocardial cells fail to function despite a normal blood supply. Among known causes are: infection (viruses, bacteria, parasites, worms), intoxication (alcohol), malnutrition (vitamin B_1 deficiency), and endocrine disease (hypo- and hyperthyroidism).

Restrictive Cardiomyopathy

The elasticity of the myocardium is decreased in diseases such as amyloidosis and fibroelastosis, where the amount of fibrous tissue in the subendocardial regions is augmented. The ventricles fail to relax adequately during diastole, and the hemodynamic findings resemble those of constrictive pericarditis (p. 74).

ARRHYTHMIAS

Altered Activity of the Sinus Node

Sinus Tachycardia

Each time the sympathetic activity to the heart augments, the heart rate increases. If the heart rate regularly exceeds 100 beats/min in resting persons, it is referred to as sinus tachycardia. This can be due to emotional disturbance, fever, or thyrotoxicosis. The PQRST complex is normal. The cardiac output decreases if the heart rate increases over 200 beats/min because of insufficient time for filling of the ventricles.

Sinus Bradycardia

Sinus bradycardia is defined as a heart rate less than 60 beats/min without conduction abnormalities in the electrocardiogram. It is caused by excessive release of acetylcholine by the vagal nerves at the sinus node. Sinus bradycardia is characteristic in athletes, occurs during vasovagal syncope, and is one of the cardinal symptoms of increased intracranial pressure (p. 266).

Sinus Arrhythmia

The heart rate increases during inspiration and decreases during expiration owing to reciprocal changes in vagal and sympathetic outflow to the sinus node (p. 150).

Sinoatrial Dysfunction

The sinus node may fail to generate an effective action potential (generator failure) or may not succeed in passing the action potential on to the atrial muscle cells (sinoatrial exit block). Unlike the three preceding changes, which are the consequence of predictable alterations in autonomic outflow, sinoatrial dysfunction is an abnormality seen in elderly people (sick sinus syndrome) or as a consequence of hyperkalemia or cardiac glycoside overdosage. The heart rate may not increase normally with exercise, and at times the sinoatrial block causes temporary cardiac arrest with acute hypotension and syncope.

Premature Systole

Mechanism

A premature systole (ectopic beat) implies that the contraction of the heart is initiated by parts of the myocardium outside the sinus node (ectopic foci). The electrocardiogram is abnormal. Such ectopic foci can occur by the following mechanisms:

1. *Abnormal pacemaker activity:* Certain cells or groups of cells, in particular Purkinje fibers, generate a pacemaker potential at a higher rate than that of the sinus node. The generation of abnormal pacemaker activity is favored by factors such as catecholamines, hypoxia, and cardiac glycosides (Fig. 10–2).

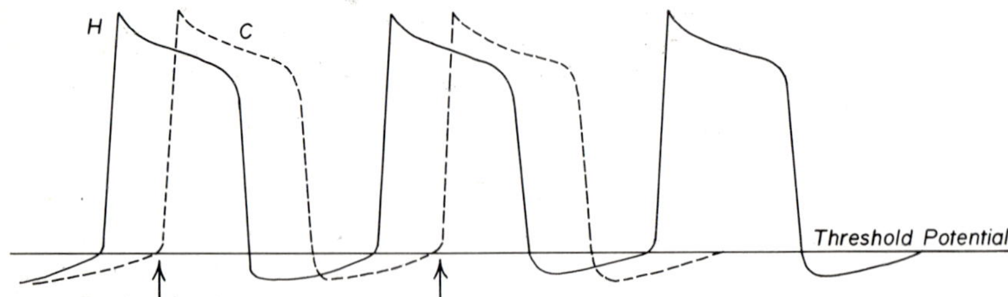

FIG. 10–2. Abnormal pacemaker activity. In normal conditions most myocardial cells outside the sinus node do not exhibit spontaneous depolarization. When present, the slow depolarization (pacemaker potential; p. 56), as shown for a Purkinje fiber (C), is not sufficient to reach threshold level before the impulse initiated in the sinus node reaches the cell and triggers the action potential *(arrow)*. When the tissue is hypoxic (H), the rate of spontaneous depolarization increases, the threshold potential is attained before the wave of depolarization originating in the sinus node reaches the fiber, and an ectopic action potential is generated.

2. *Inhomogeneity of repolarization:* If an area of the heart repolarizes faster than the surrounding areas, the depolarization of the latter may re-enter the repolarized part and induce a new action potential. This mechanism is of importance in myocardial ischemia, which causes shortening of the action potential of the ischemic parts (Fig. 10–3).

3. *Slower conduction:* In myocardial disease certain parts of the heart, particularly the atrioventricular node and the conducting tissues, transmit the action potential at a speed that is slower than normal. During episodes of acute hypoxia the conduction in the normal direction may be stopped temporarily (unidirectional block). The impulse which follows the normally conducting cells, and thus bypasses the blocked area, can cause retrograde conduction in the latter (re-entry). If the tissue is polarized at the time such a re-entering potential reaches it, an action potential can be initiated which is conducted in a retrograde way and eventually causes contraction of the atria (echo beat). The latter contraction can then be transmitted to the ventricle by the normally conducting part of the atrioventricular node (reciprocal beating) (Fig. 10–4).

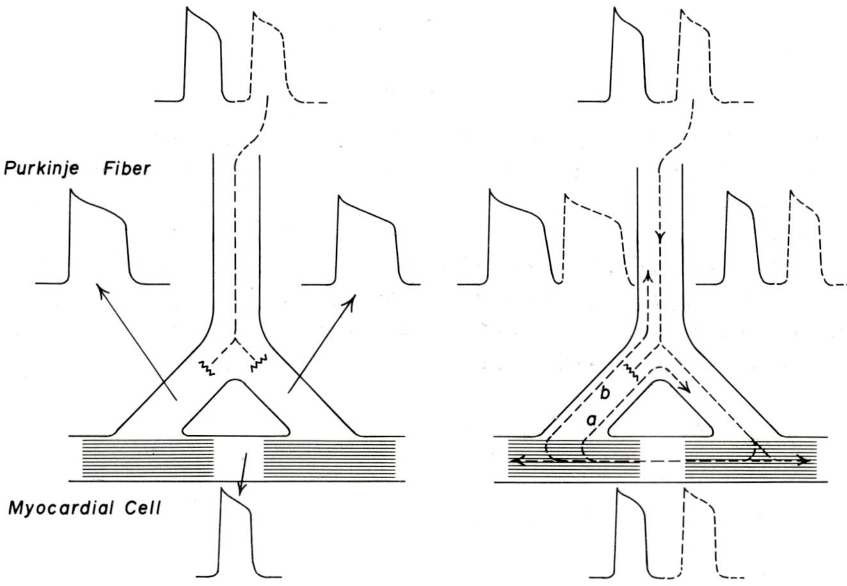

FIG. 10–3. Inhomogeneity of repolarization. In the normal heart, when a Purkinje fiber branches, the two branches have an action potential of the same duration but longer than that of the main branch or of the innervated myocardial cell. The longer action potential acts as a gate which stops the propagation of ectopic beats *(dotted lines)* reaching the branches before full repolarization has occurred **(left).** However, if a difference exists in the duration of the action potential and one branch repolarizes faster (inhomogeneity of repolarization) **(right),** one branch will halt the ectopic action potential but the other will not. The ectopic depolarization is propagated along the myocardial cells and reaches the terminal part of the gating branch at a time that it is repolarized and thus can be activated. The ensuing action potential reactivates the myocardium (a; reentry) or can be conducted to the atria and causes their contraction (b; echo beat).

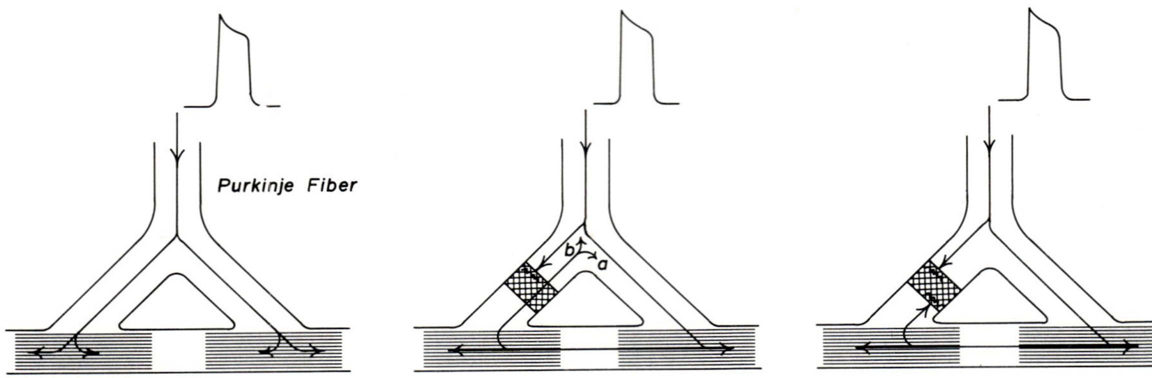

FIG. 10–4. Initiation of ectopic beats by slower conduction in Purkinje fibers. In normal conditions the conduction speed of branches of Purkinje fibers is the same. This allows for homogeneous activation of the ventricular wall **(left).** In myocardial disease the conduction in the normal direction can be stopped temporarily **(middle).** Such unidirectional block allows the retrograde spread of impulses propagated by the normal branches and leads to re-entry (a) or retrograde activation (b). When the tissue becomes more severely diseased, all conduction is blocked in both directions and re-entry cannot occur **(right).**

Consequences

If the premature beat is an infrequent event, it is referred to as extrasystole; if it is repetitive it causes tachycardia. The electrocardiographic characteristics and the hemodynamic consequences of premature beats depend on the site of the ectopic signal.

Infrequent Premature Beats

In most cases occasional premature beats have no hemodynamic consequences (Fig. 10–5).

1. *Sinus premature systoles:* If the sinus node generates an early impulse, the electrocardiogram is normal except for a shortened R–R interval preceding the premature beat.

2. *Atrial premature systole:* The ventricle is activated normally, and the electrocardiographic picture depends on the site in the atrium where the ectopic beat is generated. If this site is at a distance from the sinus node, the P wave is inverted and the QRS complex normal. Since at the time the sinus node would generate its next normal impulse the atrium is refractory, the atrial premature systole is followed by a compensatory pause.

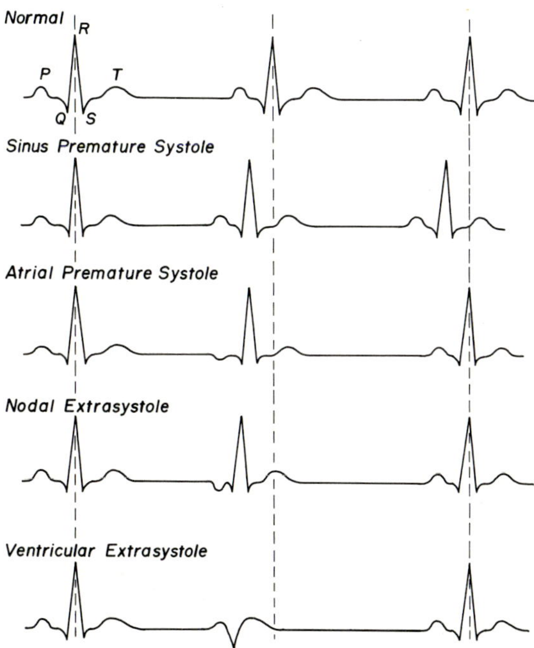

FIG. 10–5. Electrocardiographic changes with premature beats. Depending on the location of the ectopic focus, other configurations can be obtained. Extrasystoles initiated outside the sinus node usually are followed by a compensatory pause.

3. *Nodal (junctional) extrasystole:* This type of premature beat is characterized by a shortening of the P-Q interval and by the inversion or absence of the P wave.

4. *Ventricular premature beats:* Ventricular extrasystoles originate below the atrioventricular node and are characterized by the absence of a P wave and an abnormal QRS complex. The hemodynamic consequences depend on the time during diastole at which the premature beat occurs. For example, early in ventricular diastole when little ventricular filling has occurred, the pressure generated in the ventricle does not rise sufficiently to open the aortic valve (Fig. 10–1). This leads to the so-called "pulse deficit," where there is an apex beat and a QRS complex in the absence of an arterial pulse.

Repetitive Phenomena

1. *Atrial bigeminy:* If sinus premature systoles occur regularly and are coupled with normally occurring heart beats, this is called "bigeminy." It can be caused by digitalis overdose or by structural abnormalities of the sinoatrial area.

2. *Paroxysmal supraventricular tachycardia:* Repetitive atrial or nodal premature systoles can occur in bursts lasting from a few seconds to several hours. Such paroxysmal supraventricular tachycardia starts and ends abruptly. The heart rate is regular and usually exceeds 150 beats/min. In the majority of the cases the heart is otherwise normal, the cardiac output at rest is within the normal range during the episodes of tachycardia, but the maximal adaptation to exercise is reduced. In patients with heart disease, the tachycardia results in a decreased cardiac output at rest, a decline in arterial blood pressure, and angina pectoris. If prolonged, cardiac failure may ensue. If the tachycardia originates in the lower parts of the atrioventricular node, the nearly simultaneous contraction of atria and ventricles diminishes the atrial contribution to ventricular filling, whereas in tachycardia of atrial origin the normal cardiac cycle is maintained. The mechanism underlying paroxysmal tachycardia is usually unknown. A special case is the existence of abnormal strands of conducting tissue (e.g., bundle of Kent) between the atria and the ventricles, which provide a pathway for re-entry of the propagated action potential.

3. *Atrial flutter and fibrillation:* If during tachycardia the heart rate increases to above 230 to 250 beats/min, not all impulses generated by the atrium can be conducted to the ventricle because of the relatively slow conduction speed of the middle part of the atrioventricular node (Fig. 2–36). The resulting dissociation between atrial and ventricular rhythm is called atrial flutter and is characterized by normal P waves, which outnumber the QRS complexes. The ventricular rate depends on the number of impulses propagated by the atrioventricular node, and is two to four times less than the atrial rate. The major hemodynamic consequence is to reduce cardiac output at rest and during exercise mainly because the filling of the ventricles is impaired and ventricular rate is not controlled precisely. In these patients vagal activation has little effect on the atrial

rate but usually increases the dissociation between atria and ventricles because of the depressant effect of acetylcholine on atrioventricular conduction. Conversely, reduction of vagal tone (e.g., with exercise) has no effect on the atrial rate but decreases the atrioventricular dissociation. Atrial flutter is seen in conjunction with organic heart disease and thyrotoxicosis (Fig. 10–6).

Unlike atrial flutter, where the rate is fast but regular, in fibrillation the atrial rhythm exceeds 350 beats/min. The ventricular rate is irregular because not all atrial action potentials are sufficient to initiate a propagation to the ventricles. The electrocardiogram reflects the very rapid oscillations in atrial potential and the irregularity of the ventricular complexes, which have a normal pattern. Atrial fibrillation is most commonly a complication of organic heart disease, and the latter determines the hemodynamic changes. It is also observed with thyrotoxicosis and overdoses of cardiac glycosides. If normal atrial rhythm is resumed, the cardiac output at rest increases because the stroke volume is augmented by better filling of the ventricles (Fig. 10–6).

Atrial flutter may be due to hyperactivity of a single rapidly discharging ectopic focus, and atrial fibrillation to the disorganized activity of multiple ectopic foci. An alternative explanation is that flutter results from a circular re-entry movement of ectopic activation spreading over a small area of the atrium and fibrillation over a large area.

4. *Coupled ventricular ectopic beats:* Ventricular extrasystoles can be coupled

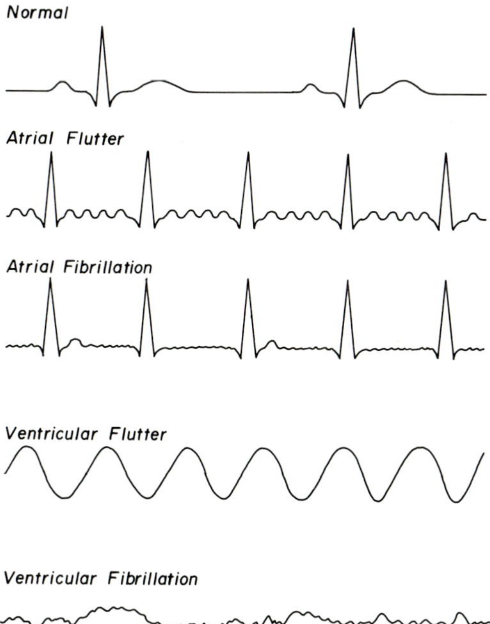

FIG. 10–6. Electrocardiographic changes with atrial and ventricular flutter and fibrillation.

repetitively with normal beats to form groups of two (bigeminy) or three (trigeminy) successive cardiac contractions followed by a pause.

5. *Ventricular flutter and fibrillation:* Repeated re-entry mechanisms in the ventricle cause regular rates over 250 beats/min (flutter) or irregular movements (fibrillation). Unless they are rapidly reversed, these situations are fatal because of acute failure of the heart to pump blood. They are caused mostly by ischemia of the myocardium (Fig. 10–6).

Conduction

Anomalous Atrioventricular Excitation

Supplementary pathways may bypass the normal atrioventricular conduction, leading to the pre-excitation syndrome (Wolff–Parkinson–White syndrome). The impulse is transmitted across the atrioventricular fibrous rings sooner by the bypass, but its further propagation depends on cell-to-cell conduction. The impulse that follows the normal pathway in the atrioventricular node is conducted slowly through the latter, but once it reaches the bundle of His its propagation is rapid. Thus the pre-excitation wave affects only a small part of the myocardium and causes a slight widening of the QRS complex. In most cases of Wolff–Parkinson–White syndrome the bypass is due to accessory connection in or around the atrioventricular node and not to the more laterally located strands of conducting tissues such as the bundle of Kent.

Conduction Block

Congenital Heart Block

In congenital heart block the myocardium is normal; the atrioventricular conducting system, however, is absent or nonfunctional, is usually proximal to the bundle of His, and there is complete dissociation between the atria and the ventricles. The atrial rate is normal and increases normally with exercise. The ventricular rate is about 40 beats/min, and the stroke volume is increased up to twice the normal value. During severe exercise the ventricular output can double. Characteristic of atrioventricular block is that, if the atria contract when the atrioventricular valves are closed, there is a marked increase in atrial pressure which is reflected in the jugular vein (canon wave) (Fig. 10–7).

Acquired Heart Block

Acute myocardial infarction or other organic heart diseases can result in necrosis and scar formation of the conducting tissues. If the bundle of His is involved, this causes total dissociation between atria and ventricles, as seen in congenital block. If the block involves the left or right bundle branch (bundle

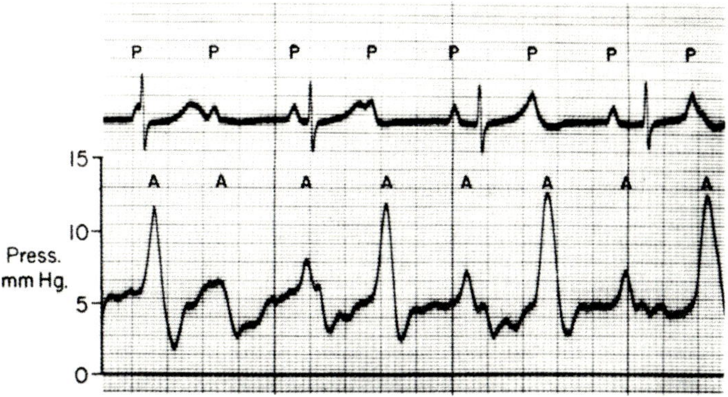

FIG. 10–7. Right atrial pressure pulse in a patient with congenital heart block. Giant "a" waves occur when the atrium contracts during ventricular systole. P = P wave of electrocardiogram. A = "a" wave of atrial pressure pulse. (From Ayers et al.: *Am. Heart J.,* 72:381, 1966.)

branch block) (Fig. 10–8), the rhythm is normal, but the QRS complex is lengthened because a larger fraction of the ventricular myocardium must be activated by cell-to-cell conduction.

The block may be temporary or partial; and according to the gravity of the impairment of conduction, the following clinical classification is used: (1) In *first degree block* the P–R interval is prolonged without hemodynamic consequences. It can also be caused by high doses of cardiac glycosides or even by increases in vagal tone. (2) In *second degree block* some but not all impulses can pass the atrioventricular node. There is usually a progressive increase in P–R interval with consecutive heart beats until one impulse is not conducted. During the asystole resulting from the block, the atrioventricular tissue recovers, and the first subsequent P–R interval is normal (Wenckebach phenomenon). When the disturbance of conduction is more severe, more impulses do not propagate, causing a temporary cardiac arrest, a drop in arterial pressure, and loss of consciousness (Stokes–Adams attacks). In yet other areas partial block occurs which allows only one ventricular contraction for each second, third, or fourth atrial contraction. (3) In *third degree block* conduction is halted completely.

Hyperkalemia

In heart muscle an increased extracellular potassium concentration decreases the resting membrane potential, the velocity of depolarization, and the overshoot of the action potential. It also decreases the duration of the depolarization plateau and the phase of rapid repolarization, thus shortening the action potential. The effects of an increase in serum potassium concentration, as observed in patients with acute renal failure, are manifest in the electrocardiogram. Initially the T

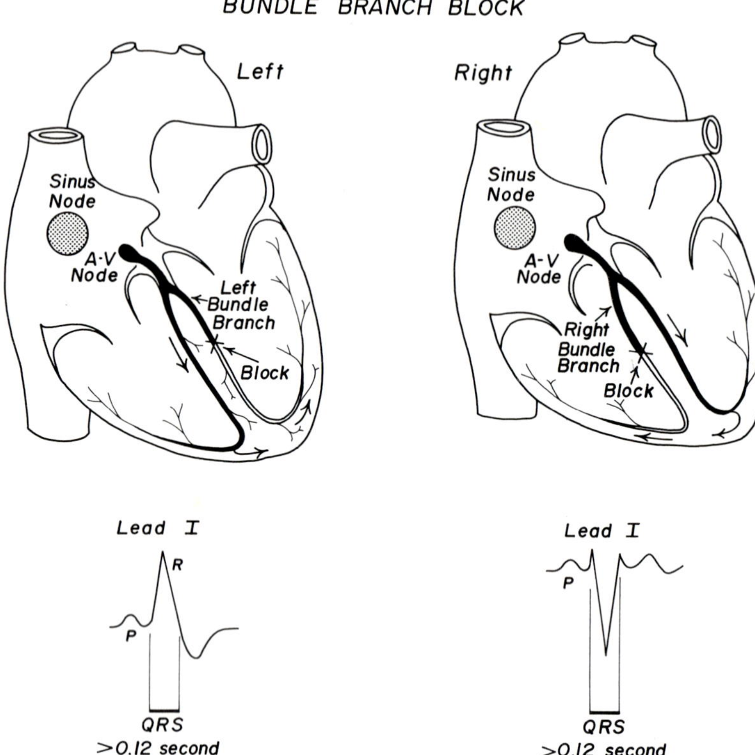

FIG. 10–8. Bundle branch block. Complete bundle branch block is present whenever the impulse migrating down from the atrioventricular node through the bundle of His is obstructed by a lesion in the left or right bundle, so its passage into the Purkinje network is prevented. When the block occurs in the right bundle branch, the impulses pass through the left bundle branch and the left ventricle is depolarized normally. The right ventricle is depolarized by propagation of the impulse by cell-to-cell conduction from the left ventricle, so the QRS complex is larger than the normal value (0.10 sec); the main deflection of the QRS is negative in the lead shown. Similar events occur when the impulses are blocked in the left bundle branch, but the main deflection of the QRS complex is positive. (Modified from Burch and Winsor: *A Primer of Electrocardiography,* 6th ed. Lea & Febiger, Philadelphia 1972.)

wave is elevated, after which conduction is blocked successfully in the atrium, atrioventricular node, and ventricles. Cardiac arrest and death result.

Principles of Therapy

Management of cardiac arrhythmias may include the following: (1) treatment of the causal disease if possible; (2) use of the appropriate pharmacological agent in the case of autonomic dysfunction; (3) electrical reversion to synchronize all myocardial cells (cardioversion, defibrillation): this is of particular use in atrial flutter and fibrillation, and can be lifesaving in ventricular fibrillation;

(4) administration of antiarrhythmic agents to decrease the excitability of the myocardial cells (p. 196); and (5) placement of an electrode catheter (pacemaker) connected to an external power supply in the right ventricle to restore normal ventricular rhythm.

HEART FAILURE

If the heart becomes unable to pump blood in sufficient quantities to meet the metabolic requirements of the tissues of the body, a complex series of derangements occur throughout the cardiovascular system, which in turn cause widespread disturbances of body function. These derangements become apparent to the clinician as the signs of heart failure and lead to the symptoms perceived by the patient. Circulatory failure can occur in the presence of an increased cardiac output, as in thyrotoxicosis or severe anemia, or be due to the inability of the heart to sustain a normal cardiac output. From the metabolic viewpoint there is no difference between "high" and "low" output failure. Occasionally low output failure can be due to abrupt malfunction of the mitral or aortic valves; the normal myocardium cannot provide an adequate forward flow. However, in most cases the heart failure is due to changes in the heart muscle itself. These changes can be secondary to a long sustained and often progressive increase in the work of the heart as a consequence of volume overload (congenital abnormalities, shunts, valvular incompetence, thyrotoxicosis) or of pressure overload (valvular stenosis, pulmonary or systemic hypertension). Primary changes in the heart muscle are most commonly due to coronary artery disease, and rapid failure is a frequent sequel of acute myocardial infarction (p. 227); other primary causes include the myocardiopathies (Fig. 10–9).

Hemodynamic Changes

When the pumping action of the left ventricle is impaired, the end-diastolic pressure rises, causing a retrograde increase in left atrial and pulmonary vein pressure. As the left atrium dilates, the posterior cusp of the mitral valve is retracted, which causes mitral regurgitation (p. 239). The pulmonary vessels become overfilled with blood. The increase in pulmonary capillary hydrostatic pressure causes interstitial edema followed by exudation of fluid into the alveoli (lung edema). As the pulmonary pressure increases the work of the right ventricle is augmented, leading to overload and eventually to right ventricular failure. When the right ventricle fails, the right ventricular and right atrial pressures rise, which leads to dilatation of the tricuspid atrioventricular ring and tricuspid incompetence. As the pressure in the atrium increases, the systemic veins become engorged, the hydrostatic pressure in the systemic capillaries is augmented, and peripheral edema ensues. It is the clinical manifestations of this engorgement that gave rise to the term "congestive heart failure" (Fig. 10–10).

In the early stage of cardiac failure the depressed myocardial contractility

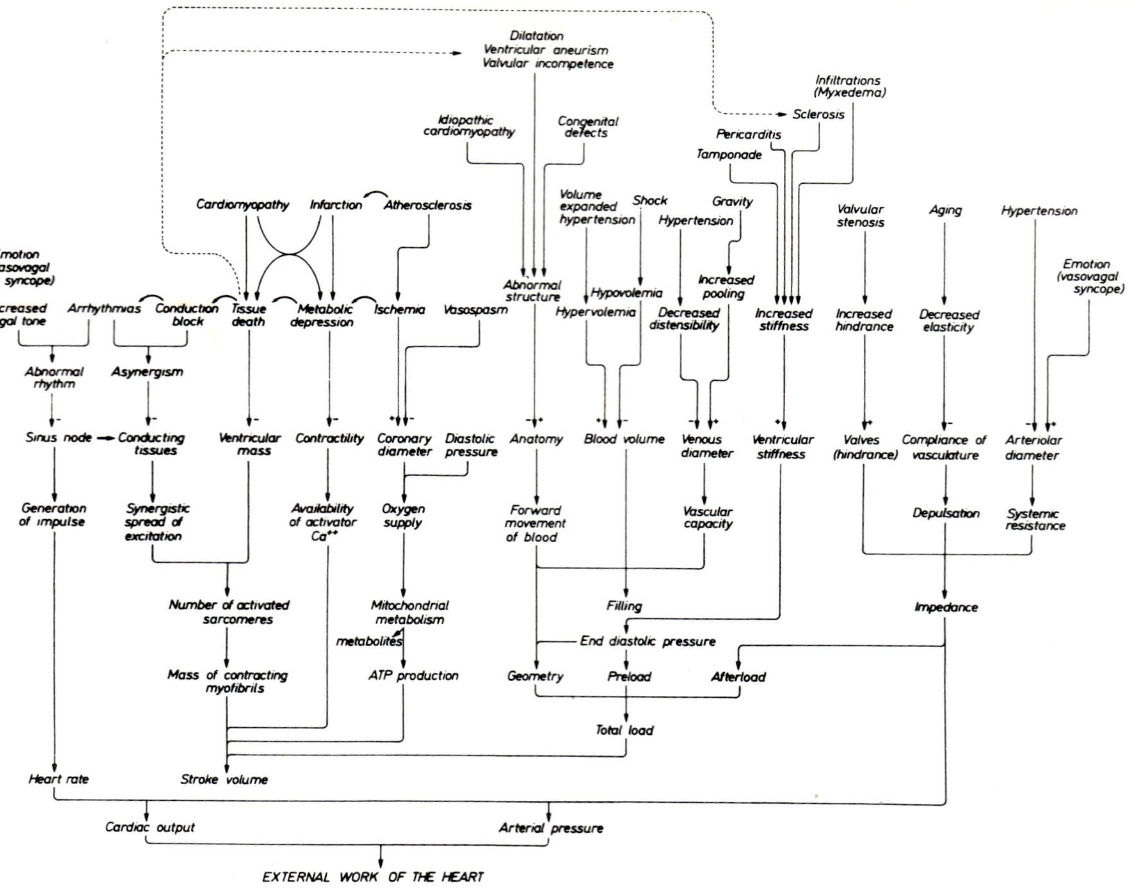

FIG. 10–9. Multiplicity of events which reduce the performance of the heart.

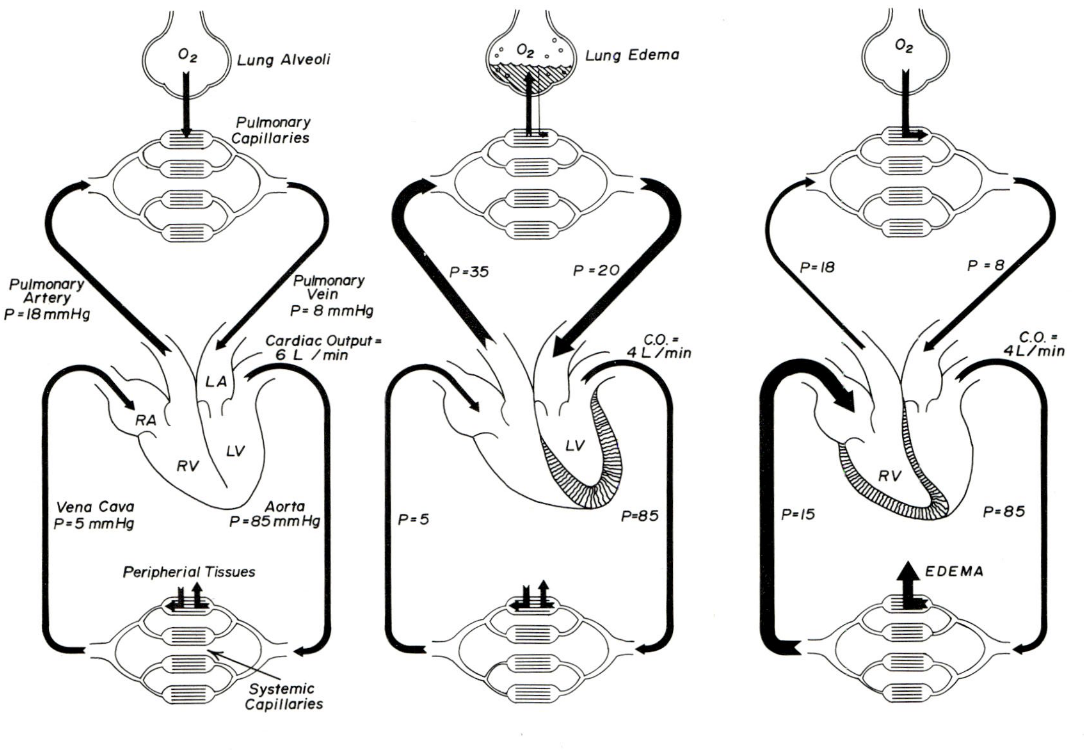

FIG. 10–10. Changes in pulmonary and systemic circulation in heart failure. As the cardiac output (C.O.) decreases, the systemic arterial pressure is maintained near normal by the arterial mechanoreceptors. P = mean pressure.

is compensated for by the increased end-diastolic pressure, which is partly due to an increase in circulating blood volume (p. 260). This results in an increased end-diastolic ventricular volume, which allows a normal peak isovolumetric ventricular wall tension to be maintained and permits the heart to achieve a sufficient level of external work at rest and for some levels of exercise (Fig. 3–7). Further compensation is achieved by cardiac hypertrophy and by increased activation of the sympathetic nerves. The manifestations of failure are not noticed until dilatation of the hypertrophied cardiac chamber has commenced with the accompanying increase in the end-systolic volume. The dilatation leads to a mechanical disadvantage; although a smaller degree of muscle shortening can eject a comparable amount of blood, more energy must be expended to achieve the same cardiac output because of the increase in wall tension (Fig. 3–8). If the failure progresses, the cardiac muscle cells cannot perform the work required to maintain stroke volume. For a time, the increase in heart rate may maintain the resting output in spite of the decrease in stroke volume.

The heart failure usually develops gradually, and a considerable depression of intrinsic myocardial function precedes any decrease in cardiac output or other impairment of the circulation in the resting subject. However, when the patients are stressed, the limitation of cardiac output becomes apparent, and compensatory mechanisms are evoked which redistribute the cardiac output to the most vital organs. When the heart failure is advanced, the cardiac output is reduced at rest and distributed preferentially to the brain and coronary vessels. Even after the resting cardiac output is reduced, the systemic arterial pressure, and hence the perfusion pressure, is maintained by the cardiovascular reflexes until the terminal stages (Fig. 10–11).

The Failing Myocardium

The most common cause of heart failure is sustained hemodynamic overloading. In an unknown way, this leads to an increased muscle mass in the overloaded chamber. The increase in muscle mass is due to an increased size of the cells (hypertrophy) and not to an increased number of cells (hyperplasia). It results from increased protein synthesis and ribonucleic acid content, and a greater number of myofibrils and mitochondria. Initially this improves the capability of the heart to meet the demands placed on it, since the distribution of the increased workload among an increased number of contractile elements reduces the energy expenditure of each. As the cell volume increases during hypertrophy, the ratio of the plasma membrane (sarcolemma and t-system) to the cell volume remains normal, mainly because of the increase in plasma membrane lining the t-system. The sarcoplasmic reticulum and the volume of the myofibrils increase proportionally, and their ratio thus remains constant. How these morphological changes relate to the dynamics of uptake and release of Ca^{2+} is unknown.

In hypertrophic cardiac muscle the ratio of capillaries to muscle fibers remains normal, which implies that the diffusion distance between each capillary and

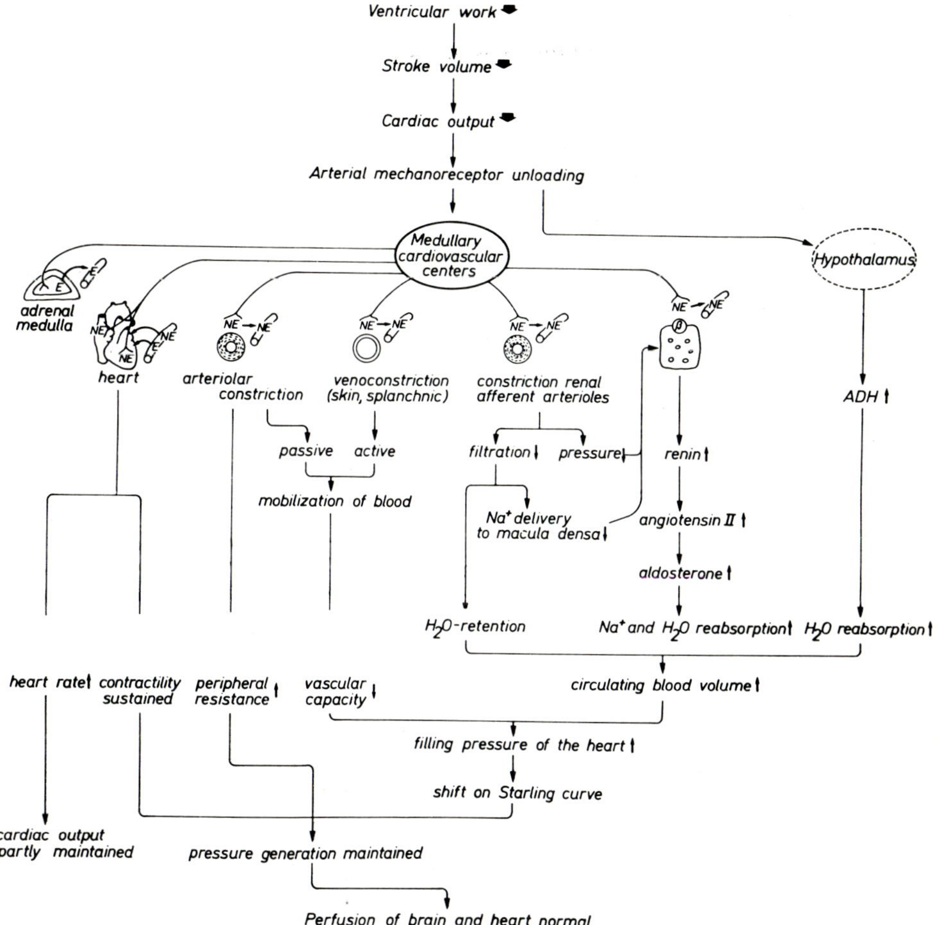

FIG. 10–11. Reflex adjustments to cardiac failure. ADH = antidiuretic hormone, β = beta-adrenergic receptor. NE = norepinephrine, E = epinephrine; ↑ = augmentation, ↓ = depression.

the center of the muscle fibers is increased. At rest the coronary resistance vessels are more dilated than normal, which ensures the proper oxygen supply to the enlarged myocardium. As the wall tension augments in the failing heart, the metabolic needs of the myocardium increase (p. 48). The coronary vessels, particularly those in the subendocardium, may no longer be able to provide sufficient blood to meet the higher metabolic demand. Thus as the cells hypertrophy, there is a delicate balance between oxygen supply and energy utilization. If the overload is maintained, the number of myofibrils increases further. The increased mass of myofibrils relative to the number of mitochondria results in an abnormally high rate of lactate production as well as metabolic inhibition of the contractile process. If this condition is maintained, it causes numerous biochemical changes in the myocardial cell. Among these there is a decrease in the ATPase activity of the myosin molecule; this enzyme splits the terminal phosphate bond of adenosine triphosphate and thereby liberates the energy for the contractile process (p. 46). When energy consumption during contraction outstrips energy production, the muscle cells gradually die and are replaced by connective tissue. When sufficient functioning cells are lost, the stiffness (p. 73) of the ventricular wall augments, its contractile potential is diminished, and the signs and symptoms of heart failure develop.

The contractility of isolated heart muscle from animals in heart failure is depressed owing to a decrease in the strength of each contractile unit in the enlarged cells. This is not due to overstretching of the muscle fibers in the failing heart since it occurs at all muscle lengths. In the human failing ventricle the pre-ejection isovolumetric phase of systole is prolonged in association with a shortening of the duration of the ejection phase but with no change in the duration of total mechanical systole (p. 68).

Adrenergic Control

In congestive heart failure the cardiac norepinephrine stores are exhausted because the synthesis of transmitter is insufficient to sustain the increased sympathetic drive to the myocardium; the defect lies with the rate-limiting enzyme tyrosine hydroxylase. However, the heart remains sensitive to the circulating norepinephrine and epinephrine. The plasma level of norepinephrine is augmented, and this plays an important role in supporting the failing heart. The increased level of circulating catecholamines is caused by the increased sympathetic outflow to the peripheral vascular beds and the adrenal medulla, probably as a consequence of decreased activity of the arterial baroreceptors when the blood pressure tends to fall. The increase in sympathetic outflow and circulating catecholamines causes pronounced vasoconstriction in the renal and splanchnic vascular beds, which in the early stages of heart failure permits the patient to engage in limited exercise even though the cardiac output does not increase normally. Eventually the muscle and skin flows also decrease reflexly.

Renal Function

Normally 20% of the cardiac output goes to the kidneys, but as cardiac output becomes decreased in heart failure, the blood flow to the kidney is reduced proportionally more than that to any other vascular bed. Abnormal renal retention is the main factor responsible for the accumulation of excessive quantities of water in chronic heart failure (Fig. 10–11). This is due to decreased glomerular filtration caused by the vasoconstriction and to increased reabsorption of sodium by the proximal renal tubules. The mechanism underlying the latter is obscure, although it may involve increased aldosterone secretion and differential changes in the caliber of the afferent and efferent arterioles, with a resultant increase in the relative amount of plasma filtered despite the lower renal blood flow. The larger filtration fraction increases the concentration of proteins in the plasma, which pass on to the capillaries surrounding the renal tubules. The resulting increase in peritubular colloid osmotic pressure creates a larger gradient for the reabsorption of water and, secondarily, of sodium. Initially the increase in circulating blood volume is beneficial because it improves the filling of the heart and shifts the myocardium along its Starling curve (Figs. 3–6 and 10–11). When it becomes excessive, it contributes to the dilatation of the ventricles.

Clinical Manifestations

In the later stage of the disease the symptoms of left ventricular failure include fatigue, breathlessness on exertion, and cough. There is dyspnea caused by the increased muscular effort necessary to maintain adequate ventilation when the pulmonary vascular bed is engorged and the pulmonary compliance decreased. Breathing is more difficult when the patient is recumbent (orthopnea) and becomes easier when sitting because of the displacement of blood from the thorax to the dependent parts. With right ventricular failure there is right heart dilatation, hepatomegaly, ascites, and peripheral edema. With combined right and left heart failure all body functions are impaired (Fig. 10–12).

The two main causes of death are: (1) pulmonary edema when fluid is forced into the alveoli, causing the patient to drown in his own fluid; and (2) hypoxia of the brain when the cardiac output decreases to such a degree that the cerebral blood flow is insufficient to meet the demands of the central nervous system. This is manifested by rapid, shallow respiratory movements which gradually deepen and become more labored before decreasing in depth and finally ceasing. After an interval the rapid, shallow breathing is resumed and the cycle is repeated (periodic breathing or Cheyne–Stokes respiration). During the apnea the arterial blood pressure decreases, and the patient becomes cyanotic and stuporose or comatose. When respiration resumes, the blood pressure increases, the cyanosis lessens, and the patient becomes responsive.

Principles of Therapy

Appropriate treatment of heart failure includes: (1) increasing myocardial contractility (cardiac glycosides); (2) reducing the preload of the heart by decreasing circulating blood volume (diuretics) and causing dilation of the systemic veins (e.g., nitrates, sodium nitroprusside, phentolamine); and (3) decreasing the afterload of the heart by causing arteriolar vasodilatation (e.g., sodium nitroprusside, hydralazine, phentolamine, prazosin).

Therapeutic agents which decrease cardiac contractility or inhibit the positive inotropic effect of catecholamines (e.g., beta blockers) are contraindicated.

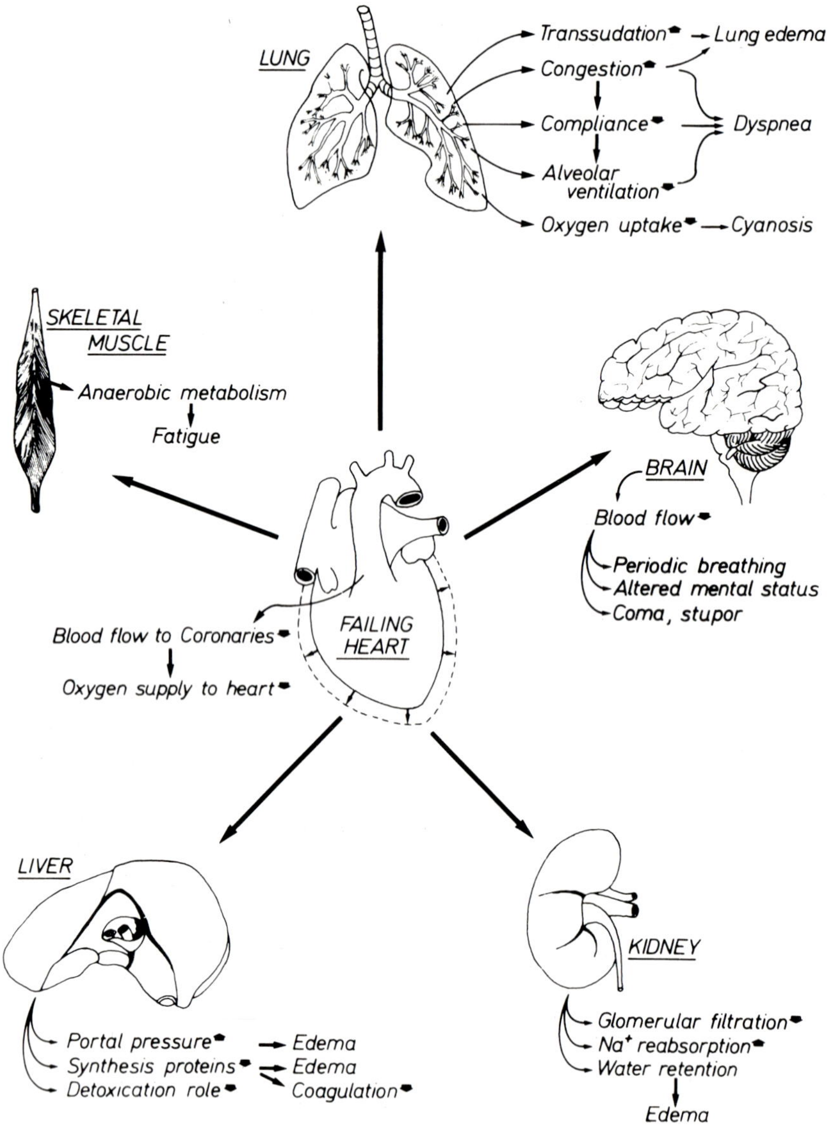

FIG. 10–12. Complications of heart failure.

CIRCULATORY SHOCK

Circulatory shock is characterized by a progressive decrease in arterial blood pressure which eventually causes profound tissue hypoxia throughout the body. If prolonged, the shock becomes irreversible.

Course

The causal factor in circulatory shock is a progressive decrease in cardiac output, which cannot be compensated for by the blood-pressure-controlling mechanisms, in particular the arterial mechanoreceptors. Initially the latter can maintain blood pressure by augmenting the systemic vascular resistance and causing reflex venoconstriction. This ensures proper perfusion of the brain and heart at the expense of other organs, e.g., the kidney and splanchnic region. In these organs the arteriolar constriction results in a decrease in capillary and venous pressure and passive mobilization of blood toward the heart. The lower hydrostatic pressure in the capillaries favors the uptake of fluid from the tissues, which maintains the blood volume.

If the cardiac output continues to decrease after the compensatory vasoconstriction is maximal, the fall in arterial blood pressure will further limit the oxygen supply to the tissues. This, together with the accumulation of metabolic products, causes dilation of the constricted arterioles and increases capillary pressure and permeability. Plasma proteins escape to the interstitial space. These factors combine to cause exudation of fluid into the peripheral tissues, which in turn reduces the circulating blood volume and decreases the filling of the heart. The extravasation of fluid is exaggerated because the postcapillary vessels remain constricted longer than the arterioles since venous smooth muscle cells are relatively insensitive to metabolic changes. The metabolic acidosis resulting from the tissue hypoxia depresses cardiovascular function even more. Ultimately the veins dilate and exaggerated pooling further reduces the circulating blood volume.

The clinical signs of circulatory shock result from the combination of increased sympathetic activity and decreased blood pressure. Among the most prominent are tachycardia, thready pulse, pale and cold skin, sweating, and dry mouth. When the perfusion of the brain becomes insufficient, the progressive cerebral hypoxia causes mental excitation followed by loss of consciousness.

Causes

Many conditions can lead to circulatory shock. They include: (1) Acute failure of the heart. (2) Decreases in venous return caused by hypovolemia. This may occur through (a) loss of blood with external or internal hemorrhage; (b) loss of plasma as seen with severe burns or massive liberation of substances which increases capillary permeability (anaphylactic shock); (c) loss of water and electrolytes as seen in progressive dehydration caused by excessive vomiting, diarrhea (e.g., cholera), or thermal stress. (3) Presence of depressor substances. Certain bacterial toxins such as *Escherichia coli* endotoxin have a pronounced depressant effect on the myocardium and cause increased capillary permeability presumably through liberation of histamine. Other myocardial depressant polypeptides can be liberated from ischemic tissues, particularly the gastrointestinal system; although they are not the precipitating cause of the shock, they may contribute to its irreversibility. (4) Insufficiency of the adrenal cortex (Addison's disease), which predisposes to shock. The corticosteroids, through their multiple actions on the body cells, including synergistic action with catecholamines, serve to increase the resistance to stress.

NERVOUS CONTROL

Cardiac Denervation

Knowledge of the performance of the heart in the absence of its nerve supply is relevant to transplantation of a human heart from a donor to a recipient. After surgical denervation, the resting heart rate in dogs is about 100 to 130 beats/min. This represents the intrinsic rate of the sinus node. Catecholamines are absent in the denervated heart, but there is no depression of the fundamental properties of the myocardium. During exercise the cardiac output increases normally in proportion to the oxygen consumption, and there is little reduction in the maximal ability to exercise (Fig. 10–13). For example, the time required for racing greyhounds to run a standard race is only slightly less after cardiac denervation than before. The heart rate increases more slowly and the maximal rate is less, so the similar cardiac output is achieved by a greater stroke volume. The increased rate after denervation is due mainly to the supersensitivity of the sinus node to the circulating norepinephrine, which escapes into the bloodstream from the sympathetic nerve endings and the adrenal medulla. After pharmacological blockade of the beta-receptors in the heart, the ability to exercise is markedly reduced; the enhanced cardiac contractility is prevented and the increase in heart rate much less (Fig. 10–14). The residual increase is due to the higher temperature of the blood caused by the exercise and the fact that the sinus node is sensitive to stretch and increases its firing as the atrial transmural pressure is augmented by the surge of blood from the exercising muscle. The increased filling of the heart is responsible for most of the increases in stroke volume (p. 72). With cardiac transplantation in humans, the sinus node of the recipient is preserved, and eventually there is some regeneration of sympathetic nerves from the recipient to the donor heart. After the operation the resting heart rate is about 100 beats/min, and two P waves are present on the electrocardiogram. The donor P wave controls the heart rate.

Long Q–T Syndrome

The long Q–T syndrome is seen in children and is characterized by electrocardiographic abnormalities and often fatal ventricular arrhythmias following emotional or physical stress. It results from an imbalance in the sympathetic innervation of the heart, probably a congenital decrease in right cardiac sympathetic nerve activity.

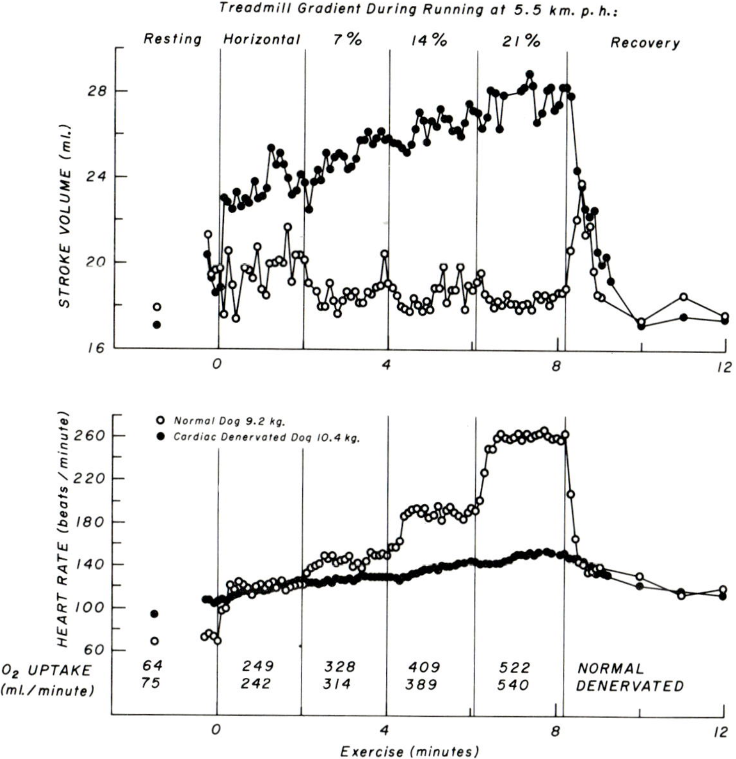

FIG. 10–13. Changes in heart rate and stroke volume during exercise of increasing severity in a normal dog and a dog with cardiac denervation. The dogs ran on a treadmill at a constant speed, and the severity of the exercise was increased at intervals by a stepwise increase in the grade of the treadmill. There were similar values for oxygen consumption and for cardiac output at each work level. In the normal dog the increase in cardiac output was due to a faster heart rate, with either no change or a slight decrease in stroke volume. By contrast, in the denervated dog subjected to moderate grades of work the increase in cardiac output was due to an augmented stroke volume; with more severe exercise the heart rate made a more substantial contribution, accounting for about half of the increase in cardiac output. (From Donald and Shepherd: *Am. J. Cardiol.,* 14:853, 1964.)

Idiopathic Orthostatic Hypotension

A few people, usually elderly men, have gradually lost the function of their autonomic nerves. This is caused by widespread degeneration of the neurons in the brain and spinal cord, the etiology of which is unknown. Less severe forms occur in diabetes mellitus due to the damage (neuropathy) of the sympathetic nerves. The condition is characterized by a marked decrease in blood pressure on standing caused by an inability to increase the heart rate and constrict the systemic resistance and capacitance vessels (Fig. 10–15). The blood pressure may fall with mild exercise even when supine. Since in this position there is

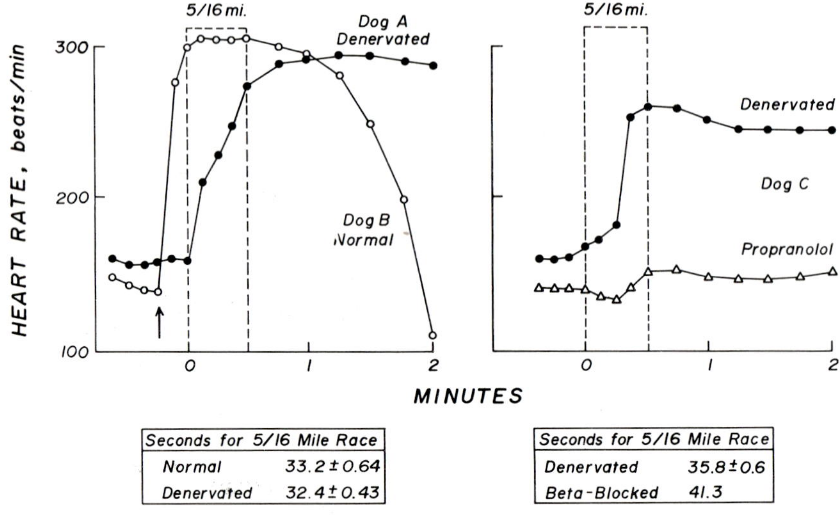

Seconds for 5/16 Mile Race	
Normal	33.2 ± 0.64
Denervated	32.4 ± 0.43

Seconds for 5/16 Mile Race	
Denervated	35.8 ± 0.6
Beta-Blocked	41.3

FIG. 10–14. Heart rate responses in racing greyhounds before and after cardiac denervation and beta-receptor blockade. **Left panel:** In the normal dog the heart rate increased almost to maximal when hearing the signal that the race was about to start *(arrow).* Immediately after the race the heart rate returned to the resting level within about 2 min. By contrast, in the dog with cardiac denervation the heart rate did not increase prior to the race, did increase throughout the race, reached a maximum which was only about 10 beats less than in the normal dog, and returned much more slowly to the resting value. The time to complete the standard 5⁄16 mile race in two greyhounds, studied before and after denervation, increased only from an average of 32.1 to 33.6 sec, indicating the adequate manner in which the denervated heart meets the circulating demands of maximal running effort. **Right panel:** Heart rate response in a greyhound with cardiac denervation before and after beta-adrenergic receptor blockade with propranolol. After propranolol there was only a very modest increase in heart rate during the 5⁄16 mile race; the dog's speed decreased progressively and slowed almost to a walk during the last third of the race. (Data from Donald et al.: *J. Appl. Physiol.,* 19:849, 1964; and *Circ. Res.,* 22:127, 1968.)

no hindrance to venous return, the fall in pressure is due to the absence of compensatory constriction of the resistance vessels.

Syncope

Fainting can occur in susceptible subjects, usually when standing, in response to pain or an emotional experience. It is due to a sudden transient fall in arterial blood pressure caused by vagally mediated bradycardia and dilation of the resistance vessels in the skeletal muscles (vasovagal syncope). The brain blood flow is reduced by about a third, and the resultant hypoxia of the brain cells causes the loss of consciousness. The clinical features include pallor, sweating, nausea, hyperventilation, and dilation of the pupils. Recovery occurs quickly and is facilitated by the subject lying down and raising his or her legs to increase the intrathoracic blood volume.

In most cases the cause of the faint is unknown. It may occur during blood

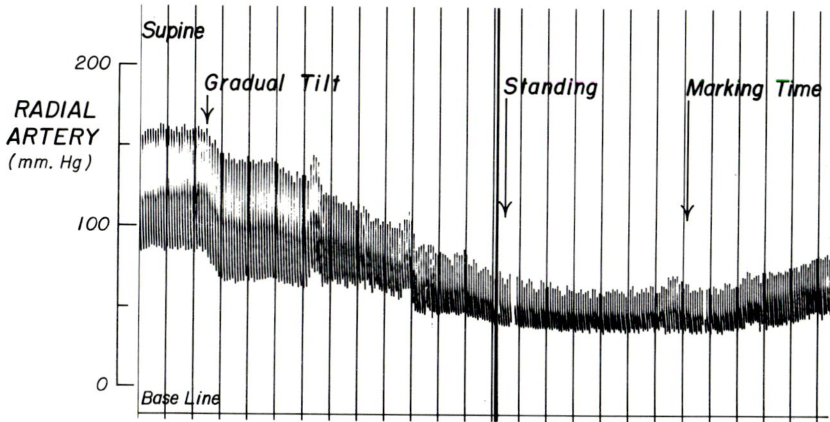

FIG. 10–15. Inability to maintain blood pressure on standing in a patient with an extensive loss of autonomic nervous function (idiopathic orthostatic hypotension). The action of the leg muscle pump in marking time, which squeezes blood into the central circulation and helps maintain the filling pressure of the heart and hence the stroke volume and cardiac output, does not restore the blood pressure. This demonstrates the importance of the reflex constriction of the resistance blood vessels in the splanchnic bed, kidney, and inactive muscles, as well as the constriction of the splanchnic capacitance vessels in maintaining blood pressure during standing in the normal subject. Vertical lines are at 10-sec intervals.

withdrawal in blood donors. During the blood loss the filling pressure of the heart decreases, the stroke volume is reduced, the heart quickens, and cardiac output falls. The arterial blood pressure is maintained through constriction of the systemic resistance vessels and veins by the reflexes originating from the mechanoreceptors in the heart and carotid sinus. The decreased filling of the left ventricle, together with the increased vigor of its contraction due to the increased sympathetic outflow to the myocardium, may excite the mechanoreceptors in the ventricle (p. 136). This could cause the sudden slowing of the heart and the dilatation of the vessels in the skeletal muscles which are characteristic of the faint. The muscle vasodilatation might be caused by a decrease in sympathetic tone or by activation of cholinergic vasodilator fibers (p. 125).

Temporary loss of consciousness also occurs in a variety of conditions characterized by an acute fall in cerebral blood flow consequent to a sudden decrease in cardiac output. This can be due primarily to the heart (e.g., paroxysmal tachycardia, heart block) or to a decreased venous return (e.g., paroxysms of coughing).

Vasoregulatory Asthenia

In vasoregulatory asthenia the working capacity is reduced although the cardiac output increases normally. This is due to faulty regulation of the distribution of the blood to the peripheral organs, presumably because the sympathetic nervous system fails in its coordinating function.

SELECTED REFERENCES

Adelman, A. G., Wigle, E. D., Felderhof, C. H., Corrigal, D. M., and Gilbert, B. W. (1977): Current concepts of primary cardiomyopathies. *Cardiovasc. Med.,* 2:495.

Braunwald, E. (1971): Mechanics and energetics of the normal and failing heart. *Trans. Assoc. Am. Physicians,* 84:63.

Carmeliet, E. (1978): Cardiac transmembrane potentials and metabolism. *Circ. Res.,* 42:577.

Cranefield, P. F. (1977): Action potential, afterpotentials, and arrhythmias. *Circ. Res.,* 41:415.

Del Greco, F. (1975): The kidney in congestive heart failure. *Mod. Concepts Cardiovasc. Dis.,* 44:47.

Dodge, H. T., and Baxley, W. A. (1968): Hemodynamic aspects of heart failure. *Am. J. Cardiol.,* 22:24.

Donald, D. E. (1974): Myocardial performance after excision of the extrinsic cardiac nerves in the dog. *Circ. Res.,* 34:417.

Ferrer, I. (1974): *The Sick Sinus Syndrome.* Futura Publishing Company, New York.

Goodwin, J. F. (1974): Prospects and predictions for the cardiomyopathies. *Circulation,* 50:210.

Hackel, D. B., Ratliff, N. B., and Mikat, E. (1974): The heart in shock. *Circ. Res.,* 35:805.

James, T. N. (1970): Changing concepts in electrocardiography. *Mod. Concepts Cardiovasc. Dis.,* 39:129.

Lefer, A. M. (1973): Blood-borne humoral factors in the pathophysiology of circulatory shock. *Circ. Res.,* 32:129.

Mason, D. T., Spann, J. F., Jr., Zelis, R., and Amsterdam, E. A. (1970): Alterations of hemodynamics and myocardial mechanics in patients with congestive heart failure: Pathophysiologic mechanisms and assessment of cardiac function and ventricular contractility. *Prog. Cardiovasc. Dis.,* 12:507.

Page, E., and McCallister, L. P. (1973): Quantitative electron microscopic description of heart muscle cells. *Am. J. Cardiol.,* 31:172.

Rabinowitz, M., and Zak, R. (1975): Mitochondria and cardiac hypertrophy. *Circ. Res.,* 36:367.

Schwartz, P. J., Brown, A. M., Malliani, A., and Zanchetti, A. (1978): *Neural Mechanisms in Cardiac Arrhythmias.* Raven Press, New York.

Waldo, A. L., Maclean, W. A. H., Karp, R. B., Kouchoukos, N. T., and James, T. N. (1977): Sequence of retrograde atrial activation of the human heart. *Br. Heart J.,* 39:634.

Wellens, H. J. J. (1975): Contribution of cardiac pacing to our understanding of the Wolff–Parkinson–White syndrome. *Br. Heart J.,* 37:231.

Wit, A. L., Hoffman, B. F., and Cranefield, P. F. (1972): Slow conduction and reentry in the ventricle conducting system. I. Return extrasystole in canine Purkinje fibers. *Circ. Res.,* 30:1.

Zelis, R., and Longhurst, J. (1975): The circulation in congestive heart failure. In: *The Peripheral Circulations,* edited by R. Zelis, p. 283. Grune & Stratton, New York.

Zweifach, B. W., and Fronek, A. (1975): The interplay of central and peripheral factors in irreversible hemorrhagic shock. *Prog. Cardiovasc. Dis.,* 18:147.

11

Circulation in the Fetus, Changes at Birth, and Congenital Heart Disease

In order to appreciate the congenital defects which may occur in the cardiovascular system and their hemodynamic consequences, it is first necessary to understand the circulation in the fetus and the changes which occur at the time of birth with the sudden transfer of the function of gas exchange from the placenta to the lungs.

PLACENTAL EXCHANGES

The functioning lung of the fetus is the placenta. After implantation of the fertilized ovum in the uterine wall, blood sinuses develop between the surface of the uterine lining (endometrium) and that of the embryo. These sinuses are supplied with arterial blood from the uterine artery of the mother and are drained by the uterine veins. As the embryo grows, specialized (trophoblastic) cells form projections into the blood sinuses, which become the placental villi into which the fetal capillaries grow. These capillaries, which receive blood low in oxygen from the two fetal umbilical arteries, are surrounded by sinuses containing oxygenated maternal blood. It is here that the transfer of gases and foodstuffs occurs. The gas exchange is less efficient than in the adult lung because more layers of cells separate the maternal and fetal blood (Fig. 11–1).

The blood returning from the placenta to the fetus in the umbilical vein has a Po_2 of only 30 mm Hg. The fetus compensates for the barrier to gas diffusion in three ways: (1) the hemoglobin concentration in the fetus is about 50% greater than that of the mother; (2) fetal hemoglobin can carry as much as 20 to 30% more oxygen per gram that maternal hemoglobin (Fig. 11–1); (3) the relative accumulation of metabolites, particularly acids, causes a shift to the right of the oxyhemoglobin dissociation curve, so that, for a given partial pressure of oxygen, more oxygen is delivered to the cells (Bohr effect; Fig. 2–1). The oxygen saturation of the maternal blood leaving the uterus decreases steadily toward the end of pregnancy, from about 65% to about 20%, indicating that as the fetus grows more oxygen is extracted and that at the end of pregnancy the maternal supply of oxygen has reached its limits.

In spite of the placental barrier to diffusion, and the small partial pressure difference for carbon dioxide, there is adequate diffusion of this gas from the fetal into the maternal blood because its solubility in the fluid of the placental membranes is about 20 times greater than that of oxygen.

FETAL CIRCULATION

About one-half of the oxygenated blood returning to the fetus in the umbilical vein passes to the fetal liver; the remainder reaches the inferior vena cava through the ductus venosus. The blood from the liver enters the inferior vena cava by the hepatic vein together with relatively unsaturated blood from systemic veins. As a result of these venous admixtures, the inferior vena cava blood has an oxygen saturation of about 67%. The majority of it is directed through the foramen ovale into the left atrium and the left ventricle, and only a minor portion enters the right ventricle together with the blood from the superior vena cava and the coronary sinus. Thus the blood in the right ventricle has a lower partial pressure of oxygen than that in the left, where the blood has an oxygen saturation of 60 to 65% and a Po_2 of about 30 mm Hg. The blood expelled by the left ventricle is distributed mainly to the heart, brain, and upper extremities. Of the blood expelled by the right ventricle into the main pulmonary artery, only about 15% reaches the pulmonary vessels. The remainder passes through the ductus arteriosus into the descending aorta, where it mixes with blood from the left ventricle to reach a Po_2 of about 20 mm Hg. This blood either is distributed to the abdominal viscera and the lower limbs or returns to the placenta through the umbilical arteries (Fig. 11–2). Thus the fetal circulation provides blood of a higher Po_2 to the heart muscle and the brain, leaving that with the lower Po_2 for the other tissues.

The placental vessels have a low resistance to blood flow and receive approximately one-half of the total left and right ventricular output of the fetus. The

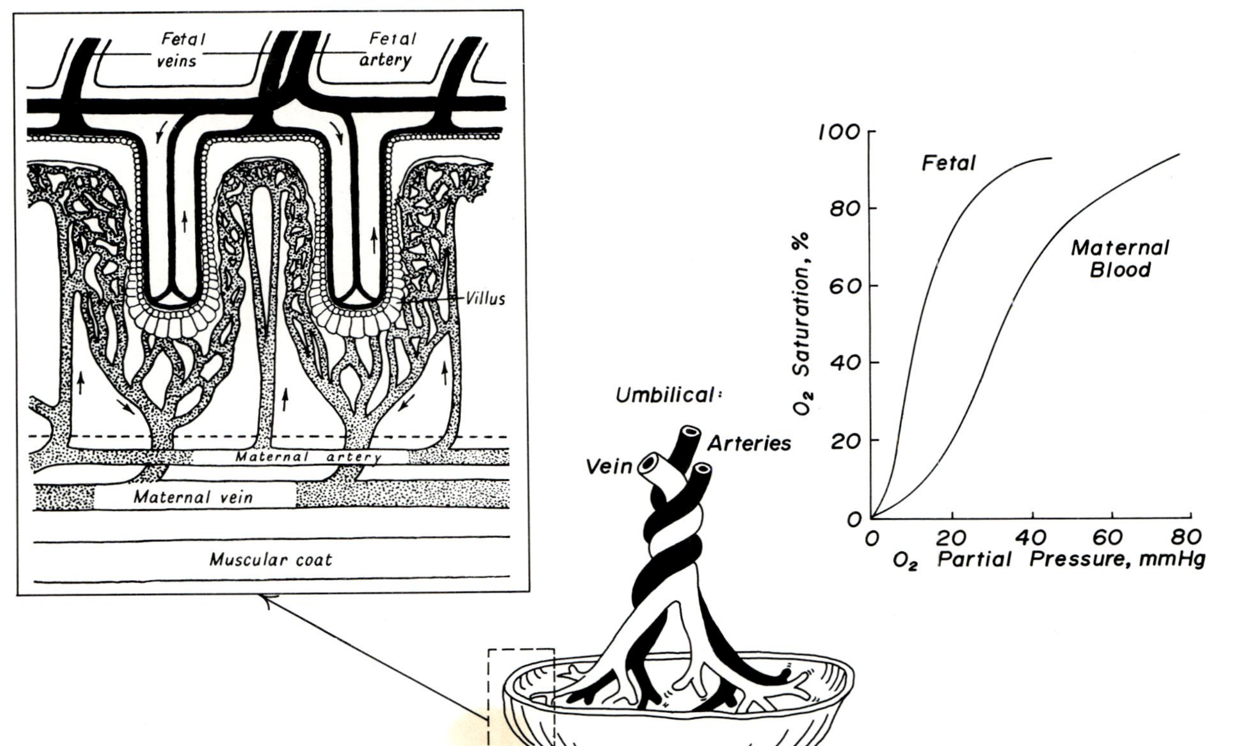

FIG. 11–1. Left: Structure of the placenta showing the relationship between fetal and maternal blood. (From Young: *Handbook of Physiology, Sect. 2: Circulation,* Vol II, p. 1619. American Physiological Society, Washington, D.C., 1963.) **Right:** Comparison of the oxyhemoglobin dissociation curve in fetal and maternal blood. Saturation is expressed as the amount of hemoglobin combined with oxygen divided by the total oxygen capacity. The curve for fetal blood is steeper and lies to the left of that of maternal blood, indicating the higher oxygen affinity in the fetus. This means that at each oxygen tension the fetal hemoglobin carries more oxygen than does maternal hemoglobin. Together with the larger amounts of hemoglobin present in fetal blood, this facilitates uptake of oxygen in the placenta.

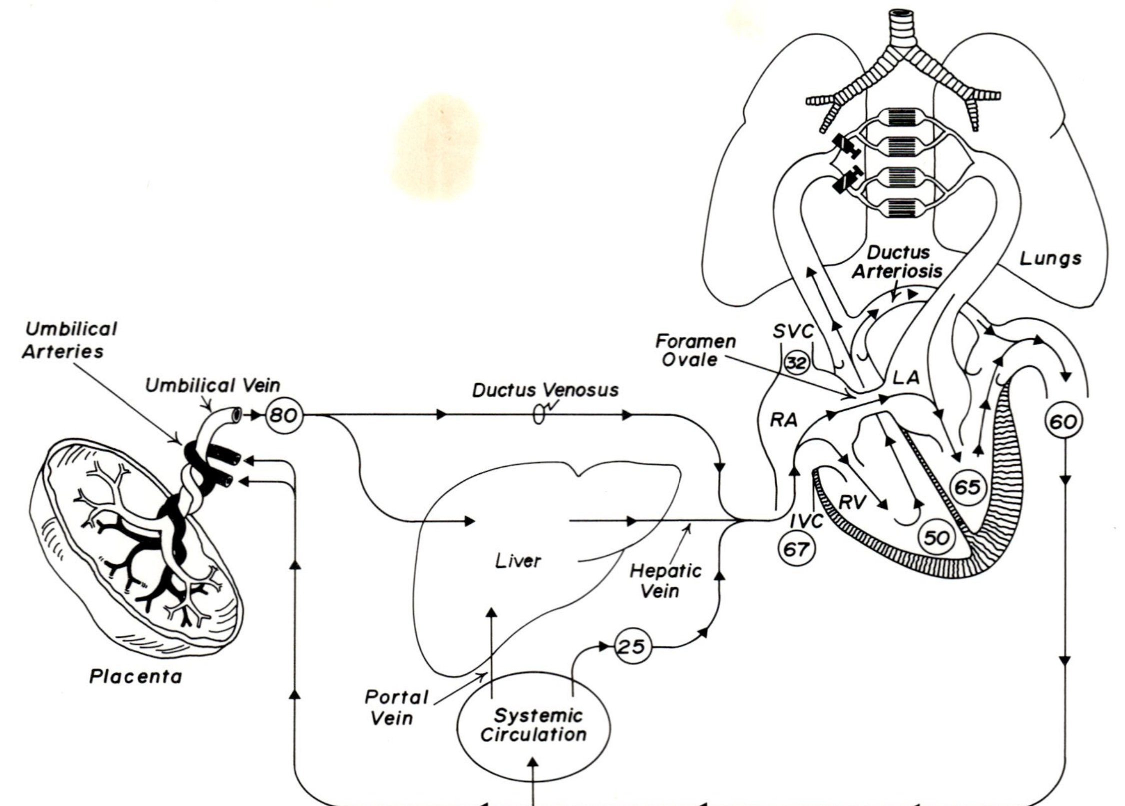

FIG. 11–2. The fetal circulation. Percentages of oxygen saturation of the blood are in circles. IVC = inferior vena cava, LA = left atrium, RA = right atrium, RV = right ventricle, SVC = superior vena cava.

fetal lungs have a high vascular resistance and receive only 5 to 10% of the output (Fig. 11–2).

CHANGES AT BIRTH

The changes at birth are outlined in Fig. 11–3.

Closure of the Foramen Ovale

The pressure in the inferior vena cava decreases when the venous return from the placenta ceases. The increased pulmonary blood flow causes an increase

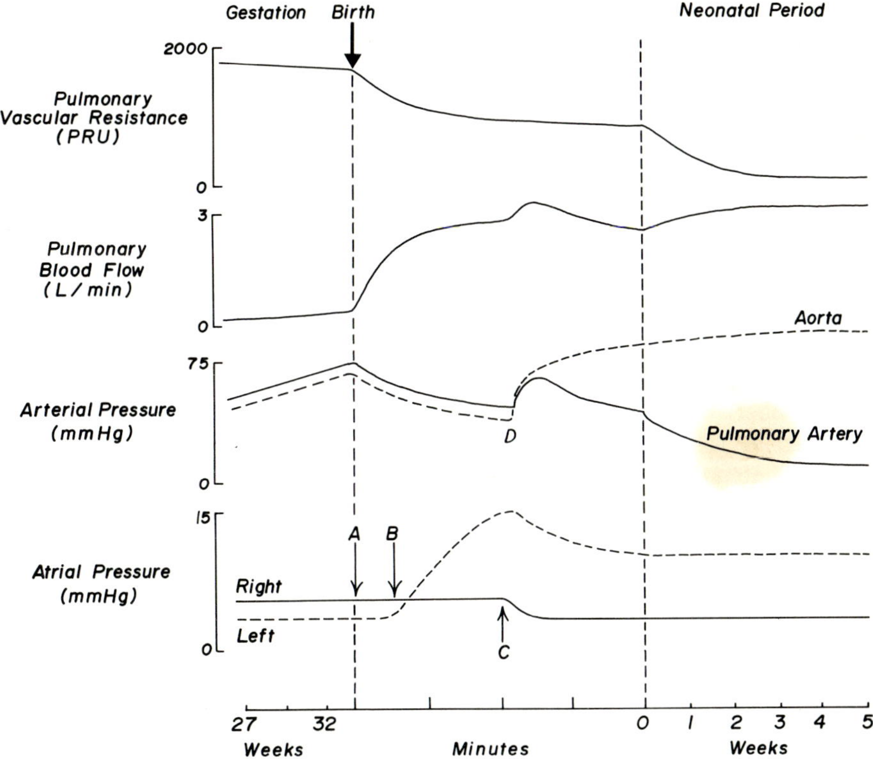

FIG. 11–3. Hemodynamic changes at birth. Note the differences in time scale *(abscissa)*. With the onset of respiration (A), oxygenation of the lung relaxes the pulmonary precapillary vessels (p. 164) with a resulting decrease in pulmonary resistance and pulmonary pressure, and an increase in pulmonary blood flow. With the increased surge of blood to the left atrium the left atrial pressure increases; when it is higher than the right atrial pressure the foramen ovale closes (B). Tying off the umbilical cord (C) decreases the venous return and hence both atrial pressures. When the pulmonary pressure falls below the aortic pressure, the flow is reversed in the ductus arteriosus (D), which causes a temporary increase in pulmonary blood flow and pressure. During the neonatal period the pulmonary resistance decreases further because of regression of the smooth muscle in the pulmonary vessels (p. 274), and the ductus arteriosus closes.

in left atrial pressure, which now exceeds that in the right atrium. This causes functional closure of the foramen ovale by the apposition of the left and right atrial flaps bordering the opening. Permanent closure occurs later.

Closure of the Ductus Venosus

Elimination of the low resistance to flow through the placental circulation is followed by a marked increase in total systemic vascular resistance and the cessation of blood flow through the ductus venosus. Fibrosis and anatomical closure of the ductus occur within about 7 days.

Closure of the Ductus Arteriosus

The ductus arteriosus normally closes within 10 to 15 hr of delivery because the smooth muscle in its wall constricts. How this is set in motion is unknown, although it has been established that high oxygen tension and substances which inhibit prostaglandin synthesis facilitate closure. The closed ductus becomes fibrosed and obliterated by the time the infant is about 2 weeks of age.

Dilatation of Pulmonary Vessels

The closure of the ductus arteriosus, the foramen ovale, and the ductus venosus separate the pulmonary and systemic circulations. The fetal situation is reversed, with the pulmonary circuit becoming the low-resistance one and the systemic circuit the one with high resistance. The pulmonary vascular resistance decreases as the smooth muscle of the pulmonary vessels relax when the oxygen tension increases. A large increase in pulmonary blood flow occurs together with a fall in pulmonary artery and right ventricular pressures. Later there is a gradual thinning of the muscle layers of the pulmonary vessels.

CONGENITAL CARDIOVASCULAR DISEASE

The incidence of congenital anomalies in the circulatory system is about 7 per 1,000 births. Of these the most common is ventricular septal defect (30%), with atrial septal defect, patent ductus arteriosus, and pulmonary stenosis each contributing about 10% to the total.

All conceivable types of structural abnormalities of the cardiovascular system have been encountered. The main perturbations they cause are obstruction to flow and abnormal shunting of blood. Only selected examples are given in this chapter.

Obstruction to Blood Flow

Coarctation of the Aorta

A coarctation of the aorta is a localized obstruction of its lumen, usually just distal to the origin of the left subclavian artery at the site where the ductus arteriosus connects to the lesser curvature of the aortic arch. The resulting circulatory disturbances differ when the ductus is open or closed, the latter being more frequent. The coarctation causes a loud systolic murmur. The cardiac output is normal, but the systemic pressure is elevated in the vessels upstream from the site of obstruction. The left ventricle is hypertrophied owing to the increased work load. The extensive development of collateral vessels from the branches of the subclavian arteries to the intercostal vessels, which arise from the aorta below the site of coarctation, provide a normal blood supply to the lower part of the body. The mean pressure and the pulse pressure in the downstream large arteries are reduced. Vascular resistance in the arms is increased but is normal in the legs. The mechanism underlying this increase in resistance in the upper limbs is unknown (Fig. 11–4).

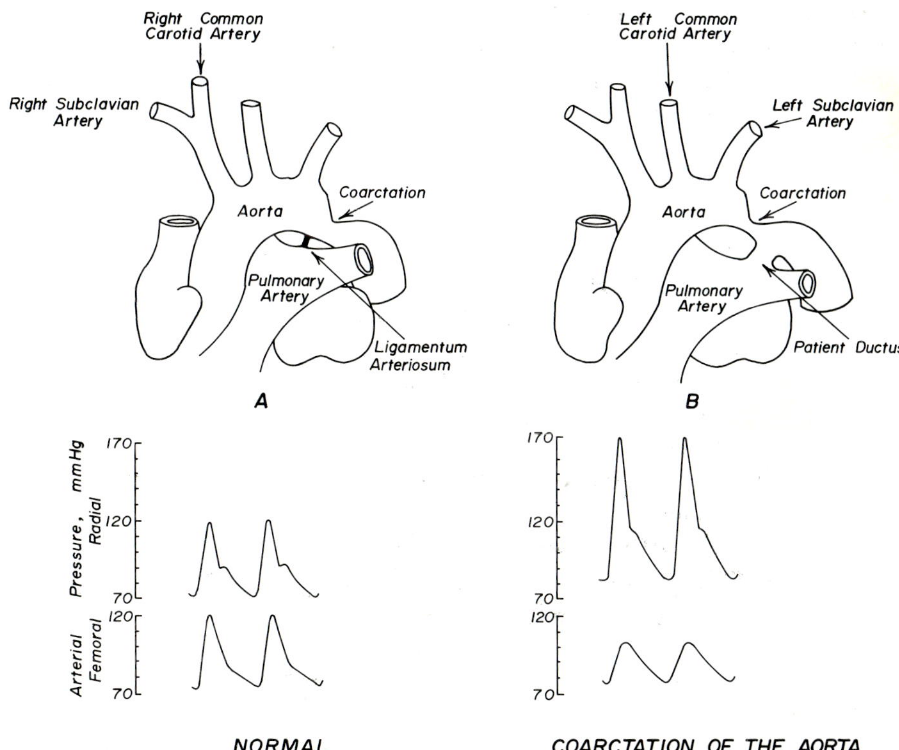

FIG. 11–4. Upper: Coarctation of the aorta is a congenital abnormality in which the lumen of the aorta is narrowed near to the site of the ductus arteriosus. The latter may be closed, with the ligamentum arteriosum as its remnant **(A)**, or it may remain patent **(B)**. If the ductus is open the hemodynamic consequences differ when the coarctation is proximal or distal to the opening of the ductus. **Lower:** Tracings of simultanous recordings of pressures in the radial and femoral arteries of a normal young adult and a patient of similar age with coarctation of the aorta and a closed ductus. In the normal subject the systolic, diastolic, and pulse pressures are similar in both arteries. In the patient the systolic and diastolic pressures in the radial artery are increased. In the femoral artery the pulse contour is reduced and has a typical sawtooth appearance. This is because the aortic obstruction is bypassed by numerous collateral vessels of varying length which dampen the pulse.

Pulmonary Valvular Stenosis

In congenital stenosis of the pulmonary valve, pressure gradients across the valve may be as high as 200 mm Hg. The normal flow through the narrowed orifice generates a loud systolic murmur. In mild pulmonary stenosis the right atrial pressure is normal. With more severe obstruction the atrial muscle hypertrophies and the forceful atrial contraction contributes to right ventricular end-diastolic pressure and hence to maintenance of the stroke volume. The cardiac output is usually maintained at the normal level, but eventually the right ventricle may dilate and fail, at which time tricuspid regurgitation occurs. If the foramen ovale is patent, blood passes from the right to the left atrium because the pressure in the right now exceeds that in the left. This causes desaturation of the arterial blood (Fig. 11–5).

Shunting of Blood Between the Two Sides of the Heart

The presence of abnormal communications within the cardiovascular system results in the shunting of blood. The shunt may cause recirculation of blood through the pulmonary circuit (arteriovenous or left-to-right shunt), diversion of blood away from the pulmonary circulation and oxygen desaturation of blood in the systemic arteries (venoarterial or right-to-left shunt), or both (bidirectional shunt).

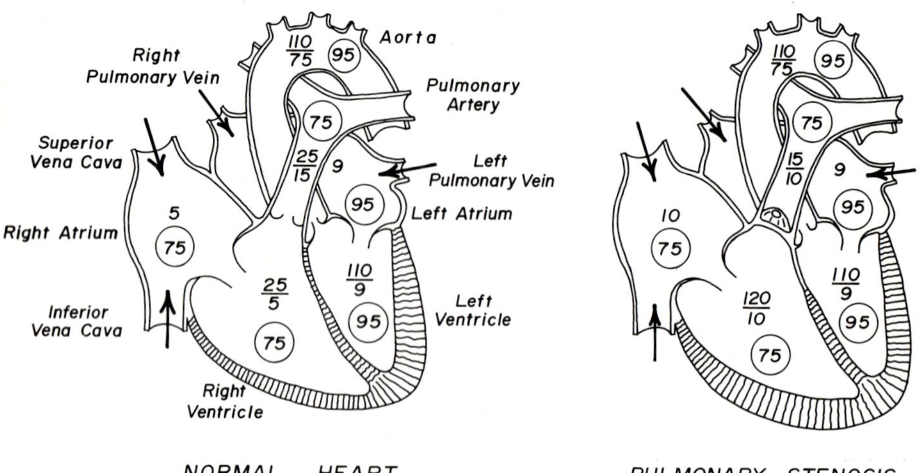

FIG. 11–5. Intracardiac and great vessel pressures and percentage oxygen saturations of the blood in a normal heart and one with pulmonary stenosis. Pressures are given in millimeters of mercury. Oxygen saturation are given in the circles.

Atrial Septal Defect

Normally the left atrial pressure is higher than the right. When a small atrial septal defect is present, this pressure difference is maintained and blood is shunted from the left to the right atrium. With large defects the pressure difference disappears, but the left-to-right shunt persists because of the greater distensibility of the right atrium and the lesser resistance to filling of the right ventricle as compared with the left. Due to the low resistance of the pulmonary vessels, there is a large increase in pulmonary blood flow, whereas the aortic flow remains normal. The large pulmonary flow causes an abnormally high pressure gradient across the pulmonary valve. Since the resting heart rate is normal, the right ventricular stroke volume is markedly augmented. The right atrium, right ventricle, and pulmonary artery are enlarged in order to accommodate the increased flow, whereas the left atrium is usually normal. Preferential shunting of blood returning from the right lung occurs because the ostia of the right pulmonary veins are situated close to the edge of the defect. The rate of ejection of blood into the pulmonary artery is increased and causes a systolic murmur. The increased rate of flow through the tricuspid valve may give rise to a diastolic murmur (Fig. 11–6).

The hemodynamic consequences of atrial septal defects can be modified by the coexistence of other shunts and/or of valvular lesions such as pulmonary stenosis. Occasionally, and for unknown reasons, the pulmonary vascular resistance increases because of hypertrophy of the media and thickening of the intima of the pulmonary arteries and arterioles. This leads to pulmonary hypertension, hypertrophy of the right ventricle, an increase in right atrial pressure, and hence a decrease in the magnitude of the shunt.

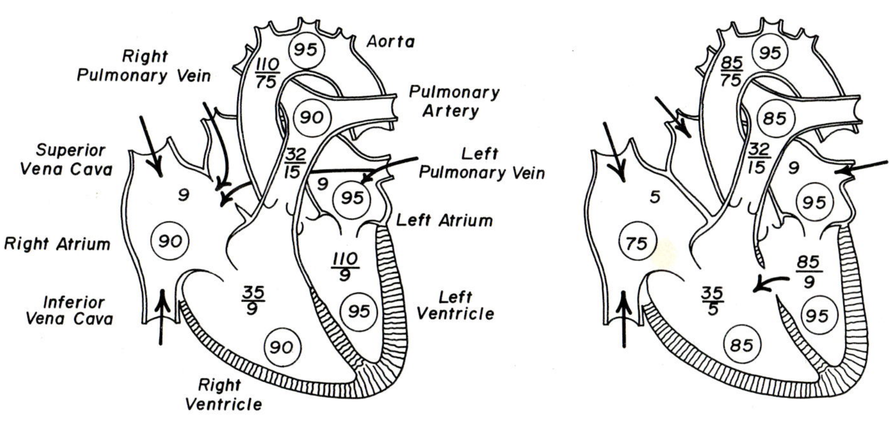

FIG. 11–6. Intracardiac and great vessel pressures and percentage oxygen saturation of the blood in a heart with an atrial septal defect and one with a ventricular septal defect. Pressures are in millimeters of mercury. Oxygen saturations are given in the circles.

Ventricular Septal Defect

The consequences of ventricular septal defects are determined mainly by their size and the state of the pulmonary vascular bed. When the defect is small and the pressure difference between the two ventricles is maintained, there is only a small left-to-right shunt and the pulmonary vascular resistance remains low. The flow of blood through the small defect causes a systolic murmur. When the defect is large, the pressure in the two ventricles equalizes, and the pulmonary vascular resistance determines the consequences. In the newborn the persistence of the fetal pattern of pulmonary vessels keeps the pulmonary vascular resistance high and limits the left-to-right shunt. If the fetal vessels become adult in type and decrease their resistance, there is a marked increase in the left-to-right shunt and thus in pulmonary blood flow. Left ventricular failure and death may occur during the first year of life unless the pulmonary vessels show a secondary hypertrophy because of the high pressure. If the pulmonary vascular resistance continues to increase and exceeds systemic resistance, the shunt may be reversed, leading to oxygen desaturation of the arterial blood (Fig. 11–6).

Patent Ductus Arteriosus

Failure of the ductus arteriosus to close after birth causes hemodynamic changes that are similar to those seen with a ventricular septal defect, and thus depend on the changes in pulmonary vascular resistance (Fig. 11–7).

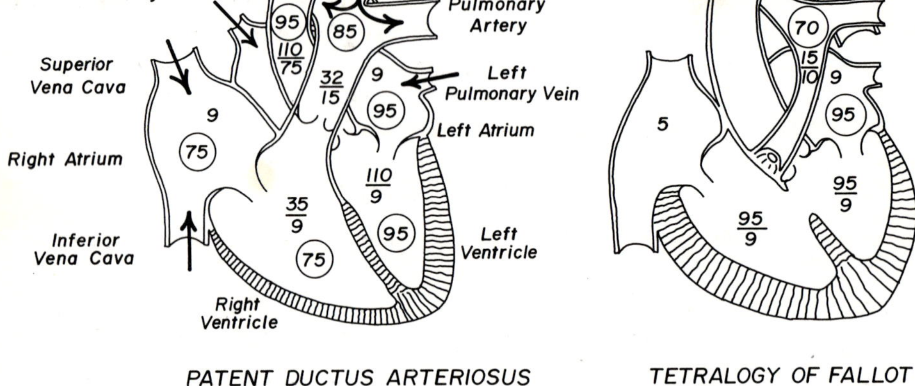

FIG. 11–7. Intracardiac and great vessel pressures and percentage oxygen saturation of the blood in a heart with patent ductus arteriosus and one with tetralogy of Fallot. Pressures are in millimeters of mercury. Oxygen saturations are given in the circles.

Arteriovenous Fistula

Direct communication between arteries and veins results in the shunting of arterial blood into the venous system. Congenital arteriovenous fistulas may occur in various sites, e.g., between the coronary arteries and the coronary sinus or between renal arteries and veins. This leads to the diversion of flow from the tissues distal to the shunt, with resultant ischemia.

Malposition of Cardiovascular Structures

Anomalous Pulmonary Venous Connections

Some or all of the pulmonary veins may drain into the right atrium or into one of its systemic venous tributaries. An intracardiac septal defect or a patent ductus arteriosus usually coexists.

Transposition of the Great Arteries

The aorta arises from the right ventricle and the pulmonary trunk from the left ventricle. The heart, brain, and the other tissues are perfused with desaturated blood. Survival after birth depends on shunts between the pulmonary and systemic circulations which allow mixing with arterial blood. A ventricular septal defect is usually present.

Combinations of Lesions

The most common combination of lesions is the tetralogy of Fallot, which is characterized by: (1) stenosis of the pulmonary outflow; (2) ventricular septal defect; (3) an aorta which overrides the septal defect so the right half of the aorta is situated over the right ventricle and the left half over the left ventricle; and (4) right ventricular hypertrophy (Fig. 11–7). The outflow of blood from the right ventricle goes partly to the pulmonary circulation and partly to the aorta. The more severe the pulmonary stenosis, the more blood there is directed to the aorta. This right-to-left shunt causes decreased oxygen saturation of the blood in the systemic arteries, which results in cyanosis.

SELECTED REFERENCES

Dawes, G. S. (1968): *Foetal and Neonatal Physiology.* Year Book Medical Publishers, Chicago.

Heymann, M. A., and Rudolph, A. M. (1975): Control of the ductus arteriosus. *Physiol. Rev.,* 55:62.

Mair, D. D., and Ritter, D. G. (1976): The physiology of cyanotic congenital heart disease. In: *International Review of Physiology, Cardiovascular Physiology II,* Vol. 9, edited by A. C. Guyton and A. W. Cowley Jr., p. 275. University Park Press, Baltimore.

Marshall, R. J., and Shepherd, J. T. (1968): *Cardiac Function in Health and Disease.* Saunders, Philadelphia.

Young, M. (1963): The fetal and neonatal circulation. In: *Handbook of Physiology, Sect. 2: Circulation,* Vol. II, p. 1619. American Physiological Society, Washington, D.C.

Zimmerman, H. A. (1959): *Intravascular Catheterization.* Charles C Thomas, Springfield, Ill.

12

Measurement of Heart Function

Knowledge of the functioning of the cardiovascular system in normal and abnormal circumstances is derived from measurement of the events within it. The interpretation of these measurements requires understanding the principles of the methods used to make them, the underlying assumptions, and the circumstances under which the measurements are made. The present chapter deals with the assessment of the function of the heart.

ELECTRICAL PHENOMENA

Electrocardiogram

The electrical activity of the heart causes the development of small potential differences which can be recorded from the body surface or the heart chambers (Fig. 12–1).

Standard Electrocardiographic Leads (Bipolar Leads)

The shape of the electrocardiogram from distant leads has little resemblance to the action potentials of cardiac muscle (Fig. 3–4). The usefulness of these leads is not based on theory but on years of correlation of the shape of the electrocardiogram with disturbances of conduction in the heart. Three leads are used. In lead I the electrodes are attached to the right and left arms, lead II to the right arm and left leg, and lead III to the left arm and left leg (Fig. 12–2).

Unipolar Limb Leads

One electrode is placed on an area of the body surface and is connected to the central terminal across a galvanometer, which records only the potential

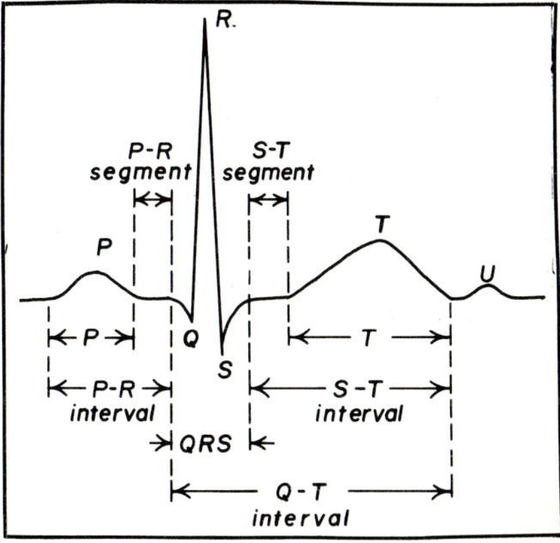

FIG. 12–1. Waves of the normal electrocardiogram. (1) The P–R interval is measured from the beginning of the P wave to the beginning of the QRS (ventricular) complex. If the ventricular complex begins with an initial downward deflection, the Q wave, the interval is sometimes referred to as the P–Q interval. The P–R or P–Q interval represents the time from the beginning of atrial muscle depolarization to the beginning of ventricular depolarization. (2) The P–R segment is measured from the end of the P wave to the beginning of the QRS complex. This represents the delay in transmission of the impulse at the atrioventricular node. (3) The S–T segment is measured from the end of the QRS complex to the beginning of the T wave. It represents the interval of time between completion of depolarization and beginning of repolarization of the ventricular muscle (4). The S–T interval is measured from the end of the QRS complex to the end of the T wave. It represents the time from completion of depolarization of the ventricular muscle to completion of repolarization (5). The Q–T interval is the sum of the QRS and S–T intervals. It represents the time for depolarization and repolarization of the ventricular muscle (6). The U-wave represents afterpotentials following repolarization of the ventricles. It is not often seen in the normal electrocardiogram. At resting heart rates in adults of about 60 to 80 beats/min the upper limit of normal for the P–R interval is 0.20 sec. The durations of the P wave and the QRS complex normally do not exceed 0.11 and 0.10 sec, respectively. (Modified from Burch and Winsor: *A Primer of Electrocardiography,* 6th ed., p. 4. Lea & Febiger, Philadelphia, 1972.)

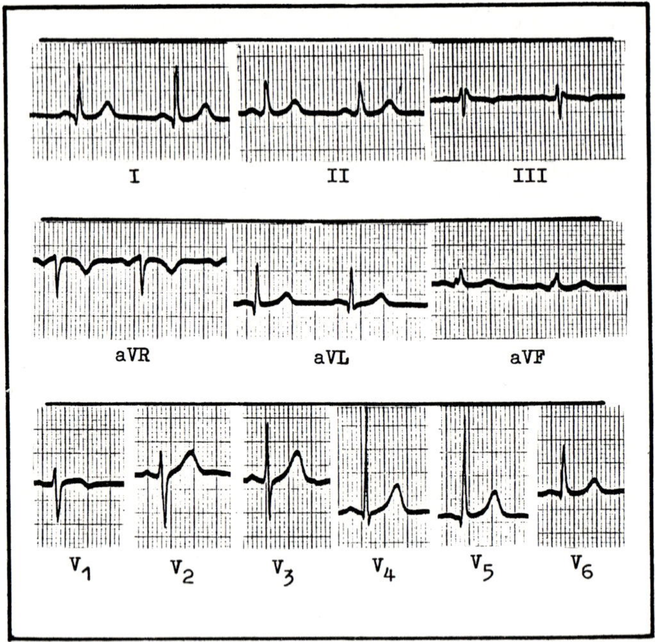

FIG. 12–2. Normal electrocardiogram showing the various peripheral leads. (From Stein: *The Normal Electrocardiogram,* p. 78. Saunders, Philadelphia, 1976.)

changes at the exploring electrode. The right arm lead (VR) records mainly the electrical activity of the ventricles, the left arm lead (VL) the upper left side of the heart, and the foot lead (VF) the base of the heart and the lower surface of the ventricles.

Augmented Limb Leads

Augmented limb leads, designated VR, VL, and VF, provide recordings between one limb and two others. This increases the size of the potentials by 50% without any change in configuration (Fig. 12–2).

Precordial Electrocardiogram

The anterior surface of the heart, comprising portions of both ventricles, lies close to the surface of the anterior chest and left axilla. Thus leads from this area resemble direct leads from the epicardial surface of the heart more than leads from other parts of the body surface, although there is a large reduction in the size of the recorded deflections. The precordial leads (V_1 to V_6) are unipolar leads which provide information concerning mainly the anterior portion of the right and left ventricles (Fig. 12–2).

Intracardiac Electrocardiogram

To record the electrical events in the atrioventricular node, the bundle of His, and the Purkinje system, a catheter containing ring electrodes at its tip is passed into the right side of the heart and placed close to the tricuspid valve. The His bundle electrogram, when recorded simultaneously with standard leads, permits the timing of conduction (1) from the sinoatrial to the atrioventricular node, (2) through the atrioventricular node, and (3) through the bundle of His and its branches (Fig. 12–3).

Vectorcardiography

An electrical vector can be represented by an arrow that points in the direction of positive current flow with a length proportional to the magnitude of the current. The vector of current flow rapidly changes in direction and length as the impulses spread through the heart, and the vectorcardiogram depicts these changes at the various stages of the cardiac cycle by integrating the simultaneous information obtained with the standard electrocardiographic leads (Fig. 12–4). It provides a measurement of the mean electrical axis of the heart. If this mean electrical axis is shifted outside arbitrarily defined limits, it is said to indicate right or left ventricular axis deviation. Vectorcardiography is a sensitive method to detect ventricular hypertrophy, intraventricular conduction disturbances, or myocardial infarction.

The vectorcardiogram reveals the influence of respiration on the orientation of the heart, since the movement of the diaphragm shifts the geometrical and electrical axes of the heart with respect to the peripheral leads. Changes during respiration in the standard limb leads caused by this shift might be erroneously interpreted as indicating changes in conduction.

ACOUSTIC PHENOMENA

Heart sounds are caused by vibrations involving the heart chambers, valves, and contents. These sounds may be heard by placing the ear on the chest wall, using a stethoscope, or by phonocardiography. The latter may be recorded externally by catheter-mounted high-fidelity microtransducers (intracardiac phonocardiography). Studies on the genesis of the heart sound have been aided by the ability of echocardiography (p. 297) to track the movements of the heart valves without significant time delay. In such studies the phonocardiogram, the echocardiogram (for echoes of the heart valves), the electrocardiogram, and an apex pulse tracing are recorded simultaneously at fast paper speed (Fig. 12–5).

Heart Sounds

The major element of the first heart sound is due to vibrations dependent on closure of the mitral and tricuspid valves; the sudden deceleration of the mass of blood within the ventricle results in vibrations in the audible range.

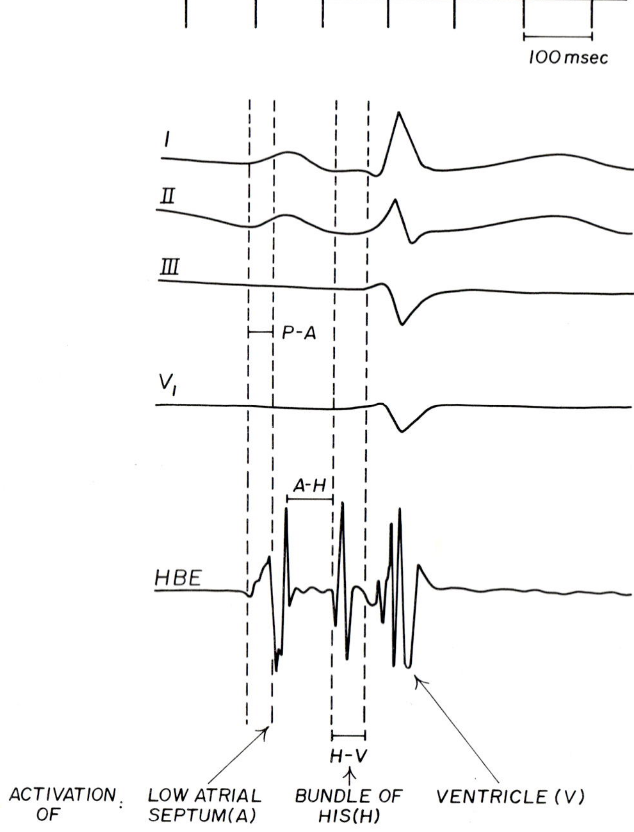

FIG. 12–3. His bundle electrogram (HBE). This is recorded from an electrode catheter passed into the right atrium and the electrodes positioned close to the tricuspid valve. The HBE tracing is composed of three bipolar complexes, corresponding to activation of the low atrial septum (A), the bundle of His (H), and the ventricle (V). Standard electrocardiographic leads (usually I, II, III, and a precordial lead V_1) are recorded simultaneously for purposes of interval measurement. (1) P–A interval: from the onset of the P wave on the surface leads to the first rapid deflection of the HBE tracing. This is a measure of conduction from the high to the low right atrium. (2) A–H interval: from the first rapid deflection of the low atrial electrogram to the onset of the His bundle deflection. This is an indirect measure of atrioventricular node conduction. (3) H–V interval: from the onset of the His bundle deflection to the onset of ventricular activation, as determined from the earliest QRS deflection or the ventricular electrogram (V) of the HBE tracing. This is a measure of the conduction time in the bundle of His and its branches. (Modified from Gallagher and Damato: In: *Cardiac Catheterization and Angiography,* edited by Grossman, p. 219. Lea & Febiger, Philadelphia, 1974.)

The initial high-frequency vibrations of the second heart sound occur simultaneously with closure of the aortic valve; the slightly longer interval between pulmonary valve closure and sound production is attributed to the increased compliance of the pulmonary arteries.

The mitral valve does not remain fully open throughout diastole. Echo- and

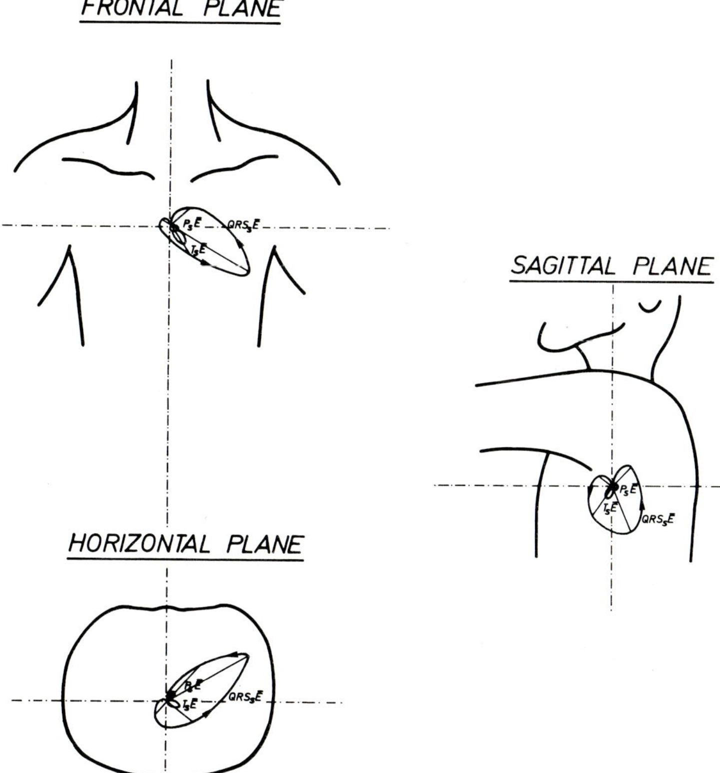

FIG. 12–4. During the contraction of the heart, changes in electromotive forces occur which can be represented by vectors. At each moment of the cardiac cycle, the direction and the amplitude of the vector results from the degree of activity of the various components of the heart. The summation of the vectors resulting from the instantaneous changes in electrical activity represent the vectorcardiogram which is displayed on an oscilloscope. The beam describes three loops in succession: depolarization of the atria ($P_s\bar{E}$), depolarization of the ventricles ($QRS_s\bar{E}$), and repolarization of the ventricles ($T_s\bar{E}$). For each loop, the direction of inscription is indicated by the arrows; they can be analyzed in terms of initial deflection, efferent limb, maximum vector, afferent limb, and terminal deflection. The loops are projected from three spatial planes: frontal, horizontal, and sagittal. Vectorcardiography is a sensitive method to detect ventricular hypertrophy, intraventricular conduction disturbances, and myocardial infarction (courtesy of Dr. J. Snoeck).

phonocardiographic records show that after the first surge of blood in early diastole a partial rebound occurs. This is associated with the third heart sound, which can be heard in circumstances of rapid ventricular filling, in certain normal youthful subjects and in some patients (e.g., mitral regurgitation). As the atrium contracts, the mitral valve "reopens" and the sudden further distention of the ventricle may give rise to vibrations referred to as the fourth heart sound. Occasionally the third, but rarely the fourth, heart sound can be detected with a stethoscope.

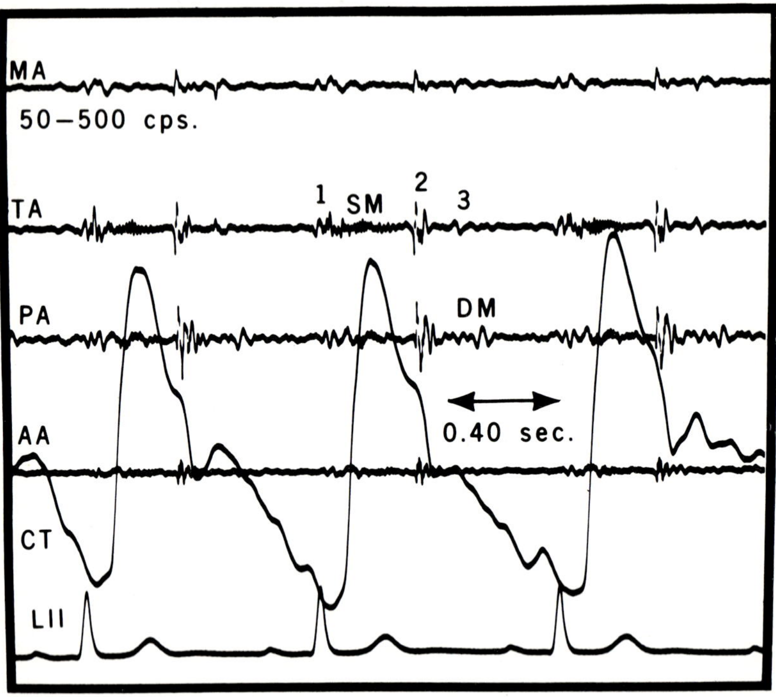

FIG. 12–5. Simultaneously recorded phonocardiogram at the mitral (MA), tricuspid (TA), pulmonic (PA), and aortic (AA) areas; a carotid pulse tracing (CT); and lead II (LII) of the electrocardiogram in a patient who was 3 months' pregnant. The first and second heart sounds are normal. A prominent third heart sound, recorded best at the tricuspid and pulmonary areas, is followed by a short, low-frequency, early mid-diastolic vibration. There is a short, high-frequency, low-amplitude systolic ejection murmur (SM) recorded best at the tricuspid and pulmonary areas. The systolic murmur probably represents increased flow due to increased blood volume during pregnancy. The short mid-diastolic murmur (DM) may represent turbulent flow across either the mitral or tricuspid valve. (From Benchimol: *Non-invasive Techniques in Cardiology.* Williams & Wilkins, Baltimore, 1977.)

Opening Snaps

An opening snap of the mitral valve is heard in patients with mitral stenosis and is attributed to the opening of the thickened deformed valve. Opening snaps also can occur with large flows during early diastole across a normal mitral or tricuspid valve. This is seen, for example, in patients with left-to-right shunts or mitral regurgitation.

Heart Murmurs

Heart murmurs can be heard in every part of the heart and great vessels when excessive turbulence occurs (p. 19). They do not always indicate cardiovas-

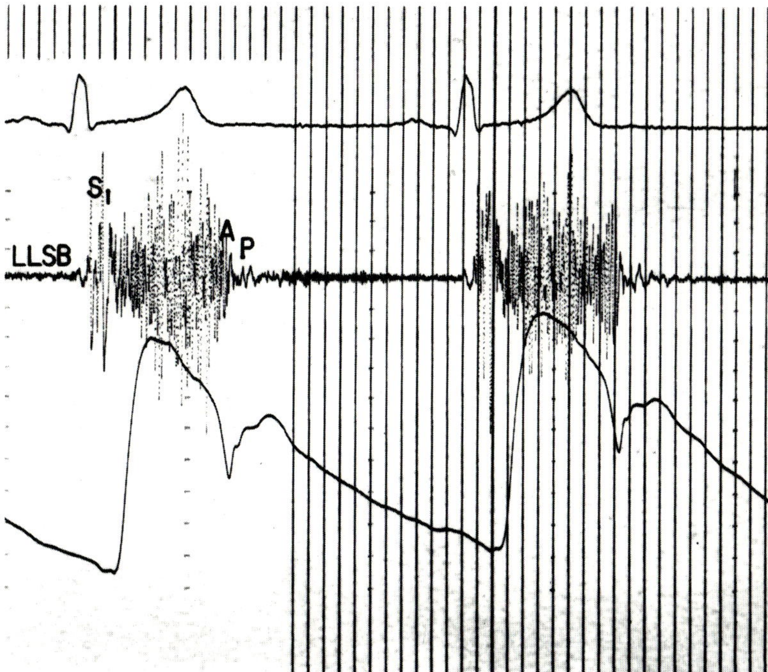

FIG. 12–6. Simultaneous recording of electrocardiogram *(top)*, phonocardiogram recorded from left lower sternal border (LLSB; *middle*), and carotid pulse tracing *(bottom)* in a patient with ventricular septal defect. Note the prominent holosystolic murmur extending throughout ventricular systole to aortic valve closure. S_1 = first heart sound. A = aortic valve closure. P = pulmonary valve closure. Time lines 40 msec. (Courtesy of Drs. J. B. Seward and A. J. Tajik.)

cular abnormalities but may be due to abnormal properties of the blood (anemic murmur) or to the presence of a thin chest wall (functional murmur). Intracardiac phonocardiography allows precise localization of the site where the murmur originates (Fig. 12–6).

MECHANICAL PHENOMENA

Pressure Changes

Measuring pressures inside the heart and circulatory system (see Appendix, Table 1) demands placing the tip of a fluid-filled catheter at the site of measurement, connecting the catheter to an appropriate manometer for transduction of mechanical energy into an electrical signal, and a recording system. High-fidelity recording of variables such as blood pressure, which has static and dynamic components, requires knowledge of the frequency and damping characteristics of the manometers used. The latter include stability, sensitivity, linearity, and an adequate frequency response. The complex wave forms can be recorded by manometers which respond accurately to the tenth harmonic of their fundamental frequency. However, when a manometer is connected to a long cardiac catheter, it is the dynamic response characteristics of the total catheter–manometer–recording system that determines the accuracy of the pressure recordings. Artifacts are produced by the motion of the catheter caused by the beating heart. In practice, an optimally damped manometer system with a uniform response up to 10 cycles per second provides adequate reproduction of the important components of intracardiac and vascular pressure pulses in man, without significant amplitude or phase distortion (Fig. 12–7). The right atrium is the most suitable zero level, with reference to atmospheric pressure, for the measurement of intracardiac and intravascular pressures. However, the depth of the right atrium in the anteroposterior plane of the thorax varies considerably from one person to another. It is customary to take an arbitrary level as a baseline for pressure measurements, such as halfway between the sternum and the back or 5 cm below the sternal angle in subjects lying supine. Strictly speaking, to measure accurately the filling pressure of the cardiac chambers the transmural pressure across their walls should be determined, since the pressure outside the heart varies with respiration.

The manometers used include: (1) Strain-gauge manometers: Strain-gauge

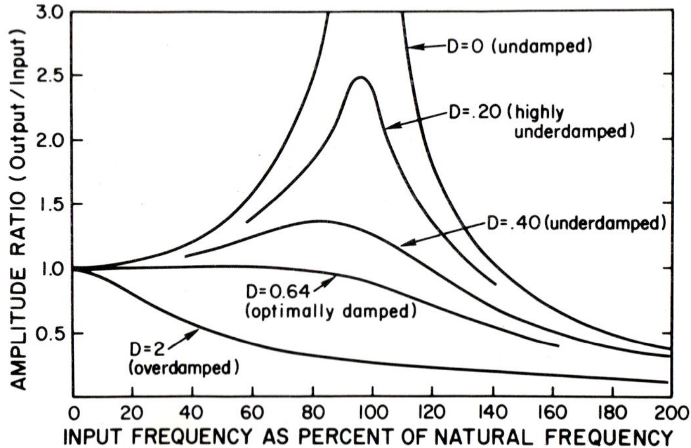

FIG. 12–7. A key property of any pressure measurement system is its frequency response. This may be thought of as a change in the amplitude ratio of the output/input over a range of frequencies of the input or pressure wave. To measure pressures accurately, the amplitude ratio must be constant over a sufficient range of frequency variation. If not, the amplitude of major frequency components of the pressure wave form may be attenuated and minor components amplified so the recorded wave form is distorted. A pressure measurement system should be employed that has the highest possible natural frequency as well as optimal damping. The amplitude of an input signal tends to be augmented as the frequency of that signal approaches the natural frequency of the sensing membrane. Optimal damping dissipates the energy of the oscillating sensing membrane gradually and thereby maintains a nearly flat natural frequency curve (constant output/input ratio) as it approaches the region of the pressure measurement system's natural frequency. D = damping coefficient. Damping may be achieved mechanically or electrically. (From Grossman: In: *Cardiac Catheterization & Angiocardiography,* p. 76. Lea & Febiger, Philadelphia, 1974.)

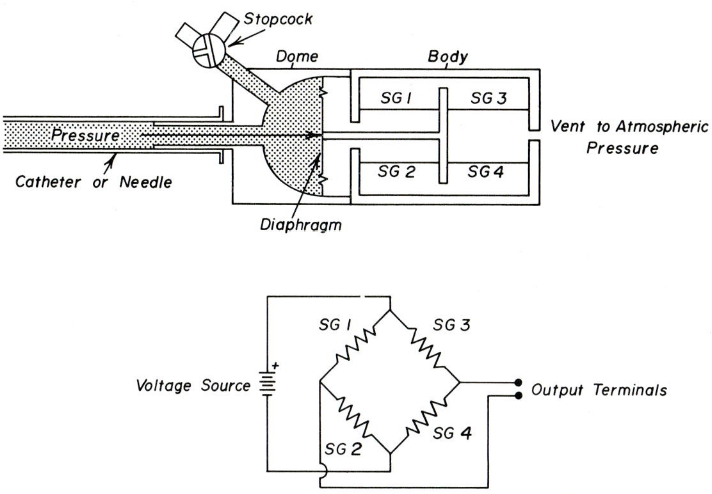

FIG. 12–8. Strain-gauge pressure transducer. The vascular pressure is transmitted via a catheter or needle to a dome and acts on a metal diaphragm, which is vented to atmospheric pressure on its opposite side. Increased pressure on the diaphragm lengthens the strain-gauge wires SG1 and SG2 and increases their electrical resistance, while having the opposite effect on SG3 and SG4. These wires form the four resistors of a Wheatstone bridge, connected as shown and attached to a voltage source. When the resistances are unbalanced by changes in pressure applied to the diaphragm, there are proportional changes in voltage and in current flow across the output terminals. A stopcock permits intermittent flushing of the catheter or needle with saline to prevent clotting and allows for withdrawal of blood samples or injection of substances.

manometry is based on the principle that when a wire is stretched its electrical resistance increases in proportion to its change in length. Wires are placed in a Wheatstone-bridge circuit so that a force unbalances the bridge in proportion to the sum of the stretching of one pair and the relaxation of the other (Fig. 12–8). (2) Capacitance manometers: In capacitance manometers the pressure is conveyed to a rather stiff metallic diaphragm which functions as one of the two plates of a condenser. Stress on the diaphragm varies the air space between the plates, changing the capacitance, which in turn is measured by means of a radiofrequency circuit. (3) Miniature manometers: Miniature strain-gauge manometers can be mounted on a catheter tip, which avoids the distortion caused by catheter movement. They are used whenever it is necessary to determine the absolute pressures at a given site, in particular the pressures generated by hydrostatic forces and by dynamic events within the circulatory system.

Cardiac Output

Many of the methods used to measure blood flow in humans are based on principles defined in 1870 by Fick, namely that the amount of a substance taken up (or released) by an organ per unit time is equal to the arterial concentration of that substance minus the venous concentration (venous minus arterial in the case of a substance released by the organ) multiplied by the blood flow through the organ. A variation involves the principle of indicator dilution, where a known amount of indicator is injected into the circulation. Provided adequate mixing occurs, the blood flow is equal to the amount of indicator injected divided by its average concentration in the arterial blood.

Oxygen Fick Method

The pulmonary blood flow, and hence the cardiac output, can be calculated by dividing the oxygen consumption by the arteriovenous oxygen difference. To calculate the quantity of oxygen consumed, the subject breathes room air through a mouthpiece. The nose is clipped, and expired air is collected for a given time. The oxygen concentration difference between the inspired and expired air is multiplied by the total quantity of air collected. To obtain mixed venous blood, a cardiac catheter is positioned in the main pulmonary artery. A peripheral artery is punctured to obtain arterial blood. Samples from both sites are obtained while the volume of expired air is being measured; the oxygen content of the samples is determined.

Indicator-Dilution Method

The indicator-dilution method is especially suited for cardiac output measurement because turbulence in the heart ensures mixing of indicator with the blood. The indicator recirculates through short circuits such as the coronary circulation before the dye curve is completed. The descending slope of the indicator-dilution curve must be extrapolated to predict the shape of the curve in the absence of recirculation (Fig. 12–9). The closer the injection site is to the sampling site, the less recirculation there is to interfere with the measurement; the most accurate results are obtained with the combination of rapid injection of indicator into the right side of the heart through a cardiac catheter and determination of the changes in concentration of the indicator in the aorta or one of its major branches.

The common indicator used is a harmless dye, indocyanine green, which is eliminated rapidly by the liver. The changes in optical density of the blood due to the dye are detected by withdrawing arterial blood at a steady rate through a cuvette–densitometer. The maximal spectral absorption of indocyanine green is in the infrared region, where oxyhemoglobin and reduced hemoglobin transmit light equally. Therefore the dilution curves are unaffected by variation in the oxygen saturation of hemoglobin, and the method can be used in patients in whom such changes may occur.

If the dye is injected at the pulmonary valve and blood from the left atrium is sampled, the indicator-dilution curve allows calculation of the pulmonary

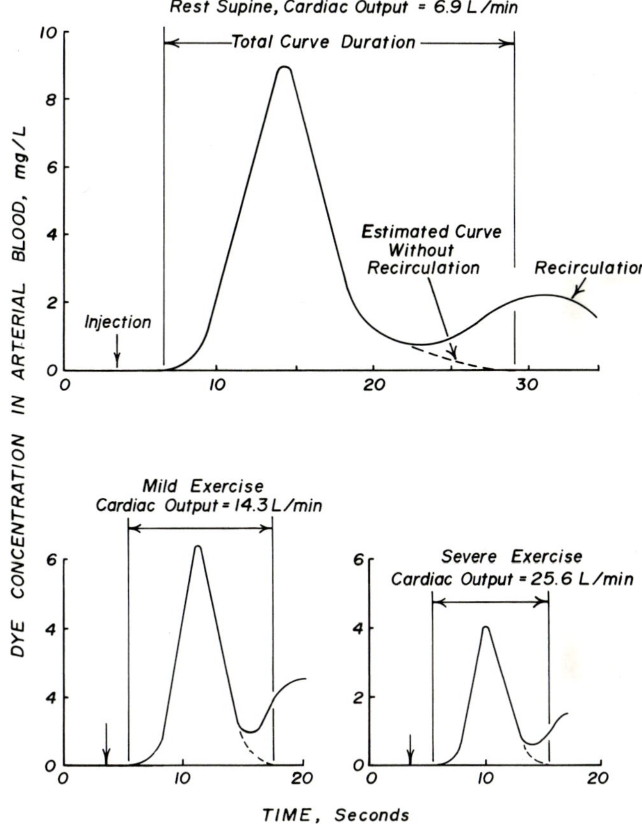

FIG. 12–9. Measurement of cardiac output by an indicator-dilution technique. The curves shown were recorded from a radial artery of a normal subject following injection of indocyanine green dye into the superior vena cava. The recirculation of dye is observable as a second peak on the curves. In order to determine the curve that would occur if there were no recirculation, the descending limb must be extrapolated to zero. The cardiac output is derived from the equation:

$$\text{Cardiac output (liters/min)} = \frac{I \times 60}{Cm \times t}$$

I = amount of indicator injected (mg). Cm = mean indicator concentration at the site of detection (mg/liter). t = total curve duration (sec). The indicator-dilution curves recorded during exercise show a diminished peak concentration, shorter duration, and more rapid recirculation.

blood volume by multiplying the output of the heart by the mean transit time of the dye through the pulmonary circulation.

Thermodilution Method

A known quantity of saline at a temperature different from that of the blood is injected rapidly into the circulation, and the temperature downstream is recorded. With this method there is no significant recirculation of indicator since dispersion occurs in the tissues of the body. However, heat is lost to the catheter during the injection as well as to the walls of the heart chambers and the blood vessels. The latter heat is rapidly recovered by the circulation, but it has a dampening effect on the contour of the dilution curves.

ASSESSMENT OF VENTRICULAR FUNCTION

Although the measurement of cardiac output provides a useful index of overall cardiac performance, it is subject to many influences. In disease, reactions such as enhanced sympathetic activity and hypertrophy compensate for the impaired contractility of the heart muscle so that normal values for cardiac output may be found under resting conditions. Studies of cardiac output and stroke volume during exercise of increasing severity demonstrate the limitations of the performance of the abnormal heart. Many other additional tests of cardiac, and particularly of left ventricular, functions are used, and some are outlined below. As with all methods, each has its advantages and limitations.

Systolic Time Intervals

Measurement of systolic time intervals is a noninvasive method for estimating the contractile state of the left ventricle. Simultaneous recordings are made of the electrocardiogram, the phonocardiogram, and the carotid pulse tracing. Three measurements are made: (1) total electromechanical systole, from the onset of the QRS complex to the closure of the aortic valve, as reflected in the second heart sound; (2) left ventricular ejection time, from the beginning of the upstroke to the dicrotic notch of the carotid pulse tracing; and (3) pre-ejection period, which is electromechanical systole minus left ventricular ejection time. The limitation of this method is the difficulty in obtaining a precise definition of the end of ventricular systole and the fact that systolic time intervals vary with heart rate (Fig. 12–10).

End-Diastolic Pressure

Inadequate systolic emptying of a ventricle leads to increases in end-systolic and end-diastolic volumes. Since the latter is usually accompanied by an elevation of ventricular end-diastolic pressure, the level of this pressure may serve as an index of ventricular function. It marks the instant when the ventricle is at its fullest. It may be necessary to stress the circulation for the abnormal increase in pressure to occur. This can be done conveniently by having the patient exercise. Isometric exercise may be used to increase the afterload on the left ventricle (p. 168).

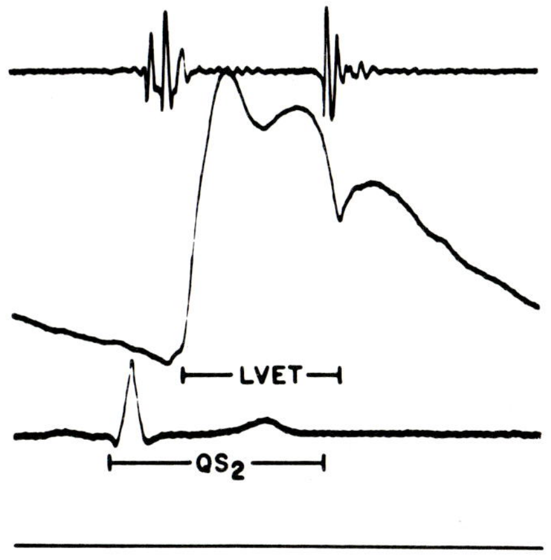

FIG. 12–10. Simultaneous tracing of phonocardiogram *(upper)*, carotid arterial pulse *(middle)*, and electrocardiogram *(lower)* at high paper speed (100 mm/sec) illustrating the measurement of three systolic time intervals. QS_2 = total electromechanical systole. LVET = left ventricular ejection time. PEP = pre-ejection phase. In patients with abnormalities of left ventricular contraction, the pre-ejection period may lengthen and the ejection time shorten. (From Weissler et al.: In: *Progress in Cardiology,* edited by Yu and Goodwin, p. 155. Lea & Febiger, Philadelphia, 1972.)

Rate of Change of Ventricular Pressure With Respect to Time

During the course of isovolumetric contraction of the left ventricle, the rate of tension development reflects the left ventricular function. The peak rate of change of left ventricular pressure usually occurs at the opening of the semilunar valves; it is a complex function depending on the loading conditions of the myocardium as well as on the contractile state. It increases with enhanced myocardial contractility and diminishes when contractility is depressed. The method necessitates a faithful measurement of ventricular pressure by a catheter-tip micromanometer. The normal range in man is so wide it is not suitable for interpatient evaluation. A variation is to measure the rate of changes in tension at a given isovolumetric pressure; this parameter is less affected by the loading condition (Fig. 12–11).

Maximum Velocity of Contractile Element Shortening

The contractile state of the human heart can be approximated by determining the maximal velocity (V_{max}) of contractile element shortening from the instantaneous relationship between rate of change in tension and isovolumetric pressure in the left ventricle (Fig. 12–12).

Angiocardiography

Knowledge of the total volume of the heart is of limited application since it provides no information relating to the size of individual chambers or the extent to which they fill and empty during the cardiac cycle. Data on ventricular

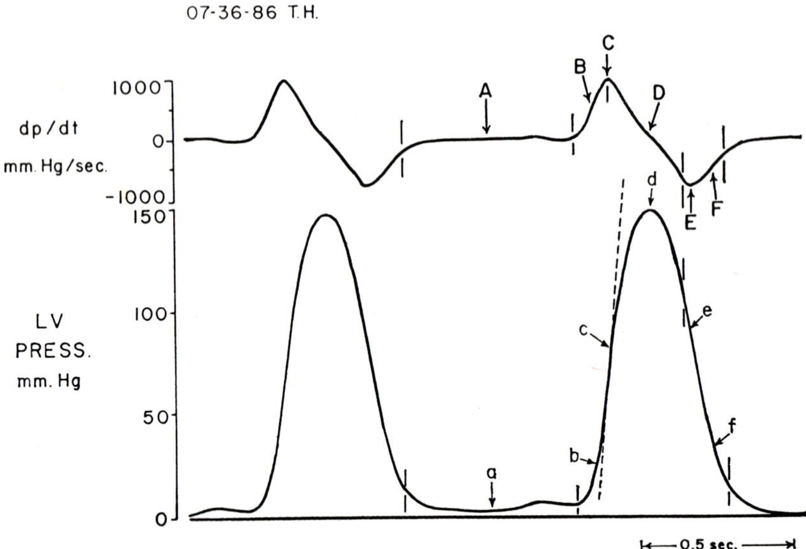

FIG. 12–11. Simultaneous recording of left ventricular pressure pulse (LV) and first derivative of left ventricular pressure (dP/dt) in a patient with an aortic valve prosthesis. The various portions of the first derivative and the corresponding segments of the pressure recording from which they were computed are labeled. During ventricular filling, when the rate of change of ventricular pressure is minimal, dP/dt is flat at a level near zero (segment A). With the onset of isovolumetric contraction, dP/dt rises slowly and then rapidly (segment B) to reach the peak dP/dt (point C) at the maximal rate of pressure rise, indicated by the slope of the diagonal broken line. Peak dP/dt usually occurs at the instant of opening of the semilunar valves—thus at peak isovolumetric ventricular pressure. During early and middle phases of ventricular ejection, dP/dt descends to the baseline; and during late ejection, as intraventricular pressure decreases, dP/dt becomes negative (segment D). The rate of decrease of ventricular pressure is maximal at point E during isovolumetric relaxation (segment F). (From Mason: *Am. J. Cardiol.,* 23:516, 1969.)

volumes are useful for a quantitative description of ventricular function, although there are discrepancies between the values obtained with the available methods. Although the indicator-dilution technique theoretically can be used to measure the volume of either ventricle, in practice it is difficult to achieve the almost instantaneous mixing of indicator with blood which is required. Angiocardiography can be used for estimating the volumes of the cavities of the left atrium and ventricle by assuming that both may be regarded as ellipsoids. To do this, radiopaque material is injected in the chambers and biplane radiography performed. The margins of the filled chambers are traced and the lengths of their major and minor axis determined (Fig. 12–13). The measurement does not account for the volume occupied by the papillary muscles and for variations in position of the mitral valve. The radiopaque media used are hypertonic and may produce extrasystoles, tachycardia, an increase in end-diastolic pressure, and hypotension.

Angiographic techniques, when combined with measurements of intraventricu-

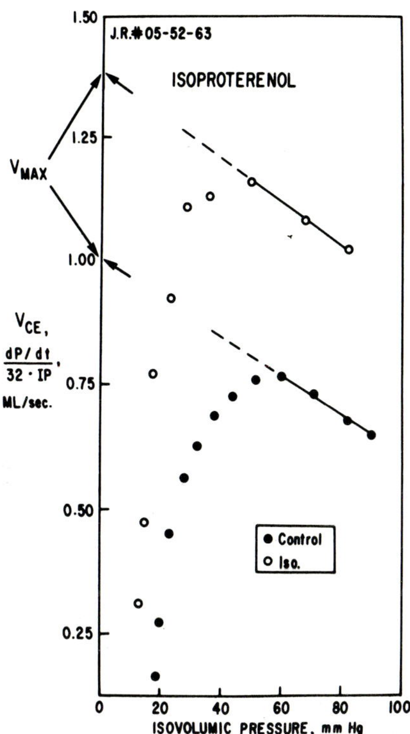

FIG. 12–12. Estimation of maximal velocity of shortening in the human heart obtained from the pressure–velocity relation during the isovolumetric contraction phase. The isovolumetric pressure *(abscissa)* is plotted against the velocity of contractile element shortening *(V_{CE})*. The latter can be estimated from the ratio between the changes in pressure with time (dP/dt) over the product of the series elastic modulus and the total isovolumetric pressure *(IP)*. In this determination the series elastic modulus, or stiffness factor, is assumed to be 32 as suggested by experiments performed on isolated cardiac tissues. The estimation assumes that the behavior of the human heart approximates that of a sphere with uniform wall thickness, and that major alterations in ventricular geometry do not occur before ejection. Extrapolation *(dotted lines)* of the pressure–velocity descending limb to zero load allows estimation of the maximal intrinsic velocity of shortening of the contractile elements (V_{max}). Note the upward shift obtained with isoproterenol, indicative of an increased cardiac contractility. (From Mason et al.: *Am. J. Cardiol.,* 26:248, 1970.)

lar pressure and cardiac output, also provide assessment of the performance of the heart as a pump. The following measurements may be made: (1) Systolic ejection fraction: The relation of stroke volume to left ventricular end-diastolic volume can be derived from contrast ventriculography; in normal hearts the ejection fraction should be larger than 60% (Fig. 12–14). (2) Ventricular pressure–volume relationships: The instantaneous relationship of left ventricular pressure and volume throughout the cardiac cycle constitutes the pressure–volume loop of the ventricle (Figs. 3–10 and 12–15). Integration of the pressure–volume loop during contraction represents the cardiac work and permits the estimation of ventricular power, which is the product of instantaneous intraventricular pressure and rate of ventricular ejection. The latter is determined from the rate of change of ventricular volume during systole. (3) Ventricular mass: The ventricular mass can be derived from knowledge of left ventricular wall thickness, chamber dimensions, and volume (see Appendix, Table 4).

Depression of the ratio of ejection fraction to ventricular end-diastolic volume, and of ventricular power relative to end-diastolic volume, indicates depressed left ventricular contractility. Inappropriately increased ventricular dilation and elevated end-diastolic volume per unit of stroke work also indicate depressed contractility.

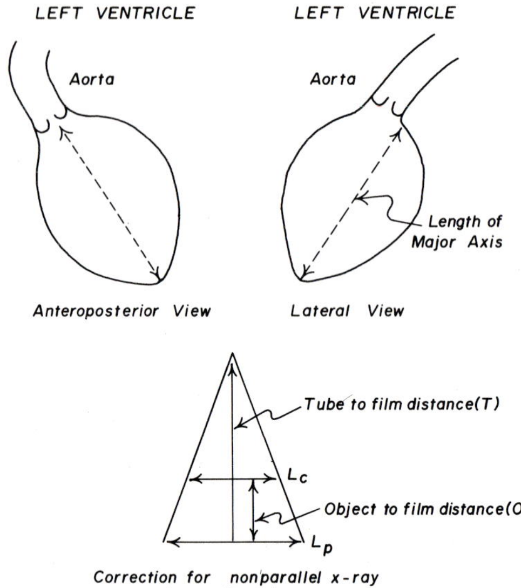

FIG. 12–13. Measurement of left ventricular volume by biplane angiocardiography. Simultaneous anteroposterior and lateral X-rays of the heart synchronized with the electrocardiogram are taken following injection of a radiopaque medium into the right heart. The volume is calculated, assuming that the ventricle has an ellipsoidal shape, according to the formula: $V = 4/3\ \pi abc$, where a = one-half the length of the major axis and b and c = one-half the lengths of the minor axes. The longest of the distances betwen the lower pole of the heart and the junction of its right border with either the aorta *(left)* or the superior vena cava *(right)* is used as the major axis. These lengths must be corrected for nonparallel X-ray distortion by the formula $L_C = L_P\ (T - O)T$. (From Yang et al.: *From Cardiac Catheterization Data to Hemodynamic Parameters,* 2nd ed. Davis, Philadelphia, 1978.)

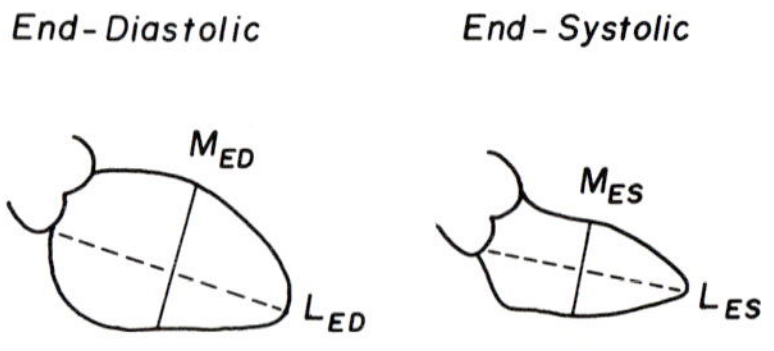

FIG. 12–14. Calculation of indices of left ventricular ejection from right anterior oblique cineangiograms. L = long ventricular axis. M = short ventricular axis perpendicular to and bisecting L. ED = end-diastole. ES = end-systole. From the area *(A)* of the pictures, the ejection fraction *(EF)* can be calculated using the formula:

End-Diastolic M_{ED} L_{ED} End-Systolic M_{ES} L_{ES}

$$EF = 1 - \frac{A_{ES}^2 \times L_{ED}}{A_{ED}^2 \times L_{ES}}$$

The mean normalized systolic ejection rate (MNSER) is obtained by dividing the ejection fraction by the ejection time: MNSER = *(EF/ET)*. The mean velocity of circumferential fiber shortening *(V_{CF})* can be estimated from the equation:

$$\text{Mean } V_{CF} = \frac{M_{ED} - M_{ES}}{ET \times M_{ED}}$$

No correction for nonparallel X-ray distortion is required for these indices. (Modified from Krayenbuehl et al.: *Cardiovasc. Med.,* 3:888, 1978.)

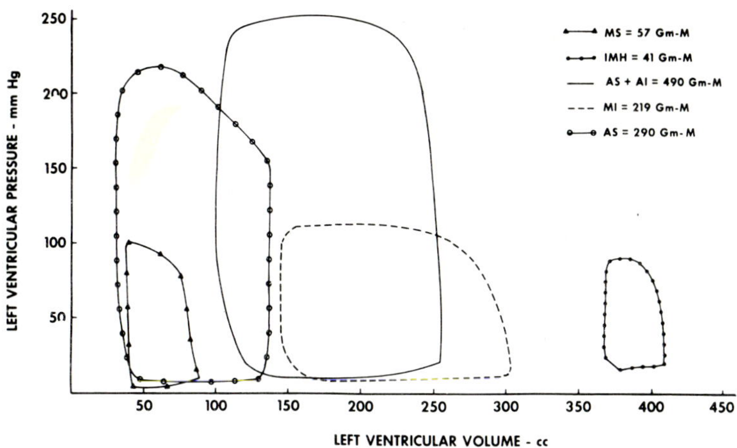

FIG. 12–15. Left ventricular pressure–volume curves from patients with mitral stenosis (MS), idiopathic myocardial hypertrophy (IMH), aortic stenosis and insufficiency (AS and AI), mitral insufficiency (MI), and aortic stenosis (AS). The volume of the left ventricle at various stages of a cardiac cycle was calculated from pictures obtained using biplane angiocardiography. Normally the heart performs about 100 gram-meters of work/stroke. In mitral stenosis and idiopathic myocardial hypertrophy the stroke volume and stroke work are reduced. In mitral insufficiency, on the other hand, the ventricle changes markedly in size during systole owing to regurgitation of blood into the atrium, and therefore the stroke work is greater than normal. Stroke work in aortic stenosis is greater than normal because of the high pressures the ventricle develops in this condition. (From Dodge et al.: *Am. J. Cardiol.,* 18:20, 1966.)

Echocardiography

The use of ultrasound for studying the human cardiovascular system has the benefits of being noninvasive, involving no discomfort to the subject, and causing no concern about radiation dosage.

Ultrasound has a frequency of greater than 20,000 cycles per second. It obeys the laws of reflection and refraction, can be directed in a beam with little tendency to scatter, and is reflected by objects of small size. The velocity at which ultrasound travels depends on the density and elastic properties of the medium. As the ultrasound wave travels through a homogenous medium, it continues in a straight line. When it reaches an interface between two media with different acoustic impedances, the beam undergoes reflection and refraction. The acoustic impedance is the density of the medium multiplied by the velocity at which an ultrasound travels through it. In humans ultrasound measurement studies are performed by means of a transducer which emits high-frequency waves when stimulated electrically. The beam should remain perpendicular to the structure under examination. The ultrasonic rays reflected at various tissue interfaces travel back to the transducer, which also acts as a receiver.

A cardiac structure is identified by assessing the appearance, position, motion pattern, and intensity of echo signals derived from it (Fig. 12–16). By making

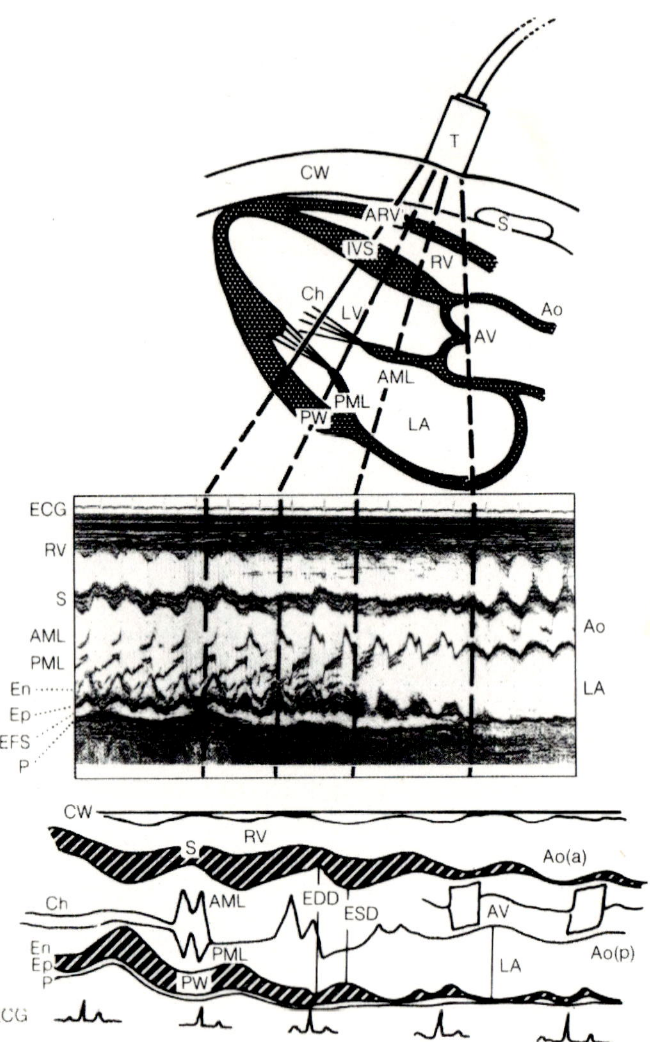

FIG. 12–16. Echocardiographic correlates of the cardiac structures. The transducer (T) is directed from the apex to the base of the heart. AML = anterior mitral leaflet. Ao = aorta. Ao(a) = aorta, anterior wall. Ao(p) = aorta, posterior wall. ARV = anterior right ventricular wall. AV = aortic valve. Ch = chordae tendineae. CW = chest wall. ECG = electrocardiogram. EDD = end-diastolic diameter. EFS = echo-free space. En = endocardium. Ep = epicardium. ESD = end-systolic diameter. IVS = interventricular septum. LA = left atrium. LV = left ventricle. P = pericardium. PML = posterior mitral leaflet. PW = posterior wall. RV = right ventricle. S = sternum. (From Krasnow and Stein: *Cardiovasc. Med.,* 3:797, 1978.)

some assumptions, left ventricular end-diastolic and end-systolic volumes, stroke volume, ejection fraction, mean velocity of circumferential fiber shortening, posterior wall velocity, and mass can be calculated. Other important uses for the technique include identification of the cardiac valves and their motion and the detection of pericardial effusion. Normally the heart is in direct contact with its surrounding structures. In the presence of pericardial effusion, the pericardial space fills with relatively echo-free fluid, and an echocardiographic separation occurs between the anterior right ventricular wall and the chest wall, and between the posterior left ventricular wall and the posterior pericardium.

ASSESSMENT OF MYOCARDIAL INFARCTION

Electrocardiogram

Usually the diagnosis of acute myocardial infarction can be made electrocardiographically with the demonstration of serial ST–T wave changes that persist for at least 24 hr and the appearance of a significant Q or QS wave (Fig. 12–17).

Serum Enzymes and Isoenzymes

When myocardial infarction occurs, protein molecules of large molecular weight escape from their normal intracellular location into the extracellular fluid, from which they may be carried into the circulation by either venous drainage or cardiac lymphatic flow. Among these are certain enzymes that are involved in the normal metabolism of the cell.

Among the enzymes which have been evaluated for their specificity and sensi-

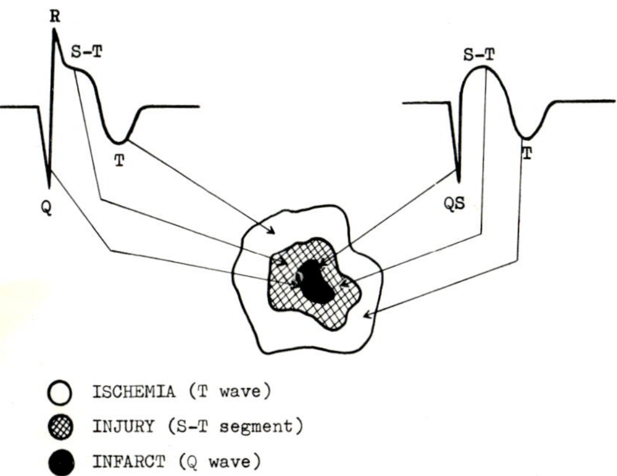

FIG. 12–17. Classic electrocardiographic patterns of myocardial infarctions with indication of the cause for the abnormal deflection. (From Stein: *The Electrocardiogram.* Saunders, Philadelphia, 1976.)

tivity in the diagnosis of myocardial infarction are lactic dehydrogenase (LDH), creatine phosphokinase (CPK), and glutamic oxaloacetic transaminase (GOT). The serum levels of LDH and CPK increase when there is damage to tissues other than the heart. Glutamic oxaloacetic transaminase is present in higher concentrations within myocardial cells than in any other tissues of the body, and almost all patients with typical electrocardiographic changes of acute transmural infarction have a significant elevation of this enzyme in their serum.

Isoenzymes are different molecular forms of enzymes that catalyze the same chemical reaction. Determination in the serum of the isoenzymes of creatine phosphokinase is a sensitive indicator of acute myocardial infarction. The M and B monomers of CPK form three dimers, designated MM, MB, and BB, which have been identified in human serum by either electrophoresis or column chromatography. The myocardium contains predominantly CPK–MM, but 15 to 20% of the total CPK activity is contributed by the MB dimer. Myocardial necrosis results in the appearance of significant amounts of the MB dimer in the serum. Thus the presence of that isoenzyme in other than trace concentrations is usually indicative of the presence of acute myocardial infarction, although occasionally false-positive results are obtained. CPK–MM and CPK–MB isoenzymes appear in the serum about 6 hr after the onset of an infarct and reach a peak within about 24 hr. CPK–MM returns to normal values within around 84 hr, whereas CPK–MB disappears from the serum more rapidly.

Myocardial Imaging

Various radioactive tracers injected intravenously can be detected with a gamma-scintillation camera and are used to define the size of ischemic regions in the heart. There are two approaches: (1) The tracer (e.g., technetium-99m stannous pyrophosphate) accumulates preferentially in the ischemic zone ("hot spot") provided some blood flow is maintained in the latter. The mechanism of uptake is obscure. Radiolabeled cardiac antimyosin fragments are concentrated specifically in ischemic myocardium. (2) Substances which exchange with the potassium ions of the normal myocardial cells (e.g., thallium-201) are distributed in the myocardium in proportion to myocardial blood flow and thus ring the ischemic zone ("cold spot").

Isotope imaging of the heart is used also to estimate the ejection portion of the left ventricle, which is an important index of left ventricular function (p. 295). The left ventricular end-diastolic and end-systolic volumes are measured during the initial passage of tracer through the heart or after equilibrium of the isotope within the myocardium. The latter provides for higher spatial resolution, since recordings are made over several cardiac cycles. The analysis by computer is synchronized to specific parts of the cardiac cycle. The relative accuracy of such measurements must be established by comparing them with those obtained with biplane contrast left ventriculography.

Precordial Electrocardiographic Mapping

Electrocardiographic mapping has been proposed as an index of changes in the size of a myocardial infarct. It analyzes changes in the S–T segment and the QRS complex, as measured simultaneously from horizontal rows of leads on the chest wall. The validity of the method depends on evidence that changes in the S–T segment correlate with regional myocardial blood flow following coronary occlusion, and with progression or diminution of the ischemic zone.

PRINCIPLES OF DETECTION AND ASSESSMENT OF VALVULAR REGURGITATION AND OF SHUNTS

Valvular Regurgitation

When an indicator is injected proximal to the regurgitant valve, the dilution curve recorded downstream from the valve shows decreased peak concentration of the indicator, prolongation of the disappearance slope, and, if the regurgitation is severe, the absence of the recirculation peak (Fig. 12–18). Most of this distor-

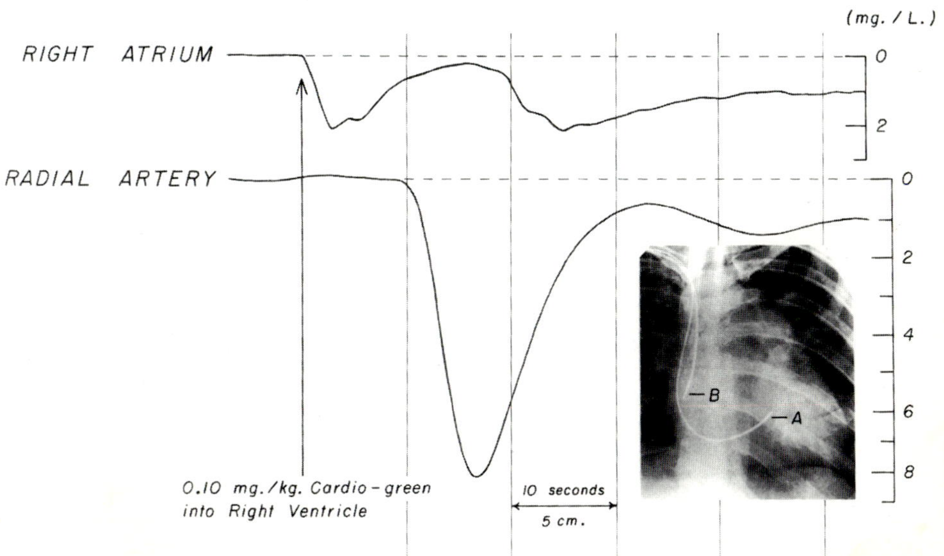

FIG. 12–18. Demonstration of tricuspid regurgitation by dilution curves. (Females, 42 years old, 51 kg, mitral and tricuspid valve disease.) At the instant indicated by the vertical arrow, indocyanine green dye was injected into the inflow portion of the right ventricle via catheter A, and the resulting dilution curves were recorded from the right atrium via catheter B and from the radial artery. Note the instantaneous appearance of dye in the right atrium, indicating that dye has regurgitated through the tricuspid valve. The regurgitant fraction calculated from these curves was 10%. (From Bajec et al.: *Proc. Staff Meet. Mayo Clin.*, 33:569, 1958.)

tion is due to the delayed clearance of indicator from the heart. To assess the regurgitant fraction, the indicator may be injected immediately distal to the regurgitant valve and the indicator concentration recorded simultaneously in the compartment upstream to the valve and in a systemic artery. Most commonly the valvular regurgitation is visualized angiographically by observing the opacification of the compartment proximal to the incompetent valve following injection of a contrast medium into the distal compartment. The estimate of the severity of regurgitation is based on the degree of opacification of the proximal compartment in terms of the area opacified and its density.

Shunts

Unusual Course Taken by Cardiac Catheter

The cardiac catheter often traverses the defect responsible for the shunt, and its course serves to define the site. For example, when an atrial septal defect

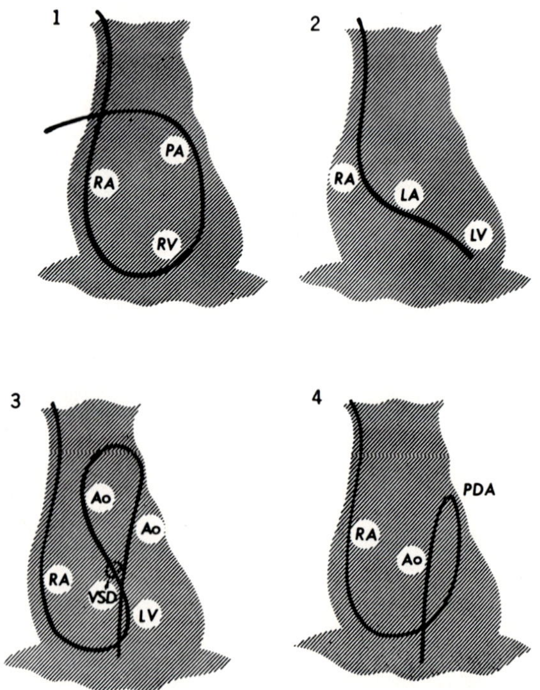

FIG. 12–19. Characteristic directions taken by catheters in a normal heart and in the presence of various congenital cardiac defects. **1:** Normal heart. **2:** Atrial septal defect. **3:** Ventricular septal defect. **4:** Patent ductus arteriosus. RA = right atrium. RV = right ventricle. PA = pulmonary artery. LA = left atrium. LV = left ventricle. VSD = ventricular septal defect. Ao = aorta. PDA = patent ductus arteriosus. (From Marshall and Shepherd: *Cardiac Function in Health and Disease.* Saunders, Philadelphia, 1968.)

is present, the catheter may pass from the right to the left atrium and the left ventricle or into a pulmonary vein. With a patent ductus arteriosus, the catheter may pass through this to enter the descending aorta (Fig. 12–19).

Measurement of Oxygen Content of Blood

In the case of arteriovenous shunts, an abnormally increased oxygen content of the blood can be detected in the right-sided chamber or vessel at the site of shunting. The approximate magnitude of pulmonary and systemic flow and thus of the flow through shunts may be estimated from the formulae:

$$\text{Pulmonary blood flow} = \frac{\text{oxygen consumption/min}}{\begin{matrix}\text{oxygen content of} \\ \text{pulmonary vein} \\ \text{blood}\end{matrix} - \begin{matrix}\text{oxygen content of} \\ \text{pulmonary artery} \\ \text{blood}\end{matrix}}$$

$$\text{Systemic blood flow} = \frac{\text{oxygen consumption/min}}{\begin{matrix}\text{oxygen content of} \\ \text{systemic artery} \\ \text{blood}\end{matrix} - \begin{matrix}\text{oxygen content of} \\ \text{mixed venous} \\ \text{blood (average of} \\ \text{samples from su-} \\ \text{perior and inferior} \\ \text{vena cava)}\end{matrix}}$$

In the case of right-to-left shunts, it is often difficult to obtain a sample of blood from the pulmonary veins or from a left-sided chamber proximal to the entry of the shunted blood. In such cases, it is assumed that the pulmonary venous blood is 98% saturated with oxygen, so that the oxygen content = 98% × oxygen capacity of the blood.

Indicator Dilution Curves

When a right-to-left shunt is present distal to the site of injection of an indicator, a fraction of the indicator traverses it, thereby bypassing the pulmonary circulation and appearing at the sampling site prior to the arrival of the portion of the indicator which passes through the lungs. The relative size of the initial part of the curve to the remainder provides an index of the magnitude of the right-to-left shunt (Fig. 12–20). The site in the heart or great vessels at which the right-to-left shunt is occurring may be localized by recording a series of dilution curves following injection of dye successively into pulmonary artery, right ventricle, and right atrium. Injection into a vessel or chamber distal to the site of the shunt results in no early appearance of dye, whereas injection at or proximal to its site results in demonstration of the shunt.

When a left-to-right shunt is present, the appearance time of the indicator at the sampling site is normal, but the magnitude of the initial peak is reduced in proportion to the size of the shunt. The disappearance slope of the dilution curve is prolonged due to repeated pulmonary recirculation of an exponentially diminishing fraction of the injected dye (Fig. 12–20).

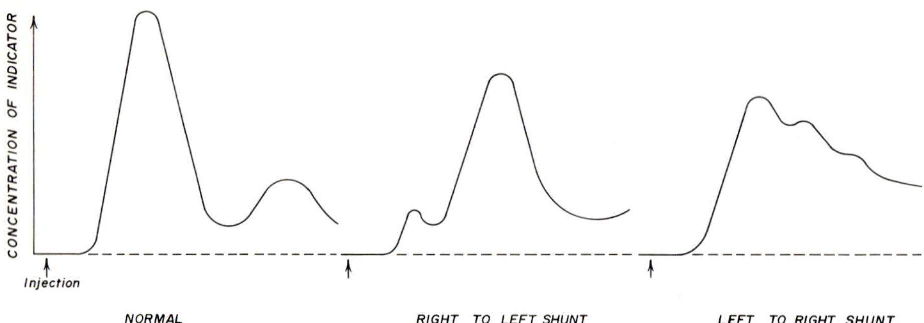

FIG. 12–20. Indicator-dilution curves in normal subjects and patients with right-to-left and left-to-right shunts. Indocyanine green dye was injected *(arrow)* into the right atrium with sampling from the brachial artery.

Angiocardiography

Selective injection of contrast media into the appropriate sites in the heart and great vessels is the most common method for localization of shunts and clinical evaluation of their magnitude. Angiography, in a sense, is an indicator-dilution technique, since it provides information concerning the temporal dispersion of an indicator, the contrast medium.

SELECTED REFERENCES

Benchimol, A. A. (1977): *Basic Principles of Auscultation and Phonocardiography. Noninvasive Diagnostic Techniques in Cardiology.* Williams & Wilkins, Baltimore.

Burch, G., and Winsor, T. (1972): *A Primer of Electrocardiography,* 6th ed. Lea & Febiger, Philadelphia.

Chung, E. K. (1977): *Principles of Cardiac Arrhythmias,* 2nd ed. Williams & Wilkins, Baltimore.

Cournand, A. (1975): Cardiac catheterization: Development of the technique, its contributions to experimental medicine, and its initial applications in man. *Acta Med. Scand.* [*Suppl.*], 579:1.

Craige, E. (1976): On the genesis of heart sounds: Contributions made by echocardiographic studies. *Circulation,* 53:207.

Federman, J., Brown, M. L., Tancredi, R. G., Smith, H. C., Wilson, D. B., and Becker, G. P. (1978): Multiple-gated acquisition cardiac blood-pool isotope imaging: Evaluation of left ventricular function correlated with contrast angiography. *Mayo Clin. Proc.,* 53:625.

Feigenbaum, H. (1976): *Echocardiography,* 2nd ed. Lea & Febiger, Philadelphia.

Marcus, M. L., and Kerber, R. E. (1977): Present status of the ^{99m}technetium pyrophosphate infarct scintigram. *Circulation,* 56:335.

Mason, D. T., Zelis, R., Amsterdam, E. A., and Massumi, R. A. (1972): Clinical determination of left ventricular contractility by hemodynamic and myocardial mechanisms. In: *Progress in Cardiology,* edited by P. N. Yu and J. F. Goodwin, p. 121. Lea & Febiger, Philadelphia.

Muller, J. E., Maroko, P. R., and Braunwald, E. (1978): Precordial electrographic mapping: Technique to assess the efficacy of interventions designed to limit infarct size. *Circulation,* 57:1.

Rapaport, E. (1977): Serum enzymes and isoenzymes in the diagnosis of acute myocardial infarction. *Mod. Concepts Cardiovasc. Dis.,* 46:43,47.

Ritchie, J. L., Hamilton, G. W., and Wackers, F. J. Th., editors (1978): *Thallium-201 Myocardial Imaging.* Raven Press, New York.

Sandler, H., and Alderman, E. (1974): Determination of left ventricular size and shape. *Circ. Res.,* 34:1.

Strauss, H. W., and Pitt, B. (1978): Evaluation of cardiac function and structure with radioactive tracer techniques. *Circulation,* 57:645.

Tajik, A. J., Seward, B., Hagler, D. J., Mair, D. D., and Lie, J. T. (1978): Two-dimensional real-time ultrasonic imaging of the heart and great vessels: Technique, image orientation, structure identification and validation. *Mayo Clin. Proc.,* 53:271.

Weissler, A. M., Lewis, R. P., and Leighton, R. F. (1972): The systolic time intervals as a measure of left ventricular performance in man. In: *Progress in Cardiology,* edited by P. N. Yu and J. F. Goodwin, Vol. 1, p. 155. Lea & Febiger, Philadelphia.

Wooley, C. F. (1978): Intracardiac phonocardiography: Intracardiac sound and pressure in man. *Circulation,* 57:1039.

Yang, S. S., Bentivoglio, L. G., Maranhao, V., and Goldberg, H. (1978): *From Cardiac Catheterization Data to Hemodynamic Parameters.* Davis, Philadelphia.

13

Measurement of Vascular Function and Blood Volume

This chapter describes how measurements are made of the events in the systemic circulation which have permitted our understanding of the function of its individual components and their role within the total system.

ARTERIAL BLOOD PRESSURE

Invasive Methods

Blood pressure is measured directly by passing a catheter into the aorta or inserting a needle into a peripheral artery (e.g., the brachial or femoral) and attaching it to a suitable manometer. This is done whenever precise values are required.

Noninvasive Method

The commonly used auscultatory method dates to the work of Riva-Rocci (1896) and Korotkow (1905). A cuff containing an inflatable bag is wrapped around the upper arm, and the bag is inflated to pressures above the systolic pressure. When the cuff is deflated slowly, characteristic sounds are heard from the brachial artery (Korotkow sounds). The cuff must be at least as wide as the diameter of the arm for the pressure to be effectively transmitted to the tissues. When the pressure in the cuff is above the systolic pressure, the transmural pressure of the brachial artery is zero. Consequently even at the height of systole the artery remains closed. When the cuff pressure falls just below the systolic pressure, there is a brief interval in each cardiac cycle when the compressed segment of artery can open against the tissue pressure, presenting a long, narrow channel through which a jet of blood flows. During the remainder of the cardiac cycle the pressure exerted by the cuff on the tissues holds the artery closed. The velocity of the jet of blood is considerably increased above any velocity that was present when the artery was not compressed; turbulence occurs which generates a short tapping sound, indicating the systolic pressure.

As the cuff pressure falls further, the proportion of the cardiac cycle in which the artery is patent increases. The sound becomes louder and longer until it reaches a maximal intensity. When it begins to diminish, there is a change in the character of the sound, known as "muffling." The muffling occurs at a cuff pressure a few millimeters of mercury above the true diastolic pressure (Fig. 13–1).

FLOW RESISTANCE

The resistance to flow offered by any part of the cardiovascular system can be estimated from the ratio between the perfusion pressure and the flow (Fig. 13–2).

VISCOSITY

The viscosity of plasma can be measured by determining the time taken for a known pressure to cause a given volume of plasma to flow through a capillary tube; the viscosity is expressed relative to the flow rate of water. This method is unsatisfactory for whole blood because of the behavior of the red blood cells (p. 17). A rotational viscometer is used for measuring whole blood viscosity. This instrument permits analysis of the rheologic properties of blood because an almost uniform rate of shear is applied to the greatest proportion of fluid. Such viscometers consist of two coaxial cylinders, one rotating and one at rest. The cylinders are separated by a narrow annulus containing the blood. As one cylinder rotates, the other tends to be dragged around with it by the torque

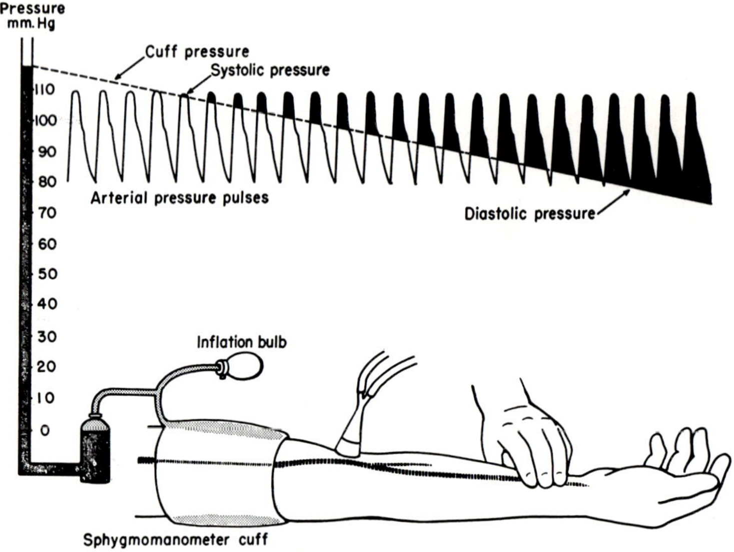

FIG. 13–1. Indirect method for measurement of arterial blood pressure. The sphygmomanometer consists of an inelastic cuff containing an inflatable rubber bag which is connected to a bulb and a mercury manometer. The cuff is wrapped around the arm. When the pressure within the sphygmomanometer cuff is increased above arterial blood pressure, the arteries under the cuff are occluded and no pulse can be palpated at the wrist. As the cuff pressure is gradually released, the systolic peaks of pressure finally exceed cuff pressure and blood spurts into the arteries below the cuff, producing palpable pulses at the wrist. The sudden acceleration of blood below the cuff produces turbulence and vibrations which are audible through a stethoscope. The pressure in the mercury manometer at the time the pulse is heard or felt indicates systolic pressure. As cuff pressure is further diminished, the sounds increase in intensity and then rather suddenly become muffled at the level of diastolic pressure where the arteries remain open throughout the entire pulse wave. At still lower pressures the sounds disappear completely when laminar flow is re-established. (From Rushmer: *Cardiac Diagnosis, A Physiologic Approach,* p. 166. Saunders, Philadelphia, 1955.)

force transmitted by the blood. At a given speed of rotation the viscosity is linearly related to the torque exerted on the resting cylinder. The instrument is calibrated with fluids of known viscosity.

MEASUREMENT OF REGIONAL BLOOD FLOWS

Brain

The inert gas technique, based on the Fick principle, is used for the measurement of total brain blood flow. The quantity of an inert gas taken up by a tissue within a given time is equal to the quantity entering that tissue via the arterial blood minus the quantity leaving the tissue in the venous blood during a given time. The method assumes free diffusion of the indicator across the

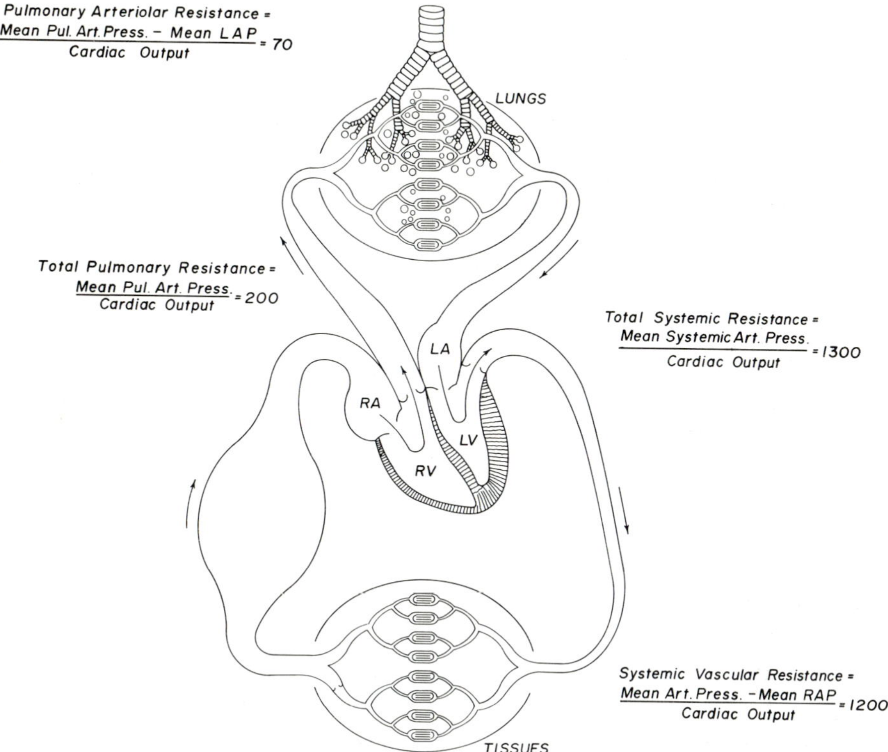

FIG. 13–2. Approximate values of vascular resistance in the pulmonary and systemic circuits. To calculate the resistance, the flow through the bed and the arterial pressure are measured, or, more correctly, the pressure difference across it. The venous pressure is usually so low it becomes an important factor in the equation only when it is in excess of a few millimeters of mercury. The resistance is expressed as dynes-sec-cm^{-5} *(figures)* as derived from the mean pressure (dynes/cm^2) divided by the mean flow (cm^3/sec). For practical purposes comparisons of resistance changes are expressed in millimeters of mercury divided by liters per minute, and are expressed conventionally as peripheral resistance units (PRU). Certain authors prefer to express the dependency of flow on the diameter of the blood vessels as the reciprocal of the resistance (conductance). Art = arterial. L = left. R = right. A = atrium. P = pressure. F = flow. R = resistance.

blood–brain barrier so the clearance of the indicator depends only on the blood flow and is not limited by diffusion (Fig. 3–17). The amount of inert gas taken up or given off by the brain cannot be determined directly but must be inferred from the jugular venous concentration. For the collection of cerebral venous samples, the internal jugular vein can be either punctured directly or catheterized from the cubital or femoral veins. Argon, krypton-85, and xenon-133 are most commonly used as tracers. The inert gas technique is based on the following assumptions, which have been shown to be reasonable: (1) The cerebral blood flow is constant during the period of measurement and is not altered by the

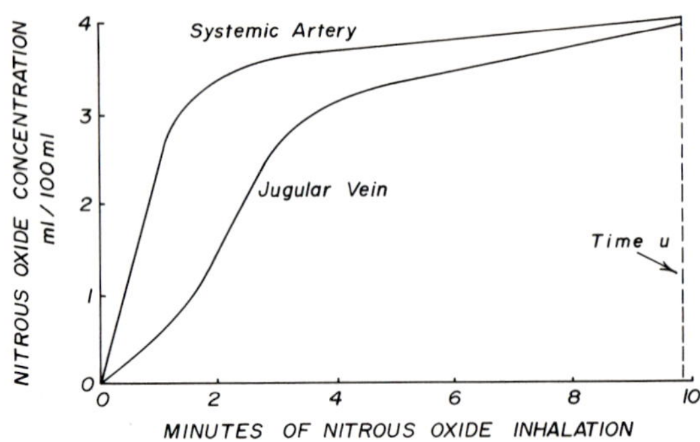

FIG. 13–3. Measurement of total brain blood flow. The accumulation of an inert gas in the brain tissue is measured during its inhalation. The gas is breathed and taken into the arterial blood via the lungs. Initially the brain takes up the inert gas from the blood, so the concentration in the venous blood leaving the brain is less than the arterial concentration. The inhalation is continued until equilibrium is reached between the arterial and the cerebral venous (jugular vein) concentration of the gas. The amount taken up by the brain is calculated from the equation:

$$\text{Cerebral blood flow (ml/100 g/min)} = \frac{\lambda[C_V]_U}{\int_0^u [C_A - C_V]\, dt}$$

C_A and C_V = the arterial and venous concentrations of the inert gas, respectively. λ = the partition coefficient for the inert gas between brain tissue and blood. $(C_V)_U$ = the venous concentration of the inert gas at time U, where the mean brain concentration is in equilibrium with the jugular venous concentration. In the example shown in the figure, nitrous oxide is used, since this was the prototype of the inert gas technique. More commonly the inert diffusible gases argon, krypton-85, or xenon-133 are employed.

inert gas used; (2) the venous samples obtained from the superior bulb of the internal jugular vein are representative of mixed venous blood leaving the brain; (3) the most slowly perfused brain tissue is in equilibrium with the jugular venous blood; and (4) the mean partition coefficient of the inert gas is representative for both gray and white matter (Fig. 13–3).

To measure local differences in brain perfusion, a mixture of xenon-133 in air is administered for 1 min by means of a face mask. When inhaled it passes rapidly from the lungs into the arterial blood and is uniformly distributed to all parts of the brain. The xenon emits gamma and X-rays. Since the X-ray activity is derived largely from the scalp and skull, subtraction of X-ray counts from gamma counts may be used to distinguish between cerebral and extracerebral blood flow, the latter comprising about 6%. Values for regional blood flow are calculated by analysis of the washout curves recorded from the head by collimated probes placed over various regions of the skull.

During cerebral arteriography a bolus of the tracer xenon-133 or krypton-85 may be injected into the internal carotid or vertebral artery. By counting the gamma activity through the intact skull, this technique can be used for regional flow measurements. It eliminates interference from extracerebral tissues.

Cerebral metabolism can be estimated for the whole brain by measuring total brain blood flow and the arteriovenous differences in oxygen, glucose, lactate, and other metabolically important substances.

Coronary Blood Flow

The standard method for delineation of the anatomy and patency of the coronary vessels is opacification of the left and right coronary arteries by selective catheterization and injection of contrast medium (coronary arteriography). There is no wholly satisfactory method for the measurement of coronary blood flow in the human.

In the nitrous oxide method, a catheter is placed in the coronary sinus and a 15% nitrous oxide mixture is inhaled while samples are taken simultaneously from the coronary sinus and a systemic artery for analysis. The coronary blood flow can be calculated from the changes in arteriovenous difference in nitrous oxide content using the Fick principle, assuming a value of 1.0 for the relative solubility (partition coefficient) of nitrous oxide between myocardium and blood. The flow measured is that through the portion of the heart drained by the coronary sinus only and thus originates almost exclusively from the left ventricle.

At the time of cardiac catheterization, diffusable radioactive tracers (e.g., xenon-133) can be injected into one of the coronary arteries, usually the left. These tracers accumulate in the myocardium. The rate of washout of the tracer provides a measurement of regional myocardial blood flow. The myocardial distribution of tracer can be visualized by means of an external scintillation camera (Fig. 13–4).

Coronary sinus blood flow has also been measured by the thermodilution method (p. 291). A 5% dextrose solution at room temperature is injected at a constant rate into the coronary sinus and the resulting change in temperature detected at a short distance downstream. This permits rapid changes in coronary flow to be studied. It has the disadvantage that it requires catheterization of the coronary sinus, and that reflux of blood from the right atrium into the coronary sinus may be a source of error. Another approach is to measure the mean transit time of a contrast medium between two sites of a coronary artery together with the radiographic determination of its dimensions. This allows calculation of blood flow as the product of the mean blood velocity multiplied by the cross-sectional area in individual coronary arteries or in aortocoronary bypass grafts.

Splanchnic Area

To measure splanchnic blood flow an indicator such as indocyanine green, which is removed from the blood by the liver, is infused intravenously at a constant rate. When its arterial concentration has stabilized, the indicator infusion rate equals the hepatic removal rate. The hepatic–venous indicator concentration is obtained from a sampling catheter placed in a large hepatic vein.

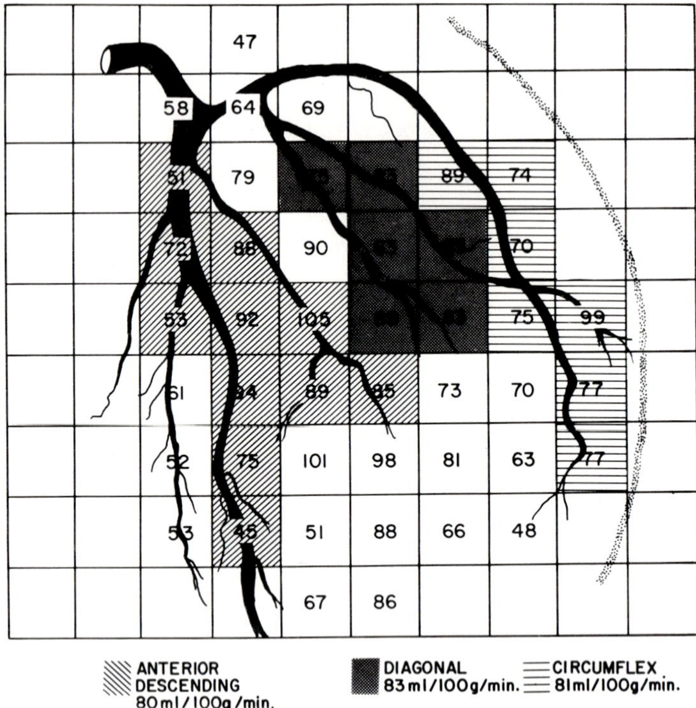

FIG. 13–4. Estimation of regional myocardial blood flow. Xenon-133 is injected selectively into a coronary artery, and the resultant initial washout is recorded precordially with a crystal scintillation camera. The regional myocardial blood flow per 100 g/min is calculated from the rate constant *(k)* in minutes derived from a semilogarithmic plot of the initial washout, the partition coefficient of the tracer in myocardial tissue (λ), and the specific gravity (P) of the myocardium. Myocardial blood flow = $k \cdot \lambda$ 100. In the example shown, the injection was made into a normal left coronary artery. Imaging was performed in the left anterior oblique projection, and the number in each square shows the calculated regional blood flow in milliliters per 100 g per minute. (From Dwyer et al.: *Circulation,* 48:92, 1973, by permission of the American Heart Association.)

The splanchnic blood flow is calculated according to the Fick principle (Fig. 13–5).

Renal Circulation

The measurement of plasma flow is another application of the Fick principle using substances that are extracted from the bloodstream by the kidney and appear unaltered in the urine (Fig. 13–6).

Extremities

Venous Occlusion Plethysmography

Venous occlusion plethysmography is the most widely used and reliable method for noninvasive measurement of blood flow in human limbs. It can be

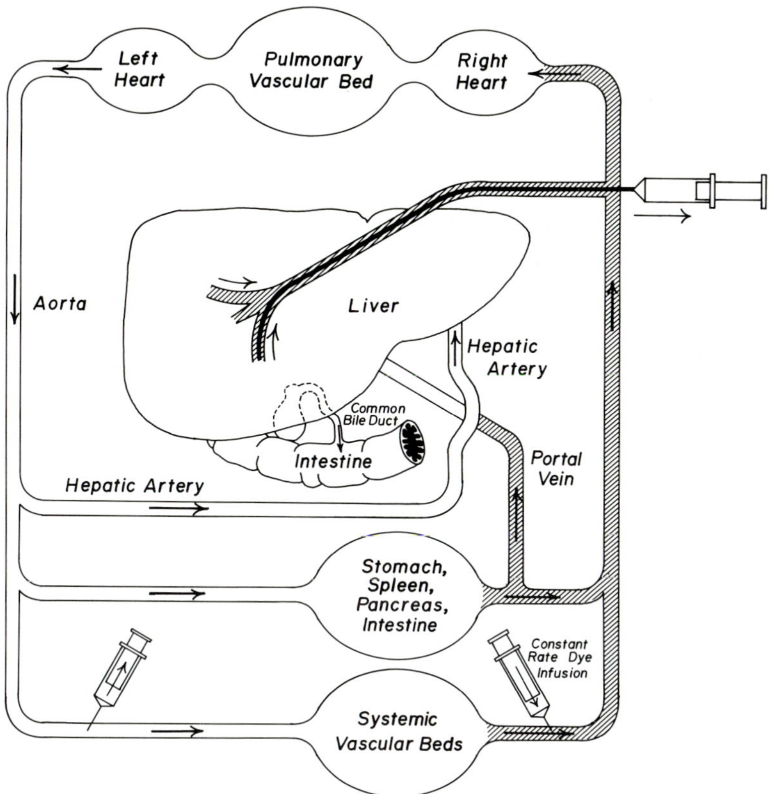

FIG. 13–5. Measurement of splanchnic blood flow. Indocyanine green dye is infused at a constant rate into a peripheral vein. After a short time the arterial concentration becomes constant as the dye is secreted by the liver into the bile and passes via the common bile duct into the small intestine at the same rate at which it is infused. The splanchnic blood flow is calculated according to the equation:

$$\text{Splanchnic blood flow} = \frac{I}{C_A - C_{HV}} = \frac{R}{C_A - C_{HV}}$$

R = the hepatic removal rate which equals the indicator infusion rate *(I)* of dye. C_A = arterial concentration of indicator. C_{HV} = hepatic -venous indicator concentration measured by means of a catheter placed in one of the hepatic veins. (Modified from Rowell: In: *Physiology and Biophysics II, Circulation, Respiration, and Fluid Balance.* edited by Ruch and Patton, p. 215. Saunders, Philadelphia, 1974.)

used for individual digits, the hand, foot, forearm, or calf. A cuff wrapped around a segment of the limb is inflated to a pressure sufficient to temporarily prevent venous outflow without interference with arterial inflow (collecting pressure). The initial increase in limb volume distal to the cuff equals the rate of arterial inflow (Fig. 13–7). The limb should be raised above the heart level to permit emptying of the veins by gravity between successive measurements. This method measures the total rate of arterial inflow to the part and does not distinguish between the rate of flow to the various tissues.

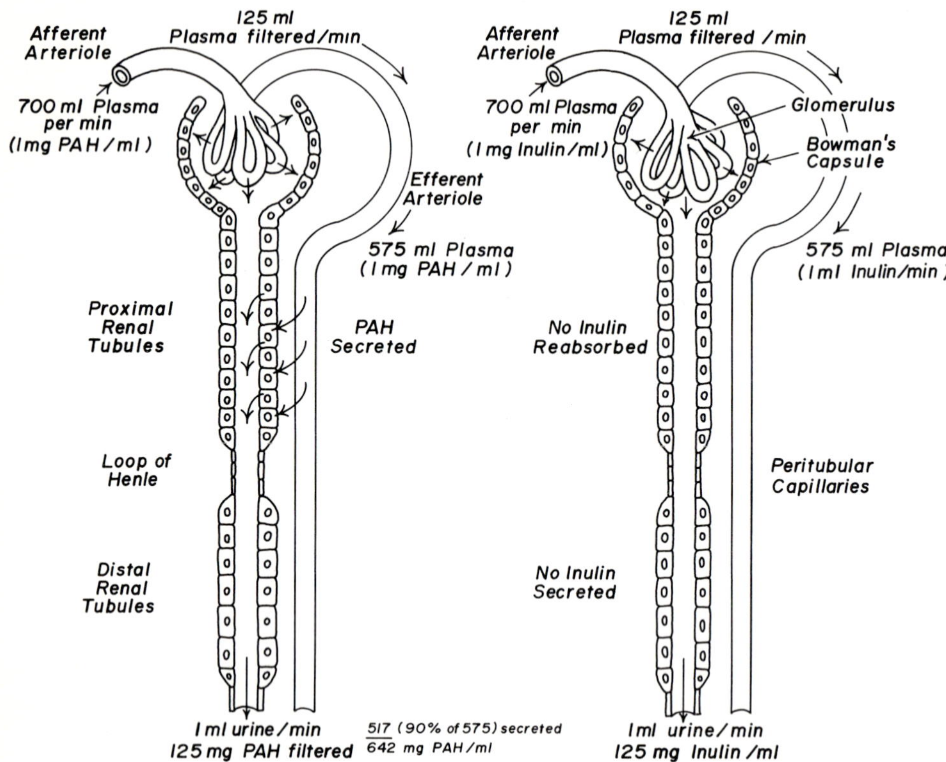

FIG. 13–6. Measurement of renal blood flow and glomerular filtration rate. **Left:**

$$\text{Renal plasma flow} = \frac{U_S \times V}{RA_S - RV_S}$$

$U_S \times V$ = the rate of excretion (mg/min) of a substance *(S)*. RA_S and RV_S = the concentrations of S (mg/ml) in arterial and venous blood, respectively. The rate of excretion divided by the arteriovenous difference gives the volume of plasma that must perfuse the kidneys each minute to supply the quantity of S excreted. The substance in common use is the organic acid para-aminohippurate (PAH), which is filtered by the glomeruli and actively secreted by the proximal tubules. The extraction of PAH in one passage through the kidney of a normal person is about 90%, so the true renal plasma flow exceeds the PAH clearance by about 10%. The renal blood flow is calculated from the renal plasma flow and the hematocrit. **Right:** Glomerular filtration can be determined using a substance which is filtered but neither reabsorbed nor secreted by the renal tubules. Most commonly inulin, a beta-glycosidic polymer of fructose (molecular weight about 5,500), is used as an indicator. The amount being filtered (glomerular filtration rate × the plasma concentration of inulin) equals the amount extracted in the urine (urine volume × the concentration of inulin in the urine.)

$$\text{Glomerular filtration rate} = \frac{U_I \times V}{P_I}$$

U_I = quantity of inulin in 1 ml urine. V = the volume of urine formed per minute. P_I = quantity of inulin in 1 ml plasma. On the average, 1,300 ml blood or 700 ml plasma perfuse the kidney each minute, and 125 ml/min is filtered through the glomeruli. The ratio of glomerular filtration to renal plasma flow indicates what fraction of the plasma entering the kidney is filtered at the glomeruli.

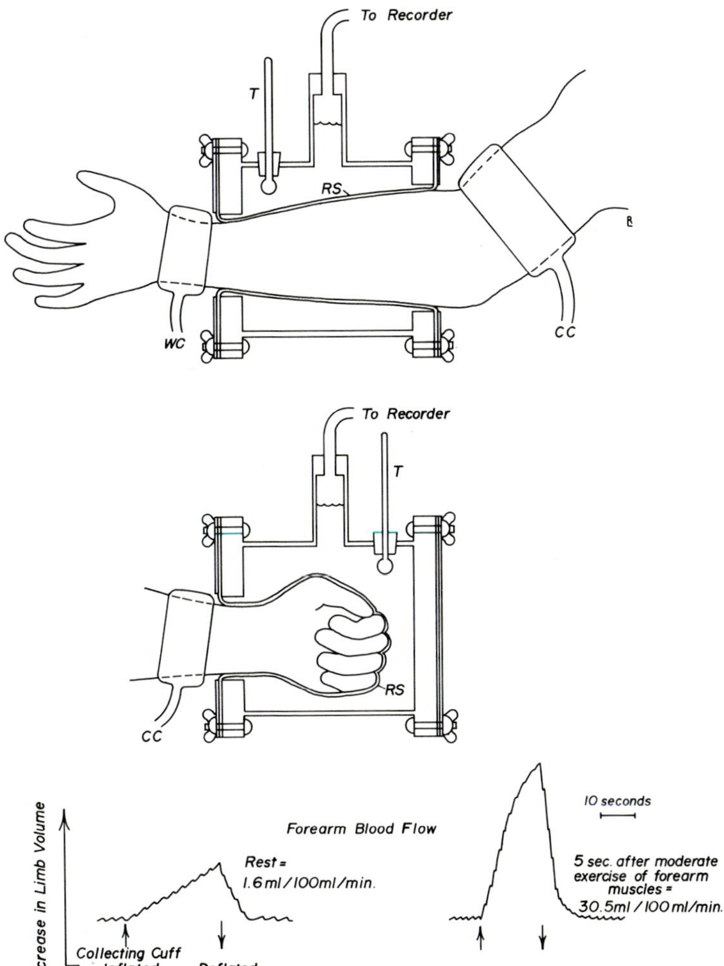

FIG. 13–7. Venous occlusion plethysmographic method for measurement of blood flow in human limbs. Water-filled plethysmographs for forearm and hand are shown. The hand or forearm is inserted into a loose-fitting rubber sleeve (RS). To measure blood flow a pneumatic cuff around the limb just proximal to the plethysmograph is abruptly inflated to a pressure sufficient to arrest the venous return temporarily (collecting cuff, CC). As a consequence, the limb volume increases as blood accumulates in the easily distensible venous system at a rate which initially equals the arterial inflow. The water temperature is maintained at about 32° to 34°C (T = thermometer). The same technique can be applied to the calf or foot. For measurement of forearm or calf blood flow, a second cuff around the wrist (WC) or ankle is inflated to suprasystolic pressures during the measurements of arterial inflow in order to arrest temporarily the circulation to the hand or foot. The volume of the segment of the limb within the plethysmograph is determined by water displacement.

The increases in volume of the extremity distal to the venous occlusion cuff can be measured with many types of plethysmographs, such as: (1) a rigid container placed around the limb or digit from which the displacement of water or air is recorded (Fig. 13–7); or (2) a strain gauge, consisting of a thin silastic tube filled with mercury, wrapped around the limb to be studied. Changes in limb volume alter the electrical resistance of the gauge.

Ultrasonic Flowmeters

The assessment of peripheral circulation with ultrasound is based on the Doppler effect. An ultrasound beam is directed through an underlying blood vessel and is back-scattered by the moving blood cells, which results in a shift in frequency proportional to the flow velocity of the red cells. The Doppler-shifted ultrasound is captured by a receiving crystal (Fig. 13–8). In a modification of the technique, short interrupted ultrasound beams are emitted at a specific frequency. The reflected echoes are received by the transducer in the interval between the two consecutive bursts. The system can measure flow velocity at selected points along the vessel diameter, whereas the continuous beam displays

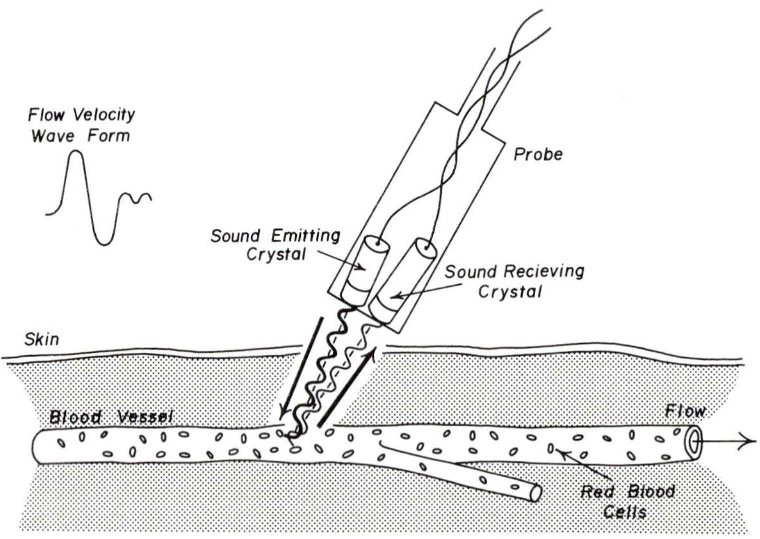

FIG. 13–8. Ultrasonic flow transducer. When ultrasound is reflected from red blood cells, it is shifted in frequency in proportion to the velocity of the bloodstream. In the transcutaneous ultrasonic detector shown, the sending and receiving crystals are placed on the skin over a limb artery or vein. Such instruments are useful for the detection of arterial and venous obstruction but do not permit quantitative measurements of blood flow in the underlying vessel since changes in frequency shift also result from changes in the angle of incidence of the beam of ultrasound hitting the flowing blood. When blood vessels are exposed during surgery, an ultrasonic flowmeter may be placed around the vessel to be studied. Since its position is fixed relative to the blood flow through it, the blood flow can be measured.

only an average of the instantaneous velocities over the whole cross-sectional area of the vessel. With the pulsed system, the velocity distribution across the vessel wall can be studied and the velocity profile mapped. The elastic properties of the arterial wall can be examined and the vessel dimensions measured, so that flow may be computed. Visualization of the anatomy of accessible vessels in various planes results in pictures comparable to a conventional arteriogram.

Heat Elimination

A calorimeter or a heat flow disk may be used to estimate heat leaving the surface of an extremity as an index of change in digital or skin blood flow. Measurement of skin temperature with thermometers, thermistors, or thermocouples is simple but of little value, since no linear relationship exists between skin temperature and blood flow.

Local Clearance of Isotopes

Isotopes that diffuse freely across cell membrances can be used to measure blood flow because their clearance from an injected depot is determined by the local blood supply only. The inert gas xenon-133 is a lipophilic substance which maintains a diffusion equilibrium between interstitium and capillary blood regardless of flow rate. When it is injected into a muscle and its disappearance rate recorded by a scintillation detector, the muscle blood flow is proportional to the slope of the disappearance curve (Fig. 13–9). This method offers the possibility of studying blood flow quantitatively in a single muscle and of measuring muscle blood flow during exercise. It also has been extended to the estimation of skin blood flow by the injection of ^{133}I-antipyrine into the skin.

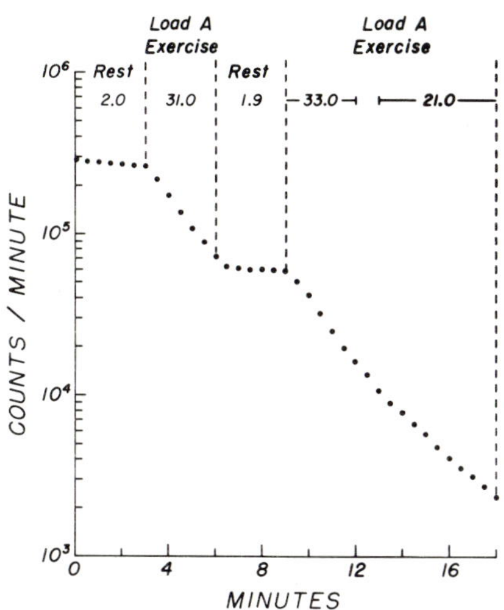

FIG. 13–9. Muscle blood flow measured by isotope clearance. In the example shown, xenon-133 dissolved in sterile isotonic saline solution (0.1 ml) was injected into one of the muscles of the forearm. The disappearance rate of the isotope is measured with a sodium iodide crystal and plotted on semilogarithmic paper. Values for muscle blood flow (F) (ml/min/100 ml tissue) are given at the top of the figure. They are calculated using the equation: $F = \lambda \cdot k \cdot 100$. λ = the partition coefficient between tissue and blood (0.7 for skeletal muscle). k = the negative slope of the clearance curve. (From Strandell and Shepherd: *Acta Med. Scand.* [*Suppl*], 472:146, 1967.)

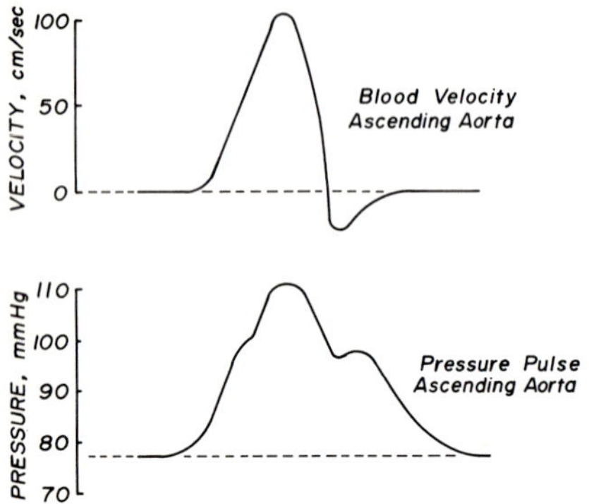

FIG. 13–10. Simultaneous measurement of pressure and blood velocity in the ascending aorta. The velocity is measured with an electromagnetic catheter tip velocity probe. The dicrotic notch of the pressure record corresponds to the reversal of velocity caused by the backflow which closes the aortic valve.

Electromagnetic Flowmeter

A field is generated by a small electromagnet embedded in a probe that fits closely around the blood vessel to be studied. Sensing electrodes in the same probe detect the potential difference induced by the movement of blood, a known conductor, across the excited field. The magnitude of the current is proportional to the average blood velocity and the intensity of the magnetic field. The instantaneous flow pattern and the mean blood flow can be recorded. This method requires surgical exposure of the vessels. Electromagnetic catheter tip velocity probes allow intravascular blood velocity measurements through percutaneous puncture of major vessels (Fig. 13–10).

CAPILLARY FILTRATION

The capillary filtration coefficient is the net transcapillary fluid movement produced by a change of capillary hydrostatic pressure, and is expressed as milliliters of fluid filtered/min × 100 g tissue × transcapillary pressure gradient (mm Hg). It is a function of the capillary surface area available for exchange and the capillary permeability, and can be measured by the change in weight or volume of the tissue caused by a known change of mean capillary hydrostatic pressure.

Extremities

An estimation of capillary filtration can be obtained in the extremities using venous occlusion plethysmography. When the distending cuff is inflated, the first rapid changes in volume are due to the filling of the veins and are determined by both arterial inflow and venous distensibility. If the occlusion cuff remains inflated, the venous pressure soon reaches cuff pressure and venous outflow equals arterial inflow. A subsequent slow increase in volume occurs owing to the filtration of water into the interstitial spaces, the rate of which may be calculated. In resting human skeletal muscle it amounts to 0.01 to 0.015 ml/min/100 g/mm Hg.

Glomerular Filtration

To measure the rate of glomerular filtration, an indicator is used which is freely filtered through the glomerular capillary membrane and does not undergo tubular reabsorption or secretion (Fig. 13–6).

VEINS

Observations on the behavior of the capacitance vessels in the human are restricted to the limbs. Common methods include the following.

Volume Measurements at a Given Venous Pressure

Changes in volume of the part under study (hand, forearm, foot, or calf) that accompany changes in venous pressure are measured at equilibrium. Shifts in such pressure–volume curves indicate alterations in the distensibility of the capacitance vessels. The changes in volume are determined by plethysmography. A catheter connected to a pressure transducer is used to measure the pressure in a large vein. Venous pressure is changed by inflation of a pneumatic cuff proximal to the site of measurement; pressures of up to 30 to 40 mm Hg are usually applied, which are not sufficient to interfere with the arterial inflow. Occasionally the pressure in this cuff is used as an approximation of the venous pressure. The limb to be studied is elevated slightly above heart level to achieve initial low venous pressure and volume (Fig. 13–11).

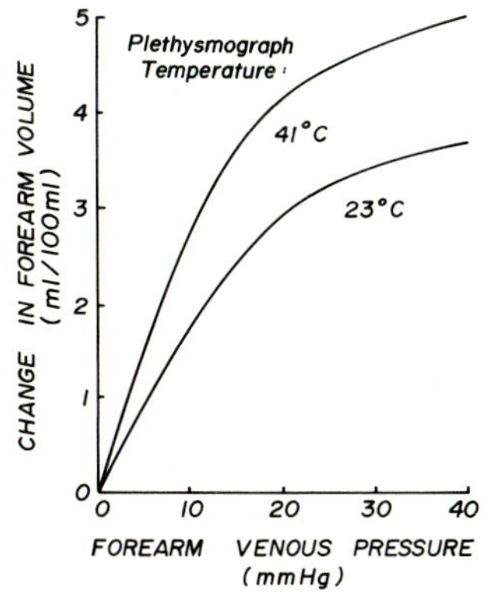

FIG. 13–11. Estimation of venous distensibility in the limbs from pressure–volume curves. The volume changes are determined by plethysmography. A catheter connected to a pressure transducer is used to measure the pressure in a large vein draining the part studied. The venous pressure is changed by inflation of a pneumatic cuff proximal to the site of measurement. Shifts in the pressure–volume curve indicate alterations in venous distensibility. In the examples shown, local warming and cooling of the forearm causes increased and decreased distensibility, respectively.

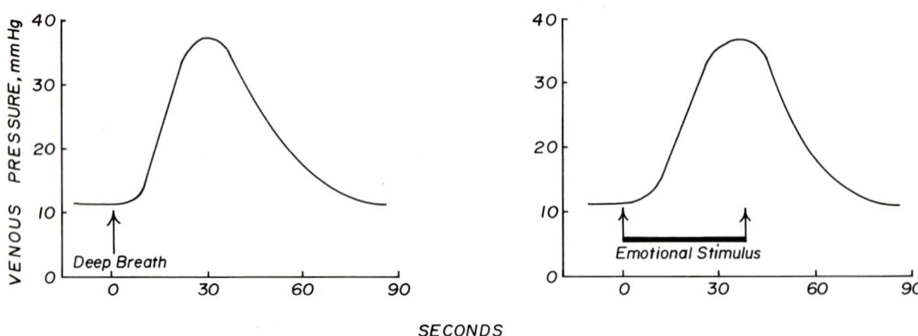

FIG. 13–12. Measurement of venous reactivity by the constant blood volume method. The circulation to the hand is temporarily arrested, and the pressure within one of its cutaneous veins is measured. Because the blood flow is arrested and no circulating vasoactive substance can enter the segment, changes in venomotor tone detected by this method are mediated by the sympathetic nerves. A deep breath and an emotional stimulus cause venoconstriction. The former activates receptors in the chest wall (p. 176).

Venous Pressure Measurement at a Given Venous Volume

The blood flow to a segment of a limb is temporarily arrested by means of a pneumatic cuff inflated to suprasystolic pressure, and the pressure within one of the large veins in the occluded limb is measured. Thus the limb veins contain a constant volume of blood and the changes in pressure are proportional to the changes in tension of the smooth muscle of the vein wall (Fig. 13–12).

BLOOD VOLUME

The total blood volume is the sum of the plasma volume and the volume of the blood cells. Its measurement is based on the principle of indicator dilution. If a known quantity of an indicator is injected into an unknown volume of fluid and disperses evenly throughout the fluid, the final concentration is proportional to the magnitude of the volume.

For determination of the plasma volume, indicators which combine with the plasma proteins are injected. This ensures that the indicator remains within the circulation long enough for measurements to be made. Usually radioactive iodinated human serum albumin (RISA) is injected intravenously, and venous samples are taken after adequate mixing has occurred. For determination of the red cell volume a sample of the subject's red blood cells tagged with a radioactive isotope of chromium (^{51}Cr), which binds to the beta-polypeptide chain of hemoglobin, is injected. A simpler but less accurate approach is to measure either the plasma volume or the red cell volume and derive the total blood volume from that measurement and the hematocrit. This is less precise because: (1) during centrifugation to determine the hematocrit, an unknown amount of plasma (about 2 to 5%) is trapped among the packed red blood cells; (2) the red blood cell volume changes with alterations in blood gases and so the venous hematocrit usually is larger (about 3%) than the arterial hematocrit; and (3) the ratio of red cells to plasma is slightly less in minute vessels than in large arteries and veins, presumably because of the axial flow and the resulting layering of plasma along their walls. To allow for these factors the value of the venous hematocrit is adjusted by multiplying the packed cell volume by 0.91 (see Appendix, Tables 8 and 9).

SELECTED REFERENCES

Greenfield, A. D. M., Whitney, R. J., and Mowbray, J. F. (1963): Methods for the investigation of peripheral blood flow. *Br. Med. Bull.*, 19:101.

Gregerson, M. I., and Rawson, R. A. (1959): Blood volume. *Physiol. Rev.*, 39:307.

Kety, S. S. (1960): The cerebral circulation. In: *Handbook of Physiology*, Section 1: *Neurophysiology*, Vol. III, p. 1751. American Physiological Society, Washington, D.C.

Lassen, N. A. (1974): Control of cerebral circulation in health and disease. *Circ. Res.*, 34:749.

Maseri, A., L'Abbate, A., Michelassi, C., Pesola, A., Pisani, P., Marzilli, M., De Nes, M., and Mancini, P. (1977): Possibilities, limitations, and technique for the study of regional myocardial perfusion in man by xenon-133. *Cardiovasc. Res.*, 11:277.

Reneman, R. S., editor (1974): *Cardiovascular Applications of Ultrasound.* North-Holland, Amsterdam.

APPENDIX

Appendix

TABLE 1. *Pressures in the cardiovascular system*

Site	Pressures (mm Hg)[a]
Right atrium	9/4 (mean 5)
Right ventricle	24/4–10 (4 early diastole, 10 end diastole)
Pulmonary artery	23/16
Left atrium	12/5 (mean 9)
Left ventricle	110/5–12 (5 early diastole, 12 end diastole)
Aorta	110/75
Femoral artery	118/70
Dorsalis pedis artery	135/68

[a] Average values for normal adult subjects resting supine. Individual values may show considerable variation.

TABLE 2. *Systemic blood flow and oxygen consumption*

Site	Blood flow (ml/min)	Arteriovenous oxygen difference (ml/100 ml)	Oxygen consumption (ml/min)
Splanchnic bed including liver	1,500	4.1	60
Skeletal muscles	1,100[a]	80	70
Kidneys	1,200	1.3	17
Cerebrum	750	6.3	48
Skin	500[b]	1.0	5
Coronary	250	11.5	28
Other organs	600	3.0	12
Total	5,800	4.0[c]	240

[a] During severe exercise it reaches 15 to 20 liters/min or up to 25 liters/min in athletes.
[b] During severe heat stress it may be 3 liters/m^2/min.
[c] Aorta minus pulmonary artery.

TABLE 3. *Measurements of normal adult hearts*

Parameter	Heart weight (g) Female	Male
Height (cm)		
161	235–295	260–340
169	245–305	275–355
176	260–320	290–370
183	275–335	305–385
	Wall thickness (cm)	
Right atrium	0.1–0.3	
Left atrium	0.1–0.3	
Right ventricle	0.3–0.5	
Left ventricle	1.3–1.5	
	Valve circumference (cm)	
Tricuspid	11.0–13.0	
Mitral	9.0–11.0	
Pulmonary	7.5– 8.5	
Aortic	7.0– 8.0	

TABLE 4. *Volume and ejection characteristics*

Volume Characteristics

Average volumes in adults determined by angiography
- End diastolic volume: 70 ml/m² body surface area
- End systolic volume: 25 ml/m² body surface area

$$\text{Ejection fraction} = \frac{(\text{end diastolic volume} - \text{end systolic volume})}{\text{end diastolic volume}} \times 100 = 65\%$$

Ejection Characteristics

Mean systolic ejection period (msec)
- Supine, at rest: 285
- Exercise (cardiac output 10 liters/m²/min): 230

Mean systolic ejection rate (ml/m²/sec)
- Supine, at rest: 185
- Exercise (cardiac output 10 liters/m²/min): 255

Rate of change of pressure with time
- Right ventricle: 350 dp/dt
- Left ventricle: 2,000 dp/dt

TABLE 5. *Heart function and exercise*

Parameter	Sedentary men	Athletes
Supine, at rest		
Cardiac output (liters/m^2/min)	3.5	3.8
Stroke volume (ml/m^2)	52	65
Heart rate	67	58
Oxygen consumption (liters/min)	0.24	0.25
Upright, severe exercise		
Cardiac output (liters/m^2/min)	10.5	13.7
Stroke volume (ml/m^2)	57	73
Heart rate	187	189
Oxygen consumption (liters/min)	3.2	4.8

TABLE 6. *Maximal exercise: comparison of nonathletic men and women*

Subject	Oxygen consumption (liters/min)	Cardiac output (liters/min)	Stroke volume (ml)
Men	4.1	24.0	120
Women	2.9	18.5	99

TABLE 7. *Blood gas values*

Site	Oxygen saturation (%)	P_{CO_2} (mm Hg)	CO_2 content (vol %)
Pulmonary veins	98		
Left atrium	97		
Systemic arteries	97		
Superior vena cava	77		
Right atrium	78		
Inferior vena cava	83		
Pulmonary artery	79		
Coronary sinus	40		
Hepatic vein	73		
Renal vein	87		
Systemic arteries		40	48–50
Mixed venous blood (pulmonary artery)		46	52–54
pH (plasma) = 7.35–7.45			
Osmolarity (serum) = 285 mOsm/liter			

TABLE 8. *Blood*

No. of red blood cells
Males: 4.5–6.2 million/mm³ blood
Females: 4.2–5.4 million/mm³ blood
Red blood cell survival (half-life by the chromium-51 method): 25–30 days
Reticulocyte count: 0.5–2.0%

Hematocrit
Males: 47% (42–54%)
Females: 42% (38–46%)

Plasma proteins

Albumin	3.3–4.5 g/dl
Alpha-1-globulin	0.1–0.4 g/dl
Alpha-2-globulin	0.5–1.0 g/dl
Beta-globulin	0.7–1.2 g/dl
Gamma-globulin	0.5–1.6 g/dl
Fibrinogen	195–365 mg/dl

Volumes

	Liters	*ml/kg body weight*
Total blood volume	5–6	60–65
Plasma volume	3.0–3.5	40–45
Red blood cell volume	2.0–2.5	24–30

TABLE 9. *Relative body composition for a 70-kg male*

Substance	% of body weight
Protein	18
Fat	15
Mineral	7
Plasma	5
Interstitial fluid	13
Intracellular fluid	40
Transcellular fluid (cerebrospinal fluid, intraocular fluid, joint fluid, gastrointestinal secretions)	2
Extracellular fluid (plasma + transcellular + interstitial)	20
Total body water (plasma + transcellular fluid + interstitial fluid + intracellular fluid)	60

Subject Index